Death in the 21st Century

**Genre Fiction and Film Companions**

Series Editor: Simon Bacon

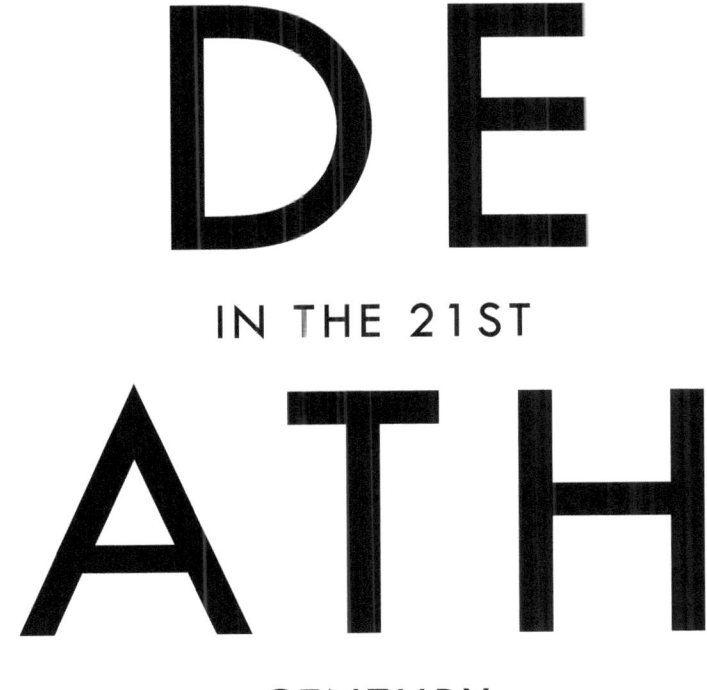

# DEATH
## IN THE 21ST
## CENTURY

A Companion

Edited by Katarzyna Bronk-Bacon and Simon Bacon

**PETER LANG**
Oxford - Berlin - Bruxelles - Chennai - Lausanne - New York

Bibliographic information published by the Deutsche Nationalbibliothek. The German National Library lists this publication in the German National Bibliography; detailed bibliographic data is available on the Internet at http://dnb.d-nb.de.

A catalogue record for this book is available from the British Library.

Library of Congress Cataloging-in-Publication Data

Names: Bronk-Bacon, Katarzyna, 1982- editor. | Bacon, Simon, 1965- editor.
Title: Death in the 21st century : a companion / [edited by] Katarzyna Bronk-Bacon and Simon Bacon.
Description: Oxford ; New York : Peter Lang Publication, [2024] | Series: Genre fiction and film companions, 2631-8725 ; vol no. 12 | Includes bibliographical references and index.
Identifiers: LCCN 2023057823 (print) | LCCN 2023057824 (ebook) | ISBN 9781800796744 (paperback) | ISBN 9781800796751 (ebook) | ISBN 9781800796768 (epub)
Subjects: LCSH: Death in literature. | Literature, Modern--21st century--History and criticism.
Classification: LCC PN56.D4 D44 2024 (print) | LCC PN56.D4 (ebook) | DDC 809.933548--dc23/eng/20240221
LC record available at https://lccn.loc.gov/2023057823
LC ebook record available at https://lccn.loc.gov/2023057824

Cover caption: Skull by Lina White (@linawhite) on Unsplash.
Cover design by Peter Lang Group AG

ISSN 2631-8725
ISBN 978-1-80079-674-4 (print)
ISBN 978-1-80079-675-1 (ePDF)
ISBN 978-1-80079-676-8 (ePUB)
DOI 10.3726/b19002

© 2024 Peter Lang Group AG, Lausanne
Published by Peter Lang Ltd, Oxford, United Kingdom
info@peterlang.com – www.peterlang.com

Katarzyna Bronk-Bacon and Simon Bacon have asserted their right under the Copyright, Designs and Patents Act, 1988, to be identified as Editors of this Work.

All rights reserved.
All parts of this publication are protected by copyright.
Any utilisation outside the strict limits of the copyright law, without the permission of the publisher, is forbidden and liable to prosecution.
This applies in particular to reproductions, translations, microfilming, and storage and processing in electronic retrieval systems.

This publication has been peer reviewed.

# Contents

| | |
|---|---|
| Acknowledgements | xi |
| Gemma Files<br>Image Intervention I: The Dying of the Light | xii |
| W. Scott Poole<br>Foreword: *The Faces of Death* (John Alan Schwartz, 1978) | xiii |
| Simon Bacon and Katarzyna Bronk-Bacon<br>Introduction | 1 |
| PART I   The War on Terror: Evil and the Inevitability of Death | 25 |
| Laura R. Kremmel<br>Image Intervention II: Skull 17 | 27 |
| Jack McCormack-Clark<br>*28 Days Later* (Danny Boyle, 2002) – Death as Insatiable Terror | 29 |
| Kevin J. Wetmore, Jr<br>*The Final Destination* Films (Various, 2000–11) – Death as Violent Inevitability | 37 |
| Dave Jeffery<br>Death (Eric Kripke, 2005–20) – The Changing Face of Death | 45 |

Anna Lüscher

The *Harry Potter* Series (Various, 2001–11) – Death Positivity — 53

Phil Fitzsimmons

*The Sleepless* (Nuzo Onoh, 2016) – Living Alongside Death — 61

PART II  Technology: Medicalisation, Ambivalence and Violence — 69

Gemma Files

Image Intervention III: Unlocking the Truth — 70

Rebecca Booth

*The Autopsy of Jane Doe* (André Øvredal, 2016) – Death as the Dissected Female Cadaver — 71

Łucja Lange

*Proof* (Rob Bragin, 2015–15) – Science as Death — 79

Stephanie Weber

*The Midnight Library* (Matt Haig, 2020) – Death and Infinite Lives — 87

Katarzyna Ancuta

*Death Note* (Various, 2003–17) – Death as Information — 95

Carl Wilson

*Death Stranding* (Kojima Productions, 2019) – Death as Interconnectivity — 105

Contents    vii

**Tom Ue**
*Ready Player Two* (Ernest Cline, 2020) – Pixelated Death    113

PART III    Climate Change: Environments and the Environmental    121

**Gemma Files**
Image Intervention IV: The King of Nature    123

**Tracy Fahey and Jennifer Moran Stritch**
Death Café (Limerick, 2015–Present) – Death in Life    125

**Mark Fryers**
*Ghosts* (Nick Broomfield, 2006) – The Sea as Death    135

**Kristy Strange**
*Geostorm* (Dean Devlin, 2017) – Death as the Eye of the Storm    143

**Ildikó Limpár**
*Mexican Gothic* (Silvia Moreno-Garcia, 2020) – Death as Mycological Rebirth    151

PART IV    Extremism: Partisanship and Identity Politics    159

**Laura R. Kremmel**
Image Intervention V: Skull 4    160

**James T. McCrea**
The Unite the Right Rally and Its Aftermath (2017–20) – The Skull    161

Nicola Young

*The Purge* Series (Various, 2012–21) – Mass Shootings and Endless Death   171

Rachael Grant

*American Horror Story: Asylum* (Brad Falchuck and Ryan Murphy, 2012–13) – Angel of Death   181

Robert Mclaughlin

Mistress Death in the Marvel Universe (Various, 1973–Present) – For the Love of Death   191

Maria Giakaniki

*Suspiria* (Luca Guadagnino, 2018) – Female Death   199

Octavia Cade

Deathface Ginny (Kelly Sue DeConnick, 2014–20) – Death and #MeToo   209

Bethan Michael-Fox and Renske Visser

*Mrs Death Misses Death* (Salena Godden, 2021) – Death as a Black Woman   215

PART V   Global Pandemics: Contagion, Mental Health and Dementia   223

Gemma Files

Image Intervention VI: The Source   224

Cath Davies

*Coco* (Lee Unkrich, 2017) – Death as Decomposition   225

Contents

Simon Bacon
*The Thing* (Matthijs van Heijningen Jr, 2011) – The Microbe as Death ... 233

Debaditya Mukhopadhyay
*Ludo* (Anurag Basu, 2020) – Death as New Normal ... 243

Heidi Kosonen
*13 Reasons Why* (Brian Yorkey, 2017–20) – Death as Controversial Suicide ... 253

Rae Hargrave
*Land of the Lustrous* (Takahiko Kyōgoku, 2017–17) – Death as Loss of Memory ... 263

Catherine Pugh
*Unus Annus* (Mark Fischbach and Ethan Nestor, 2019–20) – Death as Deletion ... 269

Lisa Morton
Afterword: The Tomorrow of Death – Dia de los Muertos ... 281

Gemma Files
Image Intervention VII: The Guardian ... 285

Bibliography ... 287

Notes on Contributors ... 313

Index ... 323

# Acknowledgements

The idea of this book came out of the immediate aftermath of the outbreak of the Covid-19 pandemic and stages where governments were deciding whether it had gone or not, often predicated on economic rather than medical factors. And although we have, in some measure, returned to the old 'new normal', Covid, and indeed its influence on the popular imagination, have not. It is in this atmosphere that everyone involved in this collection has, at various stages, helped bring it to completion, and so we like to thank everyone who – in however small a manner – have contributed to getting this collection to the point of being published. More so, we would like to thank everyone who managed to stay with us until the end, which has been no mean feat given what has been, and is, unfolding in the world at the moment and with all the stresses and strains within academia which make completing any kind of writing far more difficult than it ought to be. Many, many thanks to Laurel Plapp at Peter Lang for all her help and encouragement along the way and for the rest of the team there for their assistance in making this book look so good.

We also want to thank our two not-so-little monsters Seba and Maja for always being themselves and constantly providing distractions at the most unexpected times. And last, but not least, we want to thank Mama and Tata Bronk without whose constant help and support none of this would be possible.

# Image Intervention I: The Dying of the Light

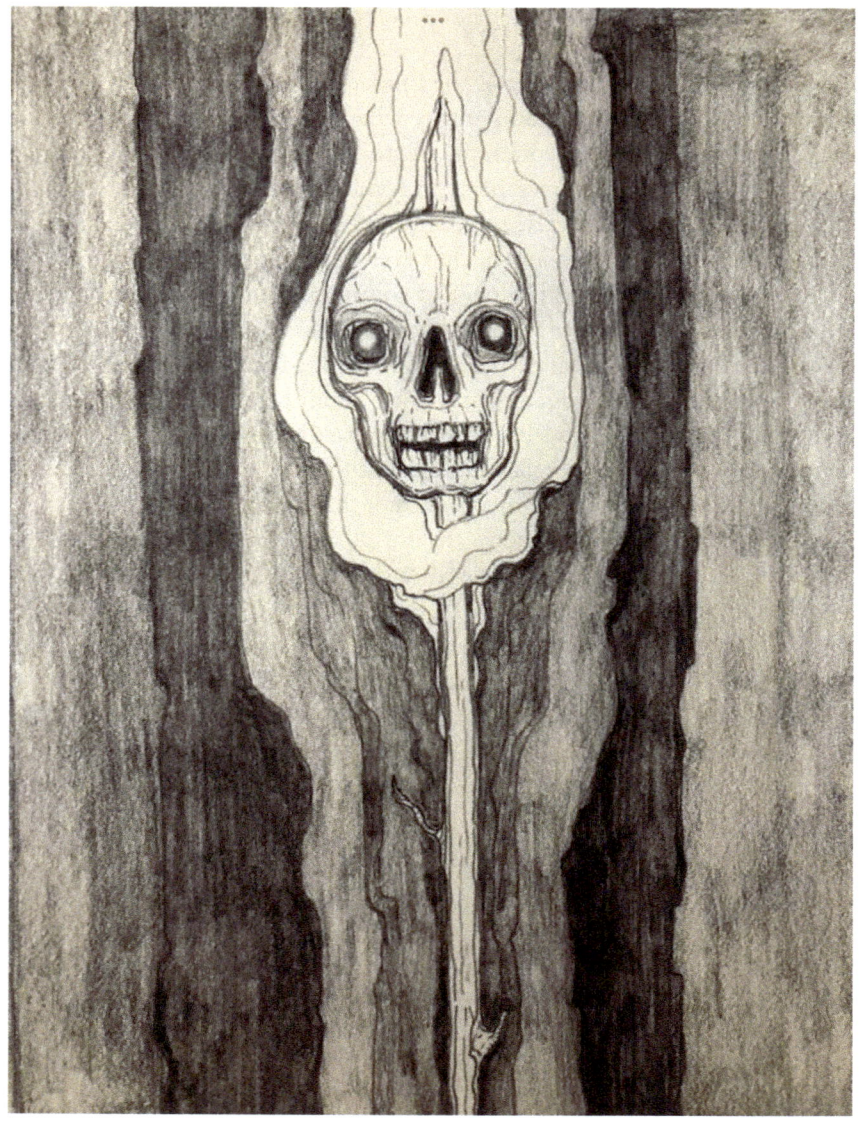

Artwork by Gemma Files
(Reproduced with the permission of the artist)

W. Scott Poole

# Foreword: *The Faces of Death* (John Alan Schwartz, 1978)

Sometime in 1988, a teen me huddled with a large group that contained a few friends, a lot of acquaintances and one or two people who bullied me. We watched a VHS marathon that included Wes Craven's 1977 *The Hills Have Eyes* and the very recently released *Predator*.

This night passed at the height of that golden age of home video during which the much-desired VCR gifted us the shocking ability to watch flicks that once had just been rumours on the wind. I recall that my high school crush was present. But it's a serious toss-up whether I was there for her or for the great white whale of Wes Craven's early work. I knew the man who frankensteined Fred Kruger from cultural nightmares once made a notorious atomic age cannibal film that I'd been too young to see. All apologies to my long-lost crush, but I'm pretty sure I showed up for the irradiated flesh-eaters.

One of my more transgressive friends brought along another tape that night: one that many in our small rural community believed to be nothing more than an urban legend. Called *Faces of Death*, the film carried a notorious reputation for supposedly showing actual human and animal death in traffic accidents, executions and purported cannibalism. It's ill-smelling reputation connected it to urban legends of 'the snuff film' that circulated since at least 1969. We know now that some of the more outlandish moments of sudden mortality are simply not-so-great SFX work.

I remember little about it because I watched under ten minutes and went home, abandoning my crush, a giant tub of popcorn and movie night, fleeing ingloriously before the pale rider and his many faces.

Why? My introduction to the macabre came early with a morbid sensibility from some of the horrific aspects of my childhood religion that entwined in strange ways with love for Universal Studio's monsters and their own unique faces of death-gruesome Frankenstein in his ersatz body of decay and the savagery of the Wolfman who tore and rent with seemingly no purpose. John Carpenter's *Halloween* held me in thrall, and in an upcoming summer I would watch it repeatedly, using my video store clerk privileges to keep it permanently, and rather criminally, on reserve for myself. My love for Wes Craven's nightmares brought me out that night to a scary hang-out with the popular kids, which in itself was a real leap into the social abyss for a not-so-popular kid already displaying the reclusive tendencies that have grown over time.

So why pull the nose up at *Faces of Death*?

There's sense in which the many brilliant thinkers you'll meet in this volume are seeking their own answers to similar questions. In various ways, each deals with how we represent death in art ... film, anime, graphic novels, literary fiction and video/PC games. The authors examine fantasies and nightmares about death through constructions of contagion, the death dealing politics of contemporary fascism and our collective suicide pact to create catastrophic climate change. Despite a diversity of purpose, there's an implicit set of questions that runs through the collection. Why do we need these representations? Why does, as the variety you see here suggests (*Harry Potter* to *The Autopsy of Jane Doe* to Moreno-Garcia's *Mexican Gothic*), mass culture need the faces of death? Another way to ask this: why would entertainment flirt so wantonly with what the Book of Job eloquently calls 'the King of Terrors?'

****

The skeletal remains of Neanderthals are, with little exception, scored and scarred, a savage archive of a brief lifetime of brutalities. These are the fragmented bones of hunters who crept up close to their prey, for whom getting dinner meant hand-to-hand combat with a prospective meal trying to make you a meal, one of nature's last fair fights. Anthropologists tend to agree that this daily reality pushed humans towards crafting the spear, arrow and sling, to imagine the possibilities of murder at a distance.[1]

---

[1] S. Mithen, 'The Hunter-Gatherer Pre-History of Human and Animal Relations', *Anthropozoos* 12:4 (1995), 194–204; more recently, see M. C. Langley et al., 'Bows and Arrows and Symbolic Displays 48,000 Years Ago in South Asian Tropics', *Science Advances* 6:24 (July 2020).

The benefits of killing your meat out of range of tooth and claw are obvious and increased the human lifespan in practical ways that went beyond increased caloric intake. You could deliver death without consequence. You could keep your own death at bay while you slaughtered other things that lived.

Perhaps these human ancestors' increasingly lethal habits gave them time to contemplate the meaning of their brief span. The small purchase that they held on to life allowed for time to ponder on graves and gifts. Considering the meaning of the dead, and their own death, led to ceremonial burial, which joined the rites of child delivery as the oldest human activity that counts as religion.

Illogic; maybe what Freud described many millennia later as our 'death instinct' took us to strange places 10,000 years ago. The building of permanent settlements meant growing food. But it also meant defending what you had grown. In what would become one of the most haunting paradoxes of human history, the ability to sustain life joined warm fingers with an icy skeletal hand, a cruel brother to progress that brought death. Agriculture allowed humans to build worlds where we could live. It also strengthened the hand of those who yearned to rule, allowing them to conscript soldiers and slaves to wall up and defend these worlds, to harness technology to our death instinct as well as to wage war on an increasingly large scale.

In her meditation on the means, ends and vocabulary of death-dealing in warfare, Elaine Scarry notes that 'reciprocal injury' is the meaning of war as it actually occurs. This is the poisonous seed of war, not the straightforward political goals of ruling classes or the grand strategies of command structures. Of course, the trip line for combat folds together a variety of causes, both in terms of historical causation and propaganda. But that's not Scarry's concern. She follows Clausewitz's argument that, once war begins, armies simply become tools to cause 'general damage' and to 'increase the enemy's suffering'. To what end? At the point of the bayonet, Clausewitz admits, the manufacture of death becomes self-justifying – a surprisingly nihilistic admission for the pragmatist best known for calling war a 'continuation of policy by other means.'[2]

---

2   Elaine Scarry, *The Body in Pain: The Making and Unmaking of the World*. (New York: Oxford University Press, 1985), 78–9, 97–100.

Clausewitz, who died in 1831, could likely not imagine the lengths to which warfare would go to 'increase the enemies suffering'. The armies of the earth gathered to harvest death on an unimaginable scale less than a 100 years later

\*\*\*\*

The twentieth century did not begin on 1 January 1900. Its real birthday was 23 August 1914, the Battle of Mons. The battle's casualties are insignificant by the standards of the Great War while being catastrophic in relation to the smaller European conflicts since the Napoleonic age. A few days after Mons, Germany annihilated a 30,000-member Russian force at Tannenberg in East Prussia (now Poland).

The months that followed saw the building of intricate rat holes stretching for hundreds of miles across Europe, an earthen tribute paid to combat tech that worked an equation of death that was incalculable and unsolvable. Machine guns delivered carnage at close to 400 rounds per minute. Bodies waded into the steel tempest, running, crawling, gibbering with war fever or complete insanity, across a landscape tangled with barbed wire, wounded by shells and rotting with corpses. Human beings died by the millions ... choked, fragmented and filleted by these terrible weapons.

This is only one resonant image of a conflict that took the lives of nearly 40 million combatants and bystanders. Hundreds of thousands died in Germany from the British naval blockade, many simply starving to death by 1917–18. Half a million civilians died in sub-Saharan Africa, caught in the crossfire of guerrilla wars waged by the British and the Germans in their colonial possessions. Across North Africa and the Middle East, the conflict drew in troops from as far away as India to die by the hundreds of thousands. The influenza strain that emerged in an American training camp late in the war swarmed like rats in the trenches of 1918, the contagion spreading across battlefields and brought home by returning soldiers while eventually killing 50 million people across the globe.

What the many fronts of the global catastrophe all have in common is the phenomenon of industrialised death, the mass production of corpses made possible by new human technologies.

These facts coinciding have made the past 100 years of human history a poignant paradox. Advances in the field of medicine and a variety of life-saving

Foreword: *The Faces of Death* (John Alan Schwartz, 1978)      xvii

techniques have not kept up with the ability of human beings to annihilate one another. The Great War introduced sanitary regimens for wounds that could go septic, medical logistics that allowed for quicker treatment and the earliest efforts at restorative facio-dental surgery for people utterly mutilated by shots or shells. Yet the weapons the world's army wielded still produced more dead bodies than ever imagined in human experience.

Humanity's paradoxical death waltz continued long after 1918. Life expectancy grew across much of the globe into the twentieth century even as nation-states created arsenals capable of executing a mass extinction event. The United States, particularly during the 1950s, late 1960s and early 1980s, contemplated and planned for a 'winnable' nuclear war against the Soviet Union.

In 2022, Europe joined east Asia as the region with the longest life expectancies on the planet, even after the wasting Covid pandemic. And yet, Russia's invasion of Ukraine employed Iskandr ballistic missiles that strike civilian and military targets at 500 kilometres with an explosive force, if not a radiation yield, similar to the first atomic weapons. Thermobaric bombs (so-called vacuum bombs) ignite a supersonic sound wave fuelled by their ability to literally siphon oxygen from the surrounding air. At the time of writing, one month into the conflict, there are 13,500 known dead on the Ukrainian side alone with perhaps 3,000 of those being civilians.[3]

****

A meditation on mass murder of modern warfare could be read as a sleight of hand, an avoidance of the reality that one can die while on a walk in the park as well as on a battlefield. Perhaps rather than policy by a different means, war is simply death performed more brutally than we would hope.

Biological and neurological death comes to human beings, in the nursery, on a highway or in peaceful sleep. 'Man is mortal', writes Mikhail Bulgakov, 'sometimes suddenly so'.

Then again, perhaps this is why war so outrages the psyche as much as it injures the body? War, what Thomas Mann called 'the coward's escape from the problems of peace', dissolves our individual experiences and the vast cultural

---

3   As of May 2023, these figures have risen to 17,500 military deaths and 8,895 civilian deaths.

histories that fuel them into wild desecrations of the human body. War outrages us, and properly so, because in it the universal quality of inevitable death doffs its hat to the power of weapons that destroy human tissue, ending the life of millions while leaving millions more in a realm of social death, besieged by trauma, clawed at by memories of violence. Even if we see our biological deaths as a process not so different from the cycle of decay that yields a surge of new life, we still revolt, hopefully in a political fashion, against states and their ruling classes seeking to turn us into compost with lethal violence and maximum suffering.

Death's ride with war, plague and famine has sometimes been a strangely saccharine confection that is neither morbid nor political. There's a tremendous amount of writing in 'death studies' that either laments or laughs at the idea of 'the good death'. This concept has received the most attention in relation to Victorian Britain but has analogues in the nineteenth-century United States and the birth of the pastoral cemetery or central Europe and the often-elaborate mourning societies of Berlin and Vienna.

Collectivised death, and how it has been guaranteed and legitimised by the national state, does make a mockery of the good death. War memorials such as France's Douaumont are simply mass graves; they are less the resting place of the 'unknown deadline and more literally a dump for the unidentifiable body parts that are the toxic waste of industrialized war'.

This is perhaps why contemporaries have replaced the 'good death' with 'the clean death'. For example, it's extraordinary how the human skull and variations of it, like the sutured and iron bolted cranium of Frankenstein's monster, became icons of the last century. Long a part of religious imagery, whether hovering on Puritan gravestones or appearing as mise en scène for thousands of portraits of and altars for the saints, the skull has held an esteemed place in Christian cosmology. The twentieth century ripped the whitened skull from this context and made it a stark reminder of death's inevitability – a symbol of blunt fact. The death's heads of expressionist art and film, the skulls on the set of a 100 horror hosts, the sugar skulls North Americans have appropriated from *dia de los Muertos* as well as the skulls that hang in classrooms for American children's Halloween might suggest a death-obsessed culture or, given their bizarrely light-hearted context, even a society that has come to accept death as part of the biological reality of the natural world.

Or perhaps this image has become a way to commodify the experience of death, to offer throwaway images of a clean death if the good death has become unattainable. Georges Bataille suggests that when 'the bones are bare and white they are not intolerable to as the putrefying flesh'. In fact, Bataille believes that 'whitened bones' act as 'a veil of decency and solemnity over death that makes it bearable'.[4]

This collection looks unflinchingly at the masks that death wears in mass culture. The scholars have taken the idea of necropolitics, how death insinuates itself into our social arrangements as much as our psyches and discovered in mass culture places where the 'veil of decency' disappears. In our time of collective death that tries to hide in tropes of a clean death fantasy and nightmare that are screened, scripted or gamed offer spaces of unexpected clarity.

In 400 BC, Sophocles completed and premiered *Oedipus at Colonus*, the story of the death of the tragic hero that had for so long haunted the dramatist. Victim of war, betrayal, the fates and, now and again, his own hubris, the blind king takes the emerging hero Theseus with him to witness his death in solitude, hiding his grave even from his closest kin.

Common readings of this play, a drama often forgotten in the grim shadow of Sophocles' other work, focus on the politics of legacy, the worry over graves and their consequences that will take centre stage in *Antigone*. There is no more Oedipus but there will be an Athens. Hans Ruin has gone further by suggesting that the drama moves beyond the power of heritage and pushes the audience to think about the meaning of literature itself. It becomes an intentional work of memory that can create a 'protective space' for considering reality beyond the power of death to destroy. In death is the emergence of historical consciousness, the simple and yet burdensome notion that our political actions in the world have consequences that long outlast us. By dying we become part of history, not as chronology of things that happened but as a human experience that will unfold either in wars waged and the powerful solidifying their status or in pursuing peace and doing justice.[5]

---

4   Georges Bataille, *Death and Sensuality: A Study of Eroticism and Taboo*. (New York: Walker and Company, 1962), 56–7.
5   For Ruin's reading, see Hans Ruin, *Being with the Dead: Burial, Ancestral Politics, and the Roots of Historical Consciousness* (Stanford, CA: Stanford University Press, 2018), 116–8, 203–6.

This collection, in so many respects, manages to carry forward the idea of historical conscious as ghost, threat and promise in ways most interpreters have not been able to imagine. Kojima's *Death Stranding* can teach you about what human responsibility can look like when facing the unyielding realities of death, even mass death, through the games he has transformed into aesthetic feasts. Danny Boyle's film *28 Days Later* can force us to forget the clean death and reimagine the apocalypse with a sense of moral seriousness rather than political nihilism.

The desire to imagine the clean death relegates the experience into the past, in its building of memorials, its rites of remembrance and the way the dead are presented to us as models to emulate or avoid. But this collection of essays will surprise you as the authors show us that mass culture forces us to ponder death in the present, to think about our moral obligations in a world where death is the ultimate event horizon. It's not only a nightmare, but also a dream, evocative of futures that we will not see. But we will become the foundation on which its built – for good or ill.

Simon Bacon and Katarzyna Bronk-Bacon

# Introduction

This book was born from the trauma of the continuing Covid-19 pandemic in 2021 when death had become all too familiar and so many had lost family members, friends and loved ones to the disease and its associated complications, many of which were man-made. At that stage, it still seemed imaginable that there would be a time when, together, we would emerge from the shadow of the global disease and enter a 'new normal': a nostalgia-laden return to a time before the disease that could still be replicated in the future. In reality, two years later, in 2023, the disease has 'officially' gone, despite warnings from the medical community claiming otherwise, and the foretold 'levelling' effects of the pandemic have produced even more divisions within society and between nations. Of note here is that the unique intersection of popular politics, environmental extremes, globalisation and technological innovation, which were identified in the proposal for this volume in 2021, remains the same in 2023 but with a shifting of emphasis on where the current anxieties lay and what 'faces' of Death they correspondingly choose to present to us. Accordingly, *Death in the 21st Century: A Companion*, will show how our fears evolving since the start of the 2000s have changed the way Death presents itself in the popular imagination and will reveal some of the faces it chooses to wear.

## Out with the Old …

Death is an inherent part of human life, and, unsurprisingly, the majority of cultures across the globe have incorporated it as an embodied entity into their own cosmologies, faiths or mythologies. Many of these contain a personification of Death that is not 'the end' in itself but facilitates or assists with the process of going from life to the afterlife, often giving form to how that culture perceives death. More often than not, Death in these configurations has very little say in who dies, although the idea of judgement of some kind does appear in individual cultures. The representation of Death often varies between cultures, which may perceive it as skeletal in nature (Western culture and the Aztecs), an angel (the Angel of Death in Judaism), a judge or bureaucrat (China and Korea) or an entity that can take many forms often dependent on the person who has died (India and Islam). These personifications can be either male or female: female versions can be found in those countries where the word 'death' is a feminine noun in their native language, such as the Romance languages as well as languages of certain Slavic countries, Hindu regions, Ireland (Banshee), ancient Aztec culture (Mictecacihuatl), Scandinavia (Hel) and Lithuania (Giltinė).

Within the Western tradition, a skeletal Death, riding a pale horse, has more popularly been seen as one of the Four Horsemen of the Apocalypse (the Book of Revelation), along with War, Famine and Pestilence, and given dominion over a large part of the earth as a signal for the end of times and the Second Coming. Alongside this is the popular figure of the Grim Reaper, which was first mentioned in the book *The Circle of Human Life* (1847).[1] The Reaper is often depicted as a skeleton holding a large scythe with which he harvests the souls of humans, an image that has since been combined with Death as one of the Horsemen. Another important aspect of the representation of Death is the notion of memento mori or reminders of death. Largely a Western tradition, although there are examples in the antiquity and parallels in Buddhism, Japanese Zen, Islam and Icelandic (Norse) mythology, memento mori has functioned from the time of early Christianity as a remembrance of not only

---

[1] Robert Menzies, *The Circle of Human Life* (Edinburgh: Myles Macphail, 1847).

those who have passed but also the brevity of life itself; as well as a reminder that one should be worthy of the time spent on earth whilst thinking of the afterlife. Skulls and skeletons have played a major part in the imagery and architecture connected to this theme as has the Danse Macabre (Dance of Death), often shown as a procession of skeletons and depicting human equality found in death. Early examples of this date from the fifteenth century, and it also served as a source for the slightly later motif of Death and the Maiden that appeared in Northern European Renaissance art from the early sixteenth century. This condenses the Danse Macabre to two figures: Death as an ugly old man (zombie/skeleton) and as a beautiful young girl known as the Maiden, once again depicting the short-lived pleasures of life and youth but with a dash of eroticism.[2]

Within this context then, representations, or visions, of Death have come to embody many aspects of our relationship with religion life and what might happen after the latter. Not unlike monsters, the figure of Death often represents that which causes society the most anxiety and which is most viewed as being an imminent threat to life. Not unlike monsters, Death often comes from the outside or the 'beyond', constructing the afterlife or the land of the dead as a place or domain outside our own rather than an inherent part of our everyday lived experience – (some of this can also be traced to the building of graveyards outside of towns and cities, which was popularised across Europe and America in the mid-nineteenth century). This removal of death from the midst of life has seen Death take on the appearance of far more abstract and varied anxieties in the twenty-first century such as: biological, cultural and technological warfare; contagion, disease and pandemics; and the ravaging hunger, poverty and the widening gap between the wealthiest and the poorest in the world.

---

2   The character of Brad Pitt in *Meet Joe Black* (1998), a rather interesting example of this imagery, says much about beauty and privilege being seen as more powerful than death in the late twentieth century.

## ... In with the New

On the cusp of the new millennium, perhaps one of the most distinctive faces of Death was the most un-Death-like, as seen in the young and beautiful Joe Black (Brad Pitt) in *Meet Joe Black* (1998). Arguably, this is a representation appropriate for an age that is increasingly obsessed with youth and beauty and a counterpoint to the monstrous bodies of rotting flesh of the burgeoning zombie horde that also created the other well-known representation of Death at the end of the twentieth century. Such contrasts are of note, as in many instances they can be inspired by the same kinds of anxieties over ageing, whilst also giving form to religious (Christian) conceptions around the corruptibility of the flesh and 'perfection' of the afterlife: here our 'heavenly' bodies are seen to change to a kind of physical perfection embodying our 'best' selves. The 2000s, however, seemed to usher in something new. Even from its very beginning, the world seemed unsure how it would transition to this new millennium with fears over computers crashing and technology failing due to the Y2K bug so severe that many airlines grounded their planes in case they crashed out of the sky at midnight on 31 December. The auspiciousness of this beginning seems to have been validated by a number of significant events occurring in seemingly quick succession: the terrorist attack on the Twin Towers on 11 September 2001 and the War on Terror that ensued; the rise of Al-Qaeda, ISIS and religious extremism and fundamentalism; the growing realisation that neo-liberalism and even democracy were not delivering the prosperity and freedom for all they had promised; the increase in populist politics and the assault on facts and science; the need, yet again, for large-scale protests around #MeToo and BLM; the realisation that climate change is now inevitable and it is just a case of how bad humanity will make it; and the pandemics that have flared across the globe – SARS (2002–4), Swine Flu (2009–10), Ebola (2013–16) and, of course, Covid-19 (2019–present). The list seems endless, and each of these events has brought its own conceptions of what Death might look like on an individual and cultural level. At the vantage point of the 2020s, some clarity is beginning to emerge on what has occurred and what continues to unfold as the twenty-first century progresses, and five things, arguably, stand out as having a significant impact on how Death is seen and experienced. As one would expect, these aspects intersect with each other, amplifying or negating certain aspects in their ongoing, and often parallel, trajectories over time. These five things are as follows: (1) 9/11 and the Subsequent War on Terror; (2) Technology and the Internet; (3) Climate Change; (4) Increasing Extremism and Populist Ideologies; and (5) Global Pandemics.

*1. 9/11 and the Subsequent War on Terror*

It is difficult to over-exaggerate the impact of the attack on the Twin Towers in New York on 11 September 2001 – on Western culture, in general, and American society, in particular – causing a communal trauma that is still working its way through the cultural imaginary. As noted by scholars such as Kevin J. Wetmore, Jr (2012) and Linnie Blake (2013), it caused a shift in popular culture and, more specifically, has had an impact on the horror genre, giving rise to entities and monsters that were unrelenting and unstoppable and often causing cataclysmic levels of destruction: disaster, action and monster movies no longer showed the collapse of the occasional building but portrayed entire cities being flattened.[3] The subsequent War on Terror and the invasion of Iraq, whilst providing a measure of symbolic retribution, did little to solve the issues of Western/American interference in the region and the rise in sectarianism and religious extremism that had caused the attacks in the first place. Indeed, in many ways this got worse, resulting in the rise of ISIS and a change in the nature of ongoing terror attacks throughout the developed world, which consequently led to increasing anxieties around such events and to a growing number of people affected by this. In the first instance, and more related to the events of 9/11 then, the terror caused by the destruction was as much about the damage to the city itself as it was to the inhabitants, and thus Death took on the form of a monstrous creature that could inflict catastrophic damage on a major metropolis. An obvious example of this is *Cloverfield* (2008) which

---

3   A common feature in post-Second World War/post-Hiroshima Japanese monsters movies like *Godzilla* (1954).

is set in New York and sees a Godzilla-type monster (or kaiju)[4] appear from nowhere and destroy huge swaths of the city and, most dramatically, skyscrapers not unlike the Twin Towers. Of note here is how we never really see the entire monster but only snippets of it, suggesting this vision of Death is only part of a much larger entity and one that we are not able to fully comprehend. A similar idea permeates films such as *Transformers* (2007), *Transformers: Revenge of the Fallen* (2009) and *Pacific Rim* (2013) – with the last more clearly making the connection to Japanese monster movies – which feature cityscapes being destroyed by huge robots (mecha) and/or monsters. Of interest here is *The Avengers* (2012) as this film also shows New York being destroyed by huge monsters from another dimension and features skyscrapers being penetrated by explosive forces – with an obvious reading seeing the act as the emasculation of the phallic nature of the vertical city space and that the monsters come from another world. This becomes a metaphorical depiction of the two hijacked planes that were flown into the Twin Towers being perceived as somehow flying to New York directly from the 'other world' of the Middle East. Monsters in these films are often depicted as originating from an alien world, having different values and extremist views as well as wanting to destroy humanity (read America). This is depicted even more clearly in *Blade Trinity* (2004) in which an ancient monster that is unearthed from a Middle Eastern desert and brought back to America causes terror and mayhem. In the final scene of the film, Blade and the monster are shown crashing through the floors and windows of a modern high-rise office building. A similar plot can be seen in the *Transformers* film, which features evil robots first appearing in a desert in the Middle East where they attack American troops stationed there. Consequently, the 'other world' of Death is closely aligned with the Middle East: a place depicted as so different and antithetical to our own that it might as well be in another dimension.

---

4   The use of monsters and, as seen later, giant robots in these films makes a direct reference to the tradition of Japanese post-Second World War monster movies which draw a parallel between the destruction and ensuing trauma of Hiroshima and that experienced during 9/11.

Closely aligned to the idea of Death being situated in a desert in the Middle East is that of dealing with returning troops who have been profoundly impacted by their experiences during the conflict overseas. This is seen in *Exorcist the Beginning* (2004), which specifically cites the desert as a place from which devils emerge, and *Osombie* (2012), which depicts Osama bin Laden, a target for much Western retribution, as a contagious undead zombie. In representing the desert as a place of such extreme otherness and as a home to Death, it is shown as affecting those who are sent there and who later return home bringing something of the Grim Reaper with them. *Mulberry St* (2006), a good example of this motif, sees a soldier retiring from the war in Iraq to her family home in New York, but both she and the world she is returning to have irreparably changed as they are overrun by monsters. A similar narrative is seen in a later film *Deliver Us from Evil* (2014), where a group of soldiers become possessed by a demonic entity in the desert, and on their return to New York, they transform into extremist death cult members who strike at the heart of the city. Interestingly, here Death does not always have a face but does have a name in such 'possession' films, positioning it more as an ideological infection than a discrete embodiment that can take on the appearance of anyone or everyone. The issue of returning soldiers also points to the perception of the War on Terror as an unending conflict, with a sense of imminent 'terror' that purposely results in configuring violence, and subsequently death, as inevitable and inescapable. In such environments, death becomes as ambivalent as it is sudden and violent, and this is portrayed in films – for example, *The Deer Hunter* (1978), *Birdy* (1984) and *Jacob's Ladder* (1990) – which often repeated tropes from an earlier era of 'war' movies on America's involvement in Vietnam.

An addendum to this, an event that is too recent to have been directly cited in any of the essays, is the conflict in Ukraine. Although seemingly tangential to the War on Terror, the conflict harks back to Cold War-era ideologies and the fall of the Soviet Union in many ways and can also be seen as a continuation of the colonial aspirations between America and Russia in the Middle East that have fuelled and manipulated extremism in the region. Alongside this, the kind of violence and destruction enacted, for its own sake, upon Ukraine (see Pomerantsev 2023) brings it vividly, both imaginatively and geographically, into the Western consciousness in a manner akin to the impact of the Twin Towers attack.

An important aspect of the danger presented by the 'land of the other' in the War on Terror and its ongoing ramifications was the use of technology, specifically social media, by the extremists to not only spread disinformation about events and the 'dark' motivations of Western governments but also groom and enlist new members from disaffected immigrant communities within those same home populations, thereby revealing the contagious nature not just of this Death from the 'East' but of technology itself.

## 2. Technology and the Internet

Technology has played a central role in the twenty-first century, not just by the increasing sophistication of and accessibility to home computers, communication devices and appliances but also through their interconnectedness. In fact, 'interconnectedness' is a crucial feature of recent technology which can be witnessed not only through the rapid increase and use of the internet and social media platforms but also by our ability to interact with our living and working spaces without having to physically be there – an aspect given even greater impetus due to the Covid-19 pandemic. In many ways, the interconnectedness provided by social media and the constant access to information of all kinds has proved to be divisive: it is unifying in its ability to bring colleagues and like-minded people together but, at the same time, can equally be used as a tool for provocation and propaganda. Now more than ever, a large proportion of the population of the developed world can be reached instantly and information of any kind, from images of kittens to advertising and from porn to political messaging, can be disseminated quickly, with little or no means of regulating the appropriateness or veracity of what was being said or sold. This has necessarily contributed to creating a range of anxieties that influence how a majority of other issues are represented and perceived by the general public, and it has consequently had a huge impact on other significant concerns of the twenty-first century, such as the environment, populism and pandemics. Part of the anxiety around technology is its ambiguous nature, how much we control it, how it is controlled by others (governments, companies and malevolent third-party actors) or even whether it is controlling us. The natural progression of this last point is not that we become too dependent upon technology but that it no longer needs us and can exist by itself. Here then robots and/or intelligent machines become both sources and embodiments of Death.

The fears presented by them can be roughly divided into two strands, with one represented by *The Terminator* series of films and the other by *The Matrix* franchise (though this also contained autonomous machines). Although the first film in *The Terminator* franchise (*The Terminator*) was released in 1984, and its third instalment (*Rise of the Machines*) in 2003, subsequent sequels have continued until 2019 (*Dark Fate*), including *The Sarah Connor Chronicles* series that ran from 2008 to 2009: all of these have a common theme that sees a future world dominated by machines determined to rid itself of humanity. Here then it was the machines themselves, originally a skeletal robot, as well as the future world (the world of the deadly other) that embodied Death. *The Matrix* franchise did something similar but gave more prominence to computers and the virtual worlds created by them. Spanning pre- and post-9/11 (1999–2003), the films show a direct link between the real and virtual worlds, and more importantly the uncontrollable nature of the internet and the impossibility of distinguishing between fact and fiction.[5] The World Wide Web and information technology are increasingly represented as a point of permeability to all manner of propaganda and radical ideologies – particularly prescient given the rise of fundamentalism and home-grown conspiracy groups such as QAnon that make much use of cyberspace to 'groom' and agitate its adherents – and such media can be perceived as inherently dangerous and as conduits of death. Films such as *White Noise* (2005), *Pulse* (2006) and *The Signal* (2007) depict media platforms such as television, computers and smart phones as a means to destabilise the mental state of those using them, often changing the users' personalities or even 'possessing' them in a way that the media interface, or screen, becomes the face of Death. Of more recent note in this regard is the sudden appearance of AI in the public consciousness. Although, as suggested above, the environment we inhabit, both professionally and recreationally, has been increasingly shaped and controlled

---

5   At the time of writing, a fourth film is currently in post-production.

by AI, the sudden realisation that this is the case and that it might not be the universal good thing for humanity, as marketed earlier, has created huge anxieties around its impact on increased discrimination, growing economic and social divides as well as the fundamental – almost sacred – notion of human uniqueness and individuality.[6]

Within this sphere is the growing idea that parts of the internet are the sole remit of nefarious activities and malevolent actors that are beyond the reach of real-world law enforcement agencies, thus establishing a new frontier reminiscent of the medieval concept of terra incognita that is full of monsters waiting to pounce on the unwary (a new home for Death). The link between such areas of the internet and ideas around the afterlife/spirit world is one that often informs cinematic representations of this motif with the keyboard doubling as a Ouija board of some kind. This 'Dark Web' is one full of terrorists, cults and predators that are looking to steal your identity or even your life for their own gain, as seen in movies such as *Friend Request* (2012), *Unfriended* (2014), *Unfriended Dark Web* (2018) and *Cam* (2018). Death in these films becomes slightly more complex than just losing your identity, as quite often it is the unreliability of the technology used or rather the skills of those manipulating them (webcams, facial recognition software, graphics programmes, deep fakes and so on) that most clearly represent the Dark Reaper: that is, the computer hacker/programmer who is never seen but can manipulate the world so that their victims effectively no longer exist. Here Death is essentially faceless and can be recognised only by the chaos, or memento mori, it leaves behind.

*3. Climate Change*

The climate crisis has obviously been a long time in the making, but it is in the new millennium that we have begun to feel its more serious effects. Melting ice caps, extreme weather, mountains of waste as well as indestructible plastic and microfibres permeating almost every environment across the planet have

---

[6] A debate that was pointed out by Walter Benjamin and the loss of aura at the start of the twentieth century in 'The Work of Art in the Age of Mechanical Reproduction' (1935).

marked the opening decades of the 2000s. Rising temperatures around the globe and increasing sea levels have been accompanied by acute weather conditions such as hurricanes, severe monsoons and unprecedented rainfall alongside drought and extensive bush/grass fires. Alongside this, the harmful effects of intensive farming methods, pesticides, chemical and human waste in addition to pollution caused by microfibres are shown to cause irreparable if not fatal damage to animals, humans and the ecosystem as a whole. Technology has not been without its influence: on the one hand, it offers greater access to information on, for example, how to decrease one's carbon footprint, and, on the other, it greatly damages the environment through the use of highly toxic materials for manufacturing smart devices, computers and so on in addition to providing a platform for climate-change denialists.

Adjacent to this is the notion that much of what is occurring is due to human, more specifically 'scientific', experimentation and interventions that have created an imbalance beyond our control. Recent conspiracy theories have given form to the pervasive distrust that the general population harbours towards 'science': a catch-all term used to cover anything from radio masts that transmit the coronavirus to bio-engineered diseases and vaccines that are under the control of malevolent forces across the globe. Within popular culture, this has produced films that are as much about dangerous human interference (science) as they are about the environment taking revenge on humanity for such meddling, as seen in examples such as the *Deep Blue Sea* trilogy (1999, 2018, 2020), *Black Sheep* (2008), *Geostorm* (2017) and *The Slender Man* (2018),[7] which portray Death as taking the form of whatever mutated monster that has been created. Nature, however, has become increasingly proactive in its response to unwanted human presence, and post-2000, as shown in several films such as *The Happening* (2008), *Splinter* (2008), *Day of the Triffids* (2009–9), *Sharknado* 1–5 (2012–18), *Annihilation* (2018) and *The Silence* (2019), these increasingly extreme reactions are depicted through 'motivated' fauna and/or flora that want nothing less than total human destruction. This environmental malevolence can equally take on the shape of the planet itself which

---

7   *The Slender Man* (2018) makes a curious link between creepypasta and the environment. The internet 'urban legend' actually appears to be a kind of ecological jouissance that emerges from woodland environments.

has decided that it can no longer tolerate humans exploiting its resources or polluting its atmosphere as in *The Day After Tomorrow* (2004), *The Day the Earth Stood Still* (2009), *2012* (2009), *Arctic Blast* (2010), *Snowpiercer* (2013) and *The Colony* (2013). These films do not always show the monster as being the true embodiment of Death but rather the catastrophic effects of the Anthropocene which has an all-too-human face – oftentimes the deranged scientist that created them – though not necessarily one person in particular but all of us collectively. Of note in many of these films is that either they often feature characters that will deny the true nature of what is occurring or show those that exacerbate what is going on for their own ends – as though Death will overlook them if they give it enough victims – which leads us to the kinds of radical partisanship and culture wars that have deepened as the twenty-first century has progressed and done little to help humanity face the huge challenges that confront it.

*4. Increasing Extremism and Populist Ideologies*

In many ways, the debates about climate change are reflective of, or part of, the increasing partisanship within society and politics. The reasons for the current extremes in viewpoints are many, but this situation is being purposely exploited by those who feel they can gain wealth and power by doing so. In part, the cultural climate of the 2020s is ripe for the rise of populism and the use of culture wars to divide and conquer. The (perceived) failure of neo-liberalism that promised an ever-increasing standard of life and individual betterment in return for supporting a system predicated entirely on exploitation and monetary worth was inevitable. It is a system where it is impossible for everyone to be winners and is heavily weighted towards those who are already wealthy and privileged, as evidenced by the widening gap between the rich and the poor. Populist ideologies then, seemingly offer a means of increasing individual self-esteem along with the spectre of financial gain by scapegoating others in the name of nationalism, 'traditional values' and/or perceived personal freedoms. Of note here is that, often, the expressed intention of such values is to bring people, and thus the nation, together; however, in reality, they create extreme divisiveness, as seen in the Brexit vote in the

United Kingdom and the Trump presidency in the United States. Curiously, a similar framing has been used in the ongoing health crisis around Covid-19 that sees it described as a great leveller and that 'we are all in it together'; however, the ongoing global experience of the pandemic strongly suggests otherwise. In fact, Covid-19 has acted as something of an apotheosis of the other pandemics that have occurred in the 2000s so far, revealing the best and the worst of a world united by a shared experience yet divided in their often-self-interested responses. One of the best examples of films expressing such populist politics is the *Purge* franchise, beginning in 2013 (*The Purge*) and spanning a series of the same name (2018–19) in addition to four further films up to *The Forever Purge* (2021). Here again it is unclear exactly what Death looks like: whether it is the wealthy politicians that organise the wholesale carnage or is it the faceless, mask-wearing thugs that roam the city streets killing anyone they find. There is much here, particularly in the final film of the series, that links to the increasing number of mass shootings and even domestic shootings – people killing 'strangers' or neighbours they do not like or stray onto their property – where extreme violence is seen as the first choice rather than the final option in everyday situations. The inevitable fanaticism and pull towards dictatorship that accompanies populist politics unavoidably leads to the seizing of power by extremist domestic groups and populist governments. Whilst many of these narratives find expression in apocalyptic movies often involving vampires and/or zombies, such as *28 Days Later* (2002), *Blade Trinity* (2004), *Hellboy* (2004), *Doomsday* (2008), *Stake Land* (2010) and *The Strain* (2014–17), others feature more overtly human protagonists, as seen in *The Hunger Games* (2012–14), *The Divergent Series* (2014–16), *The Maze Runner* (2014–18) and *The Handmaid's Tale* (2017–present). Most of these show a ruling elite, often representing a minority of the population, that maintains control via a heady brew of fake news, propaganda, physical violence and enforcement. Death in these narratives can be of two kinds thus producing two categories of movies. If they feature supernatural creatures, it is those entities that become the representation of the end of life, and if they have a leader, who appears visually different from the masses, for example, the Master Vampire, then they take on this role. If there are mainly human actors in the narrative, then it can be the right-hand person or main enforcer of the leader that fills this role. Of note in many of these examples is that the figure identified as Death is often strongly linked to historical representations of extremism such as Nazism in *Hellboy* and *The Strain* or religious extremism in *Blade Trinity* and *The Handmaid's Tale*. An important aspect of the rise of populism and right-wing groups has been the push back from the left and those advocating for greater human rights and equality. This has inevitably seen identity politics pulled into the forefront of the culture wars created specifically to bolster a society founded on 'them' and 'us' ideologies and zero-sum politics. In this configuration, there can only be winners and losers rather than equality being seen as a way to make everyone's lives better. In the 2020s, the call for more widespread individual freedoms then becomes construed as the battle cry of those, led by 'leftist extremists', wishing to destroy traditional values; a propaganda programme designed to shore-up and deepen partisan divides so that the ruling extremists stay in power. Not unlike the situation produced during the Cold War, this sees each side portraying the other as a source of ideological contagion so that those being contaminated by such ideas are subsequently infected with extremism. This makes for a convenient link to the last category to be looked at in relation to Death in the twenty-first century, namely, that of pandemics and disease.

## 5. Global Pandemics

Compared to the previous twenty years, the start of the twenty-first century has witnessed a surprisingly large number of epidemics, averaging over three outbreaks a year in various parts of the world. This statistic does not include those pandemics which spread over far wider areas across the globe. These began with SARS (Severe Acute Respiratory Syndrome, 2002–4), followed by Swine Flu (H1N1, 2009–10), MERS-CoV (Middle Eastern Respiratory Syndrome, 2012), Ebola (2013–16) and Covid-19 (Coronavirus – SARS-CoV-2, 2019–present) – it should be noted that Lassa Fever, Ebola and Yellow Fever have occurred/are currently occurring in Africa during the time of Covid-19. Much of this explosion of diseases has been attributed to environmental causes such as human incursion into the natural environments of animals that often carry these diseases and their rapid spread – locally due to poverty and lack of resources, and globally due to the increase in air travel.

What makes Covid-19 stand out when compared to most of its predecessors is not only its contagiousness but also the levels of obfuscation and disagreement as to its origin, level of spread and how best to treat it. Whilst it is something of an oversimplification to say that all the earlier pandemics in the 2000s were treated more scientifically and with a focused and shared plan of action, the fact remains that countries affected were more in tune with the nature of the disease they were dealing with and how best to contain its spread (though it should be remembered that diseases like Ebola which are far more deadly and contagious are much more limited in the area within which they can be passed on and the likelihood of asymptomatic carriers is very low). With Covid-19, this quickly went awry because the country of origin did not share vital information and was possibly lying about important aspects of its spread and the numbers infected. Countries then reacted very differently to the arrival of the disease in their nation with some immediately locking down the population and borders and enforcing mask and glove wearing, whilst others denying that it was dangerous and that achieving herd immunity as quickly as possible was the best way forward.[8] This has become increasingly problematised through the politicising of the disease and how best to tackle it or even if it actually exists – here public health demands are seen as limiting personal freedoms or as part of an elaborate plot by a secretive world elite. Even with the successful production of multiple vaccines, discord continues to prevail not only due to governmental ineptitude and groups refusing to take the vaccine but also because wealthy countries were hoarding supplies or withholding them from poorer nations.

The idea of contagious diseases and pandemics produces an obvious connection to the on-screen popularity of the vampire or zombie apocalypse, many of which can be seen to correspond with the various global outbreaks mentioned previously. Of note here are *Resident Evil* (2002–18), *Ultraviolet* (2006), *Perfect Creature* (2006), *28 Weeks Later* (2007), *I Am Legend* (2007), *Daybreakers* (2009), *Zombieland* (2009), *The Walking Dead* (2010–present), *World War Z* (2013) and *The Passage* (2019–19). Particularly interesting within

---

8    Herd immunity is the idea that once a high enough percentage of the population has antibodies to a disease, it dies out. However, as shown by viruses like influenza which are constantly mutating, this is not the case.

these films are those that specifically cite the contagion as coming from the East and/or underdeveloped nations tying it back to narratives around the War on Terror – *Ultraviolet, World War Z* and *The Passage* – and those that medicalise the contagion either by its origin or a means by which to eliminate it, intersecting with anxieties around technology – *Resident Evil, Ultraviolet, 28 Weeks Later, I Am Legend, Daybreakers, World War Z* and *The Passage*. Alongside this, and often featured in many of the cited films, is the idea of an 'outbreak narrative' that has taken hold in the popular imagination (see Ward 2009) which maps out the various stages of a contagious disease.

These phases include establishing points of origin and a patient zero; containment and quarantine; identification and vaccine; and return to normal or the establishment of a new normal. The most obvious example of the outbreak narrative is the film *Contagion* (2011), which both reiterates and reinforces the accepted contagion motif, appropriately medicalising the disease from patient zero through to its inevitable cure and re-establishment of normality. What is of special note is the importance given to 'patient zero' not just as the first person to have caught and passed on the disease but almost as an intentional actor who is both catalyst and energiser of the global outbreak. In *Contagion*, it is the unfaithful wife Beth who acts as the agent of death, if not the Grim Reaper herself. This idea has continued to gain traction in films such as *Patient Zero* (2012), *Cabin Fever III: Patient Zero* (2014) and *Patient Zero* (2018), in which 'patient zero' can be seen to represent Death itself and is shown as a far worse figure than that of the wife in *Contagion*, who actually dies of the disease, while the other 'zeros' are seemingly indestructible.

The idea of patient zero also gained early prominence in the Covid-19 outbreak, when notions of contact tracing and super-spreaders were still of importance before efforts at controlling the spread and rate of infection were largely seen as too disruptive. Other films that also follow the idea of an outbreak narrative – *Pandemic* (2007–7), *Toxic Skies* (2008), *Pandemic* (2009), *Pandemic* (2016) and *Alone* (2020) – often point to governmental/military forces as being at fault, not unlike the earlier *Outbreak* (1995) where the disease escapes from a military" to "where a diseased monkey escapes from a military. However, others have no particular or single source to blame which configures the Death of pandemics more as an adjective or a form of endless repetition.

What these films mostly do is not blame the disease itself: it is as though the virus holds no blame for the hundreds of thousands that die from it.

Of importance within this overriding narrative of the Covid-19 pandemic are other 'pandemics' that have been highlighted by aspects of the disease and its attempted containment, specifically those around mental health like Alzheimer's and dementia. The latter two in particular, which are not known to be contagious, are increasingly affecting a large number of people, predominantly the older population of the developed world – a matter brought into sharper relief due to the rampant spread of the coronavirus in retirement homes and care facilities for the elderly. In a similar manner, suicide rates persist at unprecedented levels around the world. Unlike Alzheimer's or dementia, it more obviously affects people of all ages, gender, economic and ethnic backgrounds, and the World Health Organization has noted that for every suicide, there are twenty more people have seriously considered it. The periods of extended lockdown and quarantine during Covid-19 and the associated emotional and economic struggles endured by many as well as the ongoing challenges faced by those suffering with long-Covid have had disturbingly negative effects on the mental health of a majority of the world's population. Without sufficient care or proper facilities in place to help, many choose to take their own lives, a situation which is only exacerbated by the stigma still attached to issues around mental health. In all of these (suicide, Alzheimer's, dementia), Death often presents as a loss of self, as seen in films such as *Harold's Going Stiff* (2011) or *Cam* (2018), or as an excess of identity, as in *The Matrix* (1999–2003), *Lucy* (2014) and *13 Reasons Why* (2017–20). In addition, there is the idea of assisted dying, which again speaks to a loss of one's sense of self and will to live in cases of incurable and/or terminal conditions that are often accompanied by extreme pain and worsening quality of life. This is still a contested subject, albeit one that comes up in the case of diseases like dementia and Alzheimer's, and will continue to garner increasing attention in the many Western countries with ageing populations and little or no public funding to support them.

This begins to define some of the main influences on the representation of Death in the twenty-first century. There are, of course, many other and varied manifestations that come from different intersections between the categories laid out above or just ones that are expressed differently, even whilst stemming from the same root causes. These of course are predominantly from Western popular culture, but the examples within this volume will purposely draw upon other traditions and readings as explained below. The past twenty years seem to have brought about a sea change in our perception of the world and how we exist within it. Not unlike the current pandemic, time often appears to have been stretched and not much feels different. Yet, as we look back, we discover that our understanding of life and, with that, Death has been irrevocably altered.

## The Structure and Chapter Descriptions

This volume, which is divided into five parts that roughly follow the aforementioned categories, examines the various aspects of the representation of Death across film, literature, comics, art and real-world locations to show how pervasive it is within our culture. More than just noting how death is always present within life, this collection further demonstrates how the kinds of Death we visualise are correlated to real-world events. The volume opens with 'Image Intervention I: The Dying of the Light' by Gemma Files, which is the first of seven such creative 'Interventions' throughout the volume by artists Gemma Giles and Laura R. Kremmel that act as punctum and signposts for the essays that follow them. This is followed by the Foreword titled '*The Faces of Death* (John Alan Schwartz, 1978) – The Unwelcome Faces of Death' by W. Scott Poole, who discusses how earlier representations of Death remain and how they inform those of the twenty-first century. The first part of the collection, 'The War on Terror: Evil and the Inevitability of Death', reviews the direct and indirect ramifications of a purposely created and sustained period of imminent terror. This part begins with 'Image Intervention II: Skull 17' by Laura R. Kremmel and is followed by the opening essay, '*28 Days Later* (Danny Boyle, 2002) – Death as Insatiable Terror' by Jack McCormack-Clark, which uses the figure of the zombie as Death to show how an environment of terror is created. But like the one produced by the War on Terror, it is one that feeds on the fear it engenders, seeing it turn into an insatiable monster that consumes all life around it. Following this is 'The Final Destination Films (Various, 2000–11) – Death as Violent Inevitability' by Kevin J. Wetmore, Jr, which also talks about an environment of terror, though one where Death can never be outsmarted or outrun. Here, once you are chosen, Death will quite literally hunt you down and strike in the most unexpected and violent of ways, reflecting similar qualities to those seen in fundamentalist attacks that have occurred in cities and towns across the developed world. Next, Dave Jeffery in 'Death (Eric Kripke, 2005–20) – The Changing Face of Death' discusses the figure of Death in the popular and long-running show *Supernatural*, which first appeared in 2010. Whilst originally shown as an entity above human emotions and concerns, Death slowly becomes so embroiled in the violence and machinations of the world around that, by the time of its own death, it (she) too joined in the struggle for ultimate power over the universe. The next chapter, 'The *Harry Potter* Series (Various, 2001–11) – Death Positivity' by Anna Lüscher, centres on a similar conflict-riven environment but one where death is given a politicised meaning to partisan ends. Here Death is viewed as either 'good' or 'evil' depending on one's allegiances, thus fuelling divisions within a war-torn society. The section concludes with '*The Sleepless* (Nuzo Onoh, 2016) – Living Alongside Death' by Phil Fitzsimmons, which examines strategies for surviving war, trauma and the constant presence of death and how to live a life whilst walking alongside Death.

Part II of the collection, 'Technology: Medicalisation, Ambivalence and Violence', turns the spotlight on the inherent ambivalence of technology and science, and how our relationship with it gives it ultimate meaning and the kinds of Death it embodies. This section opens with 'Image Intervention III: Unlocking the Truth', by Gemma Files, which is followed by the first essay '*The Autopsy of Jane Doe* (André Øvredal, 2016) – Death as the Dissected Female Cadaver' by Rebecca Booth. Booth's chapter centres on the medicalisation of the body which has been increasingly utilised to control and abuse the disenfranchised and maintain the existing cultural hierarchy. In response to this, Death here is shown as a female corpse providing an opposite and proportional response to centuries of masculine intrusion and violence, manifesting a call for equality in life and death. The next chapter in this section, '*Proof* (Rob Bragin, 2015–15) – Science as Death' by Łucja Lange, focuses on medical science but expands its scope to technology in general. Science here becomes the means to investigate and prove that human existence continues beyond death in some form yet convincingly asserts that science itself is the gatekeeper of such experiences and is therefore Death. The idea of the Afterlife, or afterlives, continues in '*The Midnight Library* (Matt Haig, 2020) – Death and Infinite Lives' by Stephanie Weber, which proposes that we exist not just in one life but in many. Whilst there is much of quantum existence in the infinite number of lives in Haig's story, it also speaks to our endless selves, or profiles, that 'live' online, in social media and databases, and in the periphery of the lives of others. '*Death Note* (Various, 2003–17) – Death as Information' by Katarzyna Ancuta extends the transition to online technology and focuses on the power of information where a name written on a celestial interface has the power to end someone's earthly existence. In this scenario, it becomes information itself that is the Grim Reaper and less the actors, or messengers, that fulfil its demands. '*Death Stranding* (Kojima Productions, 2019) – Death as Interconnectivity' by Carl Wilson argues that it is not just information that foretells our demise but the interconnectivity that accompanies that evokes the sense of an impending apocalypse. Here then is the apotheosis of globalism where all points are connected and brought together in a singularity that extinguishes life leaving only Death. This part closes with '*Ready Player Two* (Ernest Cline, 2020) – Pixelated Death' by Tom Ue, which discusses how the end of life is eternally deferred through the never-ending resurrection of one's consciousness in virtual avatars. However, this kind of immortality is one that has lost the 'aura' of the living person it once was and so becomes the symbol of their death; a death that is eternally re-enacted each time it is resurrected into a new avatar.

Part III, 'Climate Change: Environments and the Environmental', considers the environments of death, which attempt to create a more healthy, holistic space themselves, and then moves on to more ecological concerns. The discussion opens with 'Image Intervention IV: The King of Nature', by Gemma Files, which is followed by 'Death Café (Limerick, 2015–Present) – Death in Life' by Tracy Fahey and Jennifer Moran Stritch, who address how death has been removed from life, thus throwing our relationship to both life and death out of balance. One way of restoring this balance is through the creation of environments, such as Death Cafés, offering a more holistic approach to our shared existence in this world and the next. The next chapter in this section is '*Ghosts* (Nick Broomfield, 2006) – The Sea as Death' by Mark Fryers. Whilst the sea has always been viewed as an alien environment, more recent imbalances between humanity and the environment, both ecological and political, have exacerbated that situation in such a way that the oceans of the world are configured not just as places of danger but as embodying Death itself. '*Geostorm* (Dean Devlin, 2017) – Death as the Eye of the Storm' by Kristy Strange, the next essay in the line-up, explores climate change and extreme weather events not as instances of eco-revenge, but rather as manifestations of disaster capitalism. Here financial gain serves as the metaphorical 'eye of the storm' that engineers fiscal worth out of extreme weather and environmental collapse, sucking life and energy out of everything it touches. This part ends with '*Mexican Gothic* (Silvia Moreno-Garcia, 2019) – Death as Mycological Rebirth' by Ildikó Limpár that discusses how ecological revenge is not necessarily about death but about transformation. Here, fungal growth becomes a means of rebalancing humanity, by which Death becomes a gateway to birth into a new life beyond the limitations of the human body.

Part IV, 'Extremism: Partisanship and Identity Politics', brings to the fore ideas around fundamentalism and populist politics, discussed above, by examining ways in which various cultural wars have purposely politicised certain topics around identity and human rights in order to deepen the divides between different parts of the society for political gain. This section opens with 'Image Intervention V: Skull 4' by Laura R. Kremmel, which precedes the first essay 'The Unite the Right Rally and Its Aftermath (2017–20) – The Skull' by James T. McCrea. McCrea delves deeper into the discussion by further focusing specifically on the symbolism and meaning attached to representations of the human skull. Whilst originally signifying mortality and the brevity of human life, more recent extremist groups have used the imagery to symbolise far more specific threats of death and dominion. In the next chapter, '*The Purge* Series (Various, 2012–21) – Mass Shootings and Endless Death', Nicola Young continues the theme of extremism and the public spectacle of violence in the pursuit, and the result, of political power and in which the face of Death is the mask of the gang leader or the lone shooter. Following this is '*American Horror Story: Asylum* (Brad Falchuck and Ryan Murphy, 2012–13) – Angel of Death' by Rachael Grant, which shows that even in the most extreme of environments there is a place of calm and solace. Death here is that place, which plots a course between the chaos and violence around it. In the next chapter in this section, 'Mistress Death in the Marvel Universe (Various, 1973–Present) – For the Love of Death' by Robert Mclaughlin, Death is embodied as a beautiful woman who is pursued by two suitors over the course of many narratives. In the ensuing battle between quantity and quality for her affections, Death chooses the individual and the particular over the genocidal and the apocalyptic as sometimes even she can feel the loneliness of her position. '*Suspiria* (Luca Guadagnino, 2018) – Female Death' by Maria Giakaniki turns towards narratives more obviously centred on identity politics and, in particular, sexual equality. A topic that is largely used by 'traditionalists' as a threat against family values, the women here embrace all the qualities that men are allowed but women are denied. Consequently, Death is a vengeful, monstrous mother who claims all energies of nature and nurture for herself. If Female Death simultaneously represents the fears of the traditionalists and aspirations of the liberals, 'Deathface Ginny (Kelly Sue DeConnick, 2014–20) – Death and #MeToo' by Octavia Cade goes for straightforward revenge. Death here is the judge and executor giving the final 'reward' to all those who have abused women. The last essay in this part is '*Mrs Death Misses Death* (Salena Godden, 2021) – Death as a Black Woman' by Bethan Michael-Fox and Renske Visser, which sees death as the eponymous Black woman of the title who brings a post-#MeToo and BLM energy to her role in order to challenge what people expect of Death, and what Death might actually mean to those she comes to collect.

The final part of the collection, 'Global Pandemics: Contagion, Mental Health and Dementia', discusses the most important 'contagions' affecting the world at the moment, not just Covid-19, but also those of mental health, suicide, Alzheimer's and dementia. Whilst mental health problems are not contagious in the same way as the coronavirus – although the hereditary nature of many of such health issues suggests an equally dangerous kind of transmission – the numbers affected by it with little hope of care or support reveal this as being an even more pressing and deadly global affliction. Much of how we view death, contagion and illness is signified by the dead body, and 'Image Intervention VI: The Source' by Gemma Files leads us on our final journey through the volume, which continues in the first essay, '*Coco* (Lee Unkrich, 2017) – Death as Decomposition' by Cath Davies. Davies looks at the ways in which we cover this up to contain the porous body of Death and the contagion and disease that flows from it. Following this, '*The Thing* (Matthijs van Heijningen Jr, 2011) – The Microbe as Death' by Simon Bacon narrows the focus from the body to the microbes that infect it and float through the air to their next victim. The lack of concrete information during many stages of the Covid-19 outbreak has led to an unusual predominance and importance being given to images of the coronavirus itself as a floating, disembodied image of Death. Staying on the topic of the recent pandemic, in '*Ludo* (Anurag Basu, 2020) – Death as New Normal', Debaditya Mukhopadhyay talks about the society during and after the pandemic through the lens of popular film of the time, which metaphorically shows how local and wider governmental bodies continue to play a game with Death over those in their care. '*13 Reasons Why* (Brian Yorkey, 2017–20) – Death as Controversial Suicide' by Heidi Kosonen shifts the focus of the conversation to mental health issues, specifically around suicide. It centres on the lack of care for those in danger but also romanticises the depiction, which sees it less as a cry for help and more as a contagion infecting those around it. Moving on to afflictions such as dementia and Alzheimer's, '*Land of the Lustrous* (Takahiko Kyōgoku, 2017–17) – Death as Loss of Memory' by Rae Hargrave considers how memory is as important as the physical self. Bodies here are constructed of memories and as one goes, so does one's sense of self, and once that has gone, so has life. The final essay, '*Unus Annus* (Mark Fischbach and Ethan Nestor, 2019–20) – Death as Deletion' by Catherine Pugh, takes this a step further by bringing together several ideas regarding identities online and the essential nature of memory to life and even death. Here then identity is wiped clean leaving no traces of its existence. It is a loss of self so complete that Death becomes a deletion of all that someone was and might have been. It is the ultimate, desolate, end.

This collection comes to an end with an Afterword, 'The Tomorrow of Death – Dia de los Muertos', by Lisa Morton that returns us to the folklore of death where it was part and parcel of the rituals of everyday life that anchored us to our collective and individual pasts while allowing us to bring them with us into whatever kind of future awaited us. The revival of such traditions in the form of the 'Day of the Dead' and their ready acceptance as part of a wider 'Halloween Holiday' might point, not just to the capitalist drive to turn even death into money, but that we should (will) never fully lose sight of the fact that what makes us most human and gives all our lives their essential 'aura' of uniqueness is that they will inevitably end, as intimated in 'Intervention VII', the final and closing image in the collection.

Much of this might seem to indicate a rather bleak end to how death is seen and conceived in the first half of the twenty-first century. Yet, there is also the sense within it that if Death, as in the case of *Unus Annus*, is the blue or blank computer screen, then there is still an opportunity to reboot it; that endings are beginnings and that without Death there is no life.

Part I

# The War on Terror: Evil and the Inevitability of Death

# Image Intervention II: Skull 17

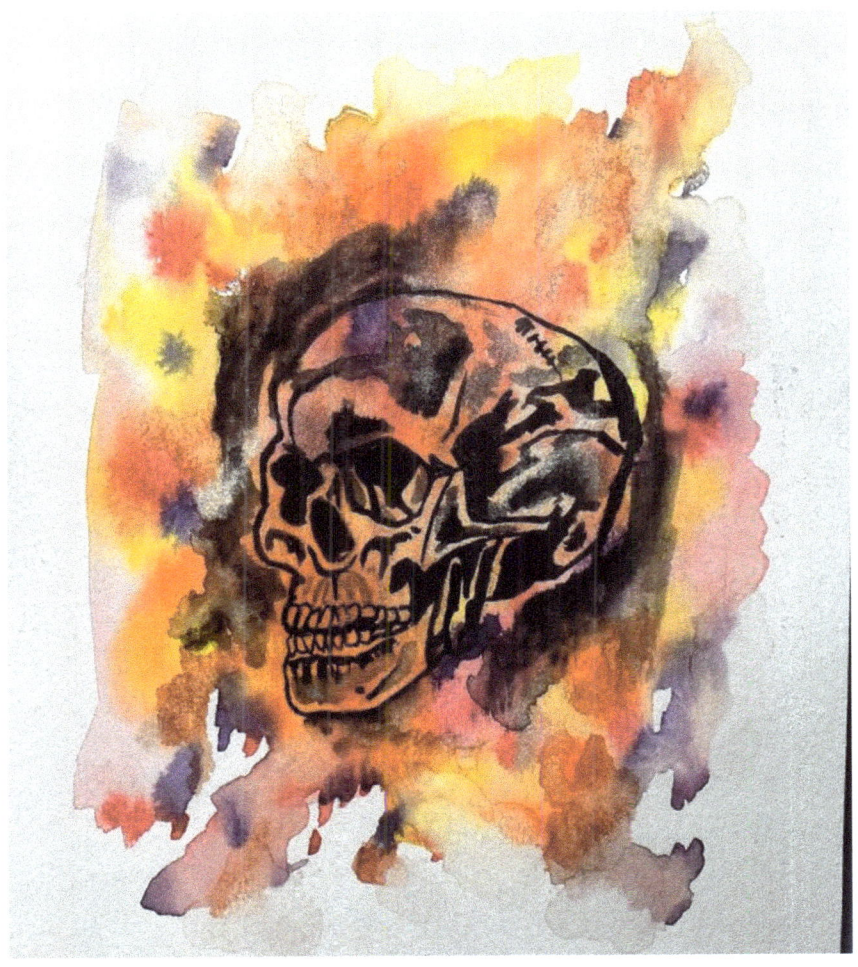

Artwork by Laura R. Kremmel
(Reproduced with the permission of the artist)

Jack McCormack-Clark

# *28 Days Later* (Danny Boyle, 2002)

## Reframing Terror and Extremism

The archetype of the zombie has become a critical point of interest for the consumer in literature, multimedia and popular culture. It has ironically spread like a virus, becoming increasingly consumed on so many different levels. Whether horror, romance or comedy, the zombie has broken into nearly every genre and remains increasingly popular among many different demographics. This level of engagement is unprecedented and has not happened to even the most prolific of Gothic monsters to the same degree. Why? What makes this creature so attractive despite its grotesque features and close relationship to humanity? This is the question for the ages but our interest in the zombie here is specifically on its rise to popularity following the 11 September terrorist attacks. Following that event, there was an unprecedented rise in interest in the zombie as an archetype with many narratives mirroring the trauma of terror, extremism and destruction. Within the sphere of twenty-first-century horror, I argue that the zombie has become a metaphor for the virality of extremism in all its mindless and destructive tendencies. This chapter will specifically analyse this within the film *28 Days Later* (2002) looking first at the infected through the rage zombie, a unique phenomenon that has not appeared as much in contemporary narratives as its slow, lumbering counterpart. My final focus is specifically on those fighting the infected. The soldiers who help the main characters, Jim, Selena and Hannah, mirror similar military responses to fighting terror, namely, fighting extremism with extremism. The soldiers, while still human, reveal themselves to be no better than the zombies. They have succumbed to their base natures and devolved to wield their power dangerously to the point where they wilfully seek to harm Jim and the others.

## 'The proletarial underclass of cinematic monsters': Why the Zombie?

As Anna Froula quite aptly stated, 'as the proletarial underclass of cinematic monsters, zombies lack the sensual cunning of the vampire and the functioning human counterpart of the werewolf or serial killer' (2010: 196). So why are they so consistently popular? What makes them attractive? The study of the zombie is not a new point of focus in academia especially in the twenty-first century where multimedia and popular culture have been saturated with an immense variety of different narratives, merchandise, themed events, music and food. The question that presents itself is why? Of all the potential monsters (many of which have become the subject of fandom over the past decade), the zombie has been the most consistently embraced since the 1980s. Nevertheless, as Richard Greene and K. Silem Mohammad state, 'zombies take up surprisingly little screen time and their presence is kind of a given. They are a plot mechanism to launch us into the character driven story' (2010: 19). Yet, despite the fact they are merely a foil or rather a part of the apocalyptic furniture, they are the most iconic image of each narrative in popular culture. Different scholars have provided potential reasons why we as a Western world have woven the tale of this monster so deeply into the fabric of our cultural expression even though they vary so much from narrative to narrative. Kevin Boon (2011) identifies a typology of eight different types of zombies: The zombie drone, zombie ghoul, bio zombie, zombies that channel the will of others, psychological zombies, cultural zombies, zombie ghosts and zombie ruse. All of these types are geared towards the zombie as the other but primarily highlight the visceral and flexible nature of the zombie. Though Boon noticeably does not identify the rage zombie, the current chapter primarily focuses on this type of zombie. Akin to Boon's identification of many different types of zombies, Laura Hubner et al. also identify the flexibility of the archetype. They state that 'the meaning of zombie texts is related to the wider social formations and specific historical circumstances in which they emerge' (2015: 4). Roger Luckhurst reinforces this through his account of zombie narratives across the twentieth and twenty-first centuries. He indicates that in the 1940s and 1950s, Dracula, Frankenstein's Monster and the Mummy were the 'unholy trinity of the undead. The zombie rotted a bit more from neglect, lurking unnoticed in graveyards, sinking into the shudder pulps and horror comics of the 1940s and 50s' (2015: 12). It was not until George Romero's *Night of the Living Dead* (1968), a film that became a cult classic, that zombies began to appear more avidly from the 1980s onwards. This interest grew especially after the sequel *Dawn of the Dead* (1978) was released. David R. Castello et al. state that 'Romero's *Dawn of the Dead* planted the suggestion that the zombies are us, insatiable masses of mindless, soulless, destructive consumers' (2016: 12). This is where zombies became a key metaphor for the effects of monstrous global capitalism and its neoliberal ideology. Annalee Newitz (2006), David McNally (2011), Jennifer Daly (2016) and Johannes Fehrle (2016) all compare zombification to Western consumerism and blind consumption, especially regarding late-twentieth-century narratives. Jen Webb and Samuel Byrnand state that 'the zombie's paradoxicality is the source of its symbolic potential – and for us, this means specifically its usefulness as a figure that grapples with the fundamental irreconcilability of capitalism and humanism' (2017: 9). The zombie is a parasitic mass which devours all, but it is unbiased, not motivated by malicious intent, nor does it think or act beyond its instinctual cannibalistic nature (Froula 2010). The other factor in the twenty-first century is zombie narratives that appeared post-11 September 2001, when the World Trade Center was attacked. Zombies have since been compared to thoughtless and mindless extremists, which is where this thesis fits within this discipline.

Previous scholarship has highlighted the event as a significant turning point in the way culture contends with the archetype of the zombie. Mark McKenna notes that 'since the dawn of the new millennium, there has been a noticeable rise in the visibility and profitability of the zombie across all media platforms with many continuing to draw political parallels with the events of 9/11' (2011: 145). This is reinforced by Froula who observes that 'the figure of the zombie in post 9/11 cinema re-animates the ramifications of US foreign policies in the Middle East in particular and is a dominant cultural metaphor within American culture in general' (2010: 195). Mckenna (2022) and Froula (2010) highlight the fact that 9/11 opened the door to a new world order that adjusted to fear caused by political, religious and cultural extremism. Stacey Abbott reflects on this by stating that, 'looking back over the past fifteen years, 11 September 2001 can be seen as such a fulcrum marking an apocalyptic moment through which so much of our experience of the 21st century has been shaped' (2016: 6). As such there has been a significant increase in interest surrounding zombies following the events of 11 September.

In the sections that follow, this discussion is continued with a specific focus on the film *28 Days Later* (2002). The film has been subject to study before its links to 9/11. Froula (2010), Mohammad (2010), Webb and Byrnand (2017) and Fred Botting (2017) analyse *28 Days Later* (2002) but focus primarily on its connection to 9/11 through the characters in the film as well as the setting. This chapter will focus on the rage virus as a metaphor for extremism and the juxtaposition of the soldiers who apply extremism to fight extremism. The main character, Jim, also applies the same rage to fight the soldiers and in doing so is not targeted by the zombies. It will be argued here that *28 Days Later* (2002) is allegorical of the spread of extremism and the lengths those fighting extremism will go to win even if that means embracing extremism.

## The Rage Zombie

The rage zombie is an important aspect of the film as it as an archetypal form and vision of death, symbolising the rapid and aggressive spread of extremism. The film actively pursues this in the opening sequences where we see experimentation on chimpanzees. One is strapped to a chair with monitors playing scenes of riots over and over again. In an act of extremism, animal rights activists break into the premises to release the animals with no regard for the future of the animals, the reason they are locked up or the harm they may inflict on others. This blind political activism is the first instance of extremism which is then followed by rage. As the activists attempt to free the animals, a scientist on duty tries to stop them. He states that they are infected and are being used in the endeavour to find a cure:

## 28 Days Later (Danny Boyle, 2002)

SCIENTIST: In order to cure. You must understand.
ACTIVIST: Infected with what?
SCIENTIST: Rage. (Boyle 2002)

The activists do not listen and release the animals, and as a result, they become infected by rage. The metaphor of the activists being infected aligns with this notion of extremism. They are converted to mindless rage in a moment of activism, which Harry M. Benshoff states is reflective of 'a paranoid fear of mindless … conformity, wherein poisonous ideology spreads like a virus, silently turning one's friends and relatives into monsters' (1997: 128). In keeping with Benshoff's assessment, the infected activist then attacks her friends. Twenty-eight days after the first infection, the film introduces the audience to a dystopic world overrun by the raging dead. The main character, Jim, awakens in a recovery ward at the hospital to discover the zombie apocalypse which occurred while he was in a coma. Initially, he encounters no life and is depicted walking deliriously through the empty streets of London as a metaphor for anxiety in the face of extremism. This is until he enters a church waking some of the dead who are piled there. The next overt allusion to extremism happens when Jim is attacked by an infected priest in the church. The image of the infected priest portrays religious extremism which is emphasised via scenes of the mass of bodies of the congregation who have died due to the plague and who can be seen still in their seats facing the altar.

The film highlights different forms of potentially devout and zealot belief through disease or plague to emphasise extremism in two instances: political and religious. It is important to note that this is not the first example in history of this happening in culture. In Albert Camus' book *The Plague* (1947), the epidemic was a 'symbol of Nazi occupation (and incidentally the prefiguration of any totalitarian regime, no matter where), and … the concrete illustration of a metaphysical problem, that of evil' (Twindle 2021: 29). In a scenario similar to a zombie narrative, five men are the survivors of an epidemic which has wiped out the population of their town. Each dead person is meant to personify the swelling ranks of both collaboration with Nazism and the victims of the regime (Camus 1947). Extremism in the book is depicted as a non-human entity which spreads and infects unbiasedly. This is how the zombie virus is interpreted now and the reason why they are so effective and terrifying. As Gregory A. Waller describes, 'the fear that zombies inspire originates in uncanny confrontation with people we know and perhaps love who want nothing but to feed on us and pull us into their own ranks' (2010: 195). Jim as the 'paranoid wandering subject whose experience is one of terror' is faced with the fall of a once seemingly impenetrable symbol of empire that has been overrun internally with rage and cannibalism which symbolises indoctrination (Botting 2017: 278). The allusion to the aesthetic terror seen and felt on 11 September is undeniable but so is the rage. While one act of extremism toppled the World Trade Center, the other was one of vengeance that appeared when the dust had settled: military intervention in the Middle East following the attack (Carlisle 2007).

## 'The answer to infection': Fighting Extremism with Extremism

The second focus of this chapter is military extremism and the juxtaposition of the blind extremism of the zombies and the military response to the infection. This is where themes arising from 9/11 connect to *28 Days Later*. A group of soldiers offer Jim, Selena and Hannah sanctuary which is first seen as a saving grace for this band of survivors. However, it becomes clear that the soldiers are just as dangerous, if not more so, than the undead. Major Henry West admits to giving into terror and hopelessness, but to keep his men alive and working, he allowed them to devolve into a base-instinctual, desire-driven state which has led to an extreme reaction to the rage virus:

> Major West: Eight days ago, I found Jones with his gun in his mouth. He said he was going to kill himself because there was no future. What could I say to him? We fight off the infected or we wait until they starve to death … and then what? What do nine men do except wait to die themselves? I moved us from the blockade, and I set the radio broadcasting, and I promised them women. Because women mean a future. (Boyle 2002)

The soldiers have been luring survivors to their fortified mansion with military broadcasts promoting sanctuary, killing the men and using the women to attempt to repopulate the earth. This highlights the impulses at the root of extremism within the film's narrative. The zombies desire flesh, conversion and repopulation. The soldiers require the same thing – just in a different context. One wants to eat human flesh, while the other wants to satisfy sexual urges. As Froula states, 'the uninfected humans are as brutal and violent about satisfying their biological appetites as the infected ones' (2010: 203). They represent two sides of the same coin, fighting extremism with extremism. Even the surname of Major 'West' speaks to Western policies around fighting terror and what the West has been willing to do through military force with regard to counterterrorism and extremism. He symbolises the fantasy that 'terrorism can be contained and defeated by superior military power without addressing its root causes' (Froula 2010: 200). Major West is not interested in a cure but in fighting those who are infected. As West says to Jim before divulging his plan to use Selena and Hannah,

> The answer to infection. Well, as I said before, it's here – though it may not be quite what you imagined. (Boyle 2002)

To ensure Jim does not get in the way of their plan to use the women in sexual servitude, the soldiers attempt to kill him by dragging him into the woods and shooting him. But Jim escapes and lures West away from the mansion. Once he returns to the mansion, he releases the infected soldier being kept in the basement who then attacks the rest of the soldiers in the house. What is interesting in this scene is that Jim is not attacked. He moves with the undead as he exacts his vengeance. As is pointed out by Webb and Byrnand,

> Jim performs as a zombie yet is able ... [to] pull back and return to the human condition ... because [he] has not yet crossed the boundary that marks the end of self awareness. [It is a] removal of the human subject from the symbolic order [but] returns to the real. (2017: 122)

Because of Jim's submission to rage and vengeance, the zombies do not trouble him. It is this part of the film which I believe speaks directly to this theme of rage and extremism as it does not make sense within the world that Boyle and screen writer Alex Garland have brought to life. Regardless of Jim's intentions, the zombies should have attacked him, but because he has given into his rage and vengeance, he has become like the creatures he was once terrified of when he wandered the streets of London.

## Conclusion

The popularity of the zombie is based on its pliability as a metaphor and dissonance as the living dead. Although it is not as sexy as the vampire, technologically prophetic as Frankenstein's monster or as exotic as the Mummy, it provides an allegory of human-like beings who can be rationalised as realistic. Without the caveats that define the other creatures, zombies become a nondescript force of the unnatural, a foil that is easily assigned with meaning which humanity easily responds to. In the case of *28 Days Later*, we see the juxtaposition of extremes in a post-9/11 world. One of rage, cannibalism and conformity; the other of desire, vengeance and brutality. In the context of the war on terror, *28 Days Later* utilises these thematic threads to create an allegory that offers commentary on extremism and the futility of combating such rage and hate with devolution, brutality and war. As a zombie film, it is often overlooked in the shadow of the likes of *The Walking Dead* (2010–present) or cult films such as *Night of the Living Dead*, but as an allegory, it still has much to offer in this post-9/11, pandemic-dominated world that we live in.

Kevin J. Wetmore, Jr

# *The Final Destination* Films (Various, 2000–11)

'The mortician said death has a design'

In the *Final Destination* films (2000–11), death is not so much personified or embodied as constructed as a presence with agency, called 'a force' in the third film in the series, but a force with awareness, agency and an agenda (Wong 2006). The series' narratives are in the mode of a slasher film with death itself as the killer. In slasher films, the object of the killer is to kill, to bring death to as many individuals as possible. The *Final Destination* films eliminate the middleman of the murderous slasher, so to speak, and has death itself as a killer, utilising various machinations to kill people so that they would have died in the very accident which they escaped. Death is a slasher killer, but one whose existence implies a universe of predestination, design and, ultimately, vicious, merciless suffering (both physical and psychological) before death, after which comes nothing. Ian Conrich terms the *Final Destination* (and *Saw*) series as 'grand slashers':

> In the grand slasher, death appears all-pervasive and generally cannot be escaped or defeated. The victims are part of a scheme or preordained plan, and the deaths are often hyper-elaborate. These are essentially survival horrors and puzzle films, in which death itself can be manipulating a situation and in which victims have to second-guess a system in which the horror that awaits can be protracted and torturous. (2015: 106)

In other words, these films out-grim the Grim Reaper by revealing Death to be 'out to get you'.

This model evokes death not as merely the end of life and certainly not a natural process but rather Death as antagonist; death as 'a shadowy figure, unwilling to draw attention to itself but unrelenting in its endeavors', according to Alexandra West (2018: 147). Death is relentless, yet hidden, and will eventually come for everyone, which is in and of itself a very medieval notion of death. As Glynne Wickham observes, emerging out of the (new) Feast of Corpus Christi in the fourteenth century, medieval visual and performing arts focused on the idea that death came for all, including 'the frivolous rich and the covetous tradesman' as well as clergy and magisterium (1987: 67):

> The Danse Macabre survives to us in innumerable graphic representations depicting this time and this messenger: the spectral figure of Death, sometimes on foot, sometimes on horseback, armed always with his scythe and summoning pope, emperor, king, queen, merchant, lawyer, artisan, artist and peasant for follow him to the grave grew out of time and gave force to the message.

Emerging out of the medieval theology and aesthetic comes the figure of Death personified (with a capital 'D') and the notion that Death will come for everyone. As Wickham discerns, the dominant medieval depiction of death was not simply the natural end of life but a personified force, often in the form of a skeleton: 'Death as a harvester and leading a procession of men and women from every walk of life to their inevitable graves' (1987: 111). The most obvious example of this being the medieval morality play *Everyman*, in which God summons the personification of Death to summon 'Everyman' to his death, and Death carries out a conversation with the eponymous character, letting him know, 'I am Death', and Everyman responds, 'O Death, thou comest when I had thee least in mind' (Lester 1990: 68–9). *The Final Destination* series continues this Danse Macabre, wherein Death is no longer a robed skeleton but an invisible yet intelligent force that leads a procession of (in the case of the first film) high school students and teachers from every walk of life to their inevitable graves.

Ironically, despite following the model of medieval morality plays (which instruct how to achieve salvation before one's death and thus concern how to live a life guaranteed to bring life everlasting within Christian belief), there is no salvation or divinity present in these films. Alexandra West argues the film (and its sequels) models a world without God: 'Death becomes an omnipresent figure in the survivor's lives but God does not' (2018: 147). Death replaces God in these films as the mechanism by which we live and die. Death becomes a kind of God in the *Final Destination* films.

The first film was originally written as an episode of *The X-Files* (1993–2002); however, the script was developed by writers Glen Morgan, James Wong and Jeffrey Reddick into a stand-alone feature: *Final Destination* (Wong 2000). That feature then produced five sequels: *Final Destination 2* (Ellis 2003), *Final Destination 3* (Wong 2006), *The Final Destination* (Ellis 2009) and *Final Destination 5* (Quale 2011). The series of films, taken together, creates its own shifting mythology about what death is and how death works in addition to why people die as well as when and how they die.

The five films (to date) all follow the same pattern: a group of individuals (sometimes part of the same group, sometimes random individuals who happen to be in the same place at the same time) is mobile, moving somewhere at velocity or adjacent to fast-moving vehicles (plane, cars, roller coaster, by a NASCAR track, on a holiday bus). One character then receives a vision, unprompted, at the start of the film that shows a terrible disaster with a number of the individuals present dying horribly in a specific order. The individual then returns to the moment before the accident and moves to get the individuals around them out of harm's way, prophesying the disaster they have just witnessed. The tragic event then occurs and the individuals who avoided the accident are alive, despite the vision, and now find themselves marked by death, who was somehow cheated of their demise at the designated time of death. The rest of the film shows the slow stalking and killing of the individuals in the order in which they would have died in the accident.

Ian Conrich observes how this plot transforms the films from simple slashers into something more complex:

> The appeal of the *Final Destination* films has little to do with knowing which victim is next or what the killer looks like. The *Final Destination* films instead foreground attempts to prolong life, with the screen at times structured around the futile creation of 'death-free' zones, but with the knowledge that the individual cannot escape his or her grisly fate. The films promise that when that moment of death occurs, it will be a highly elaborate sequence of cause and effect, a fantastic arrangement that is rooted in a seemingly innocuous situation. (2015: 114–15)

In other words, viewers watch the films as if they were slasher cinema, but rather than guessing who will die next or why the killer is stalking the victim, the viewer attempts to guess how they will eventually die, with the knowledge that the films (particularly from the second one on) foreground a number of different ways each individual could die when it is their 'turn'.

In the first, third and fifth films the victims all know each other and are part of a group – students on a class trip to France, teens from the same school at an amusement park and employees going to a company retreat, respectively; whereas in the second and fourth ones, set on a highway and at a NASCAR track, respectively, the victims are strangers to one another, who then bond over (or unite against) their coming demise. In each film, however, the narrative unfolds similarly. A large accident kills dozens, and those who listened to the one who received the vision live. But, as each group then learns, death will not be cheated, resulting in a series of spectacular accidents to replace the one that was supposed to kill them. Key to this mechanism, the vision is never questioned by the people. How and why was the individual who saw the accident happen chosen? Who or what gave them that vision? Does that entity or property also have agency and want to cheat death. The vision is always present at the start of the film, always a mystery and always starts a chain of events that results in the slow but inevitable demise of the cast.

The first film foregrounds death throughout its opening credits and first scenes. While panning past protagonist Alex's (Devon Sawa) desk during the credits, the frame centres a copy of *Death of a Salesman* and a photo of Jim Morrison (who is buried in Paris, the destination of the flight that explodes) with the words 'This is the end' written on it is shown; the camera then focuses on the word 'Terminal' as the families pull up to the airport while 'Rocky Mountain High' plays in the departure lounge as a character observes, 'John Denver – died in a plane crash' (Wong 2000). All of these images and moments foreground the explosion of the plane in the first ten minutes of the film. Alex has a vision of it and is kicked off the plane, along with a teacher and five other students. The plane explodes and then one by one, over the following week, those who leave the plane begin to die, too. Eventually, Alex and Clear (Ali Larter), a young woman who believed his vision and got off the plane, break into a funeral home to learn about the death of their friend. They are surprised by Bludworth, a mortician (played by horror staple and Candyman himself, Tony Todd), who tells them, 'You have to realize that we're just a mouse that a cat has by the tail, every single move we make from the mundane to the monumental, the red light that we stop at or run, the people we have sex with or want with us, the airplanes that we ride or walk out of, it is all part of Death's sadistic design. Leading to the grave' (Wong 2000). This statement is the series' first indication that death is an intelligence with agency and design. Death is not a natural part of life. It is 'sadistic'. This statement also suggests a philosophical/theological belief in predetermination, not from any divinity per se, but from death itself. Death decides when one dies, and if one does not die, then death makes sure one dies soon after in an even more painful and sadistic manner.

When Alex asks Bludworth how death's design might be changed, he replies as follows: 'You already did that by walking off the plane. Now you gotta figure out when and how it'll come back at you. Play your hunch, Alex. If you think you can get away from it. But beware, the risk of cheating the plan, disrespecting the design … could initiate a horrifying fury that would terrorize even the Grim Reaper – and you don't even want to fuck with that MacDaddy' (Wong 2000). Again, the mortician (an expert on death with a name to match) tells the students that death has a plan and a design and when its (his?) plans are upset, it responds with 'horrifying fury' that 'terrorizes' the Grim Reaper, itself a personification of death. So Death in the films is even above and more powerful than any personification of death.

Several times throughout the film, when the survivors attempt to figure out who will die next and how, Alex repeats the phrase, 'The mortician said that Death has a design' (Wong 2000). Eventually, he begins to reason that the design is not set in stone, and there are actually rules Death must follow: 'Now, what if you, me, Tod, Carter, Terry, Billy, Mrs. Lewton messed up that design. For whatever reason, I, I saw Death's plan. We cheated him. But what if it was our time? What if we were not meant to get off that plane? What if it still is our time? If it is, then it's not finished, and we will die – now, not later – unless, unless we find the patterns and cheat It again' (Wong 2000). They learn that if the next person to die according to Death's design is able to evade the next death planned for them, Death will 'skip' them and go on to kill the next person. Eventually, when it makes its way through the list, Death will return again for the survivors it skipped, but if they can continue to avoid dying, they can live long lives.

The second film begins a shift in the mythology of Death in the series. The film opens with a credit sequence that recaps the first film through a television interview on the one year anniversary of the crash of the plane in the first film. The host asks, 'So I'm surrounded by death?', to which the guest responds, 'Absolutely! Absolutely! Everyday, everywhere, all the time. That's what I want people to understand: that death has this grand design that we all fit into. So when Alex Browning got off that plane and took the other survivors with him, he basically screwed up death's plan' (Ellis 2003). Thus, the sequel opens with a succinct summary of the first film's conceits: Death is intelligent and has agency, Death is everywhere all the time and Death has a plan, a 'grand design'. This design can be altered by accident or intent, but it only postpones the inevitable as death will immediately set in motion a new design to kill those it missed.

The people who survive the highway pileup that opens the second film go to see the lone survivor of the first film, Clear Rivers, who has committed herself to an asylum to protect herself from Death's design, claiming that by exiting the plane, she and her friends created a 'rift'. She describes it as 'death is working backwards. It's tying up all the loose ends and sealing the rift once and for all' (Ellis 2003). She tells them that their accident has opened another rift: 'If you put them on the list they're already dead.' Kimberly asks her, 'What list?' Clear responds, 'Death's list' (Ellis 2003). The second film echoes what Conrich terms 'the inevitability of death' in the *Final Destination* films (2015: 114). The characters are all on 'Death's life', but what is that if not a metaphor for the human condition. We are all indeed on 'Death's list'. The films, however, ascribe much more intelligence and malevolence to Death.

It is the third film, in which a roller coaster accident kills a dozen but spares another eight who should have also died, that Kevin (Ryan Merriman) describes death as 'a force' with awareness (Wong 2006). Ian (Kris Lemche), who does not believe the Final Destination mythos that the other characters have worked out, questions it, similarly arriving where the characters of the first film do:

> Ok. Let's go with what you guys are saying: let's just say, you know, that Death does have a conscious plan, and that it's been set into motion. Great. So, Newton's Third Law of Motion and well, look, I'm just guessing that it goes for Death, too, when he's working in our world. Newton says that every action has an equal and opposite reaction. So, that means that if Death has taken action, so can we. And that, that action may thwart Death's intent. (Wong 2006)

To which Erin (Alexz Johnson) replies, 'Death is fucking complicated' (Wong 2006). Ian attempts to 'thwart Death's intent', but, as the series repeatedly shows, he is just killed in an even more spectacular and painful manner a few moments later.

Bludworth reappears in the fifth film, in which an bridge undergoing repairs collapses, killing everyone on it, including employees in a bus on their way to a corporate retreat. He tells the survivors, 'Death does not like to be cheated' (Quale 2011), yet again, ascribing agency and intelligence without anthropomorphising death. The fifth film, however, introduces the idea that one can get someone else to take one's place on death's list. 'Then the books are balanced' (Quale 2011). If the person who is to die kills someone else, they receive all the years that person was going to live. This is a new idea, demonstrated ironically when the protagonist, Sam (Nicholas D'Agosto), kills his best friend who was trying to kill him, but who, unbeknownst to anyone, was going to die from a medical condition in a few days. At the end of the film, believing that he has cheated death and been removed from the list for decades to come, Sam climbs onboard a plane which is revealed to be the flight from the first film that explodes a few minutes after take-off, killing Sam when his friend would have died.

*The Final Destination* films thus posit a medieval view of death: death comes for us all, and will not be stopped, cheated or diverted. What is new, however, is the idea that Death is actually a sadistic sociopath of an entity that wants us to suffer before we die and wants those of us left behind to suffer as well. Death has a design. It can be briefly altered, but Death itself will then come to repair the alteration and ensure that all who could die in that moment do, in fact, die, and die horribly. These films are entertaining pop horror, but they contain a vision of death that is disturbing, harrowing and that remains positively medieval.

Dave Jeffery

# Death (Eric Kripke, 2005–20)

## The Presentation of Death in *Supernatural*

In 2005, American scriptwriter and TV producer Eric Kripke launched the television show *Supernatural*. By exploring the effect different legends brought to local communities, *Supernatural* emerged as a perfect vehicle for a road trip format. Starring Jensen Ackles and Jared Padalecki as brothers Dean and Sam Winchester, respectively, *Supernatural* featured the monster hunter brothers tracking down various creatures and entities in order to rid the world of evil. Kripke had expanded the show to five seasons before leaving as showrunner in 2010. The show persevered for another ten seasons, switching to the CW Network, and ending in 2020. At 327 episodes, it is now regarded as the longest-running live-action fantasy show in US TV history (Porter 2020).

However, the relationship between Sam and Dean was never intended to be front and centre as the brief was to focus only on the confrontation with the antagonist of a particular episode. Yet Kripke and producer Robert Singer saw a chemistry between Ackles and Padalecki and expanded the storylines beyond the notions of folklore into theology and philosophy. During this creative shift, the Winchesters become immersed in the eternal battle between good and evil, Heaven and Hell, and the interdimensional beings associated with such tropes, including God, Lucifer and, of course, Death.

In literature, Death symbolises the finality of the human condition. Writers can tap into a wealth of human emotional responses, combining them to challenge and probe, and determine meaning. When ascribed to Dean and Sam, the human aspects of love, grief, human frailty and the ongoing desire for immortality are all subtexts. These are given greater clarity when they come into contact with Death as an entity.

In *Supernatural*, Death has many roles. Neill (2019: 52) suggests that these manifest as 'a narrative catalyst, omnipresent threat, an ally, an end and a beginning, a force for good and a tool for evil'.

Therefore, this essay will work through the presentations of Death, first as a male representation, followed by the female iteration. It will then identify and explore the idea that, in a quest for originality, the show may have sacrificed some of its own established laws when introducing an amoral, female incarnation of Death, leaving it open to criticisms of gender bias and discrimination. The essay will call for further critical analysis of the subtext of a female Death with a view to understanding the role and context in both the series and popular culture.

The lore surrounding Death's abilities is discussed on several occasions in the earlier seasons, especially when the show involves 'Reapers' or 'Angels of Death' who do Death's work by proxy. As mortality is an ongoing theme, Reapers, and subsequently Death, feature heavily in the plotlines.

In Season 5, the episode titled 'Two Minutes to Midnight' Death (played by British-Canadian character actor Julian Richings) features for the first time as a tall and cadaverous figure, wearing a black suit and long coat, with a walking cane hitting the streets in slow motion. While this representation is a play on the traditional imagery of Death as a black-swathed skeletal entity, it serves as an opportunity to introduce the intricacies of the character. For example, Dean and Death are shown in a pizza parlour, implying Death as someone with a penchant for fast food; this provides a blueprint for interactions in subsequent seasons, including meetings in one restaurant or another. Interactions between The Horseman and Dean are primarily used to establish Death's role in the show's ongoing narrative.

In this context, Death is established as being older than God and when the time comes, he intends to reap Him too. This degree of omnipotence over all living beings is a constant in Death's appearance but is perhaps cemented in the Season 6 episode 'Appointment in Samarra' where Dean has to become Death as part of an agreement to save Sam. Here, Death is used as a vehicle to impart notions of love, loyalty and honouring responsibilities, all aspects that fuel the show's prerequisite focus. Another important aspect of this episode is

Death's role in the perpetuation of the Natural Order. This notion of cosmic balance is an ongoing feature of most of the story arcs of Richings' tenure.

Not only does Death continue to provide the narrative flow to each season, but his appearances also provide opportunities for character development, thus ensuring that the iteration is divorced from traditional constructs of Death. In the Season 7 episode 'Meet the New Boss', we are reminded of Death as a theological historian, which gives rise to the idea that as an entity Death has always existed, creating the paradox that life cannot exist without the existence of Death.

These philosophical concepts provide a significant subtext for subsequent seasons, especially the Season 9 premier episode, 'I think I'm Gonna Like It Here', where Sam Winchester wrestles with the decision as to whether he should fight to stay alive or succumb to his coma. The Horseman waits patiently for Sam to make his decision. Unlike other encounters, Death has not been summoned to attend; he has gone to Sam of his own volition, to bear witness to his passing, out of reverence to the Winchester's work.

In this dynamic, we are reminded of the true philosophical purpose behind Death's existence, namely, that of maintaining a kind of cosmic status quo. This is underpinned in Episode 23 of Season 10, 'Brother's Keeper', which sees the final outing from Richings as Death is killed with his own scythe (up to now, the only time the archetypical weapon has featured in the show) by Dean instead of sacrificing Sam to an irrepressible entity known as The Darkness.

Further theological significance in this episode is that Dean is marked with the Sigil of Cain, thus holding The Darkness at bay. However, Cain as the first murderer in Christian faith ultimately becomes the destroyer of Death himself, thereby paving the way for replacing The Horseman in subsequent seasons.

As we have seen thus far, Death has been presented within the traditional context, and it is often seen as an advocate, and, in some instances, a sympathiser of Dean and Sam, fundamental to the laws of natural order and cosmic balance. Such tenets have been integral to the narrative flow of story arcs and established Death as a purveyor of emotion elements that are key to fundamental storytelling and character development. Yet, as we shall see, this focus is about to change with the advent of a new iteration.

The Season 11 episode 'Form and Void' serves as a transitional segment in Death's chronology in the show. Here we are introduced to the Reaper known as Billie (played by Canadian actor Lisa Berry) who serves as exposition to the consequences of Dean's execution of Death. Billie informs Sam that should the brothers ever die, they will not be saved. However, this notion is challenged in the Season 12 episode 'First Blood', which results in Dean making a blood pact with Billie to kill and resurrect the Winchesters to escape indefinite imprisonment. In return, at the stroke of midnight of that very same day, she will reap one of them permanently, only to die at the hands of Castiel at the end of the episode. In this story arc, we can see hints of how laws concerning the nature of Death which were already established earlier in the show's universe are becoming fluid thus foreshadowing how the writers intend to tackle future episodes.

When Billie inexplicably returns in the Season 13 episode 'Advanced Thanatology', we are introduced to her as the new incarnation of Death, and it is here that modifications are made to the fundamental philosophies established in the early seasons. There is an immediate change in Billie's appearance. Gone is her red jacket and sour demeanour. Now she wears only black, including a long coat and the tell-tale scythe of Death. Her temperament is cooler and more calculated, and there is no proclivity for fast foods. This is New Death, and these less-than-subtle nuances are enough to make the switch clear to the audience. When questioned by Dean as to how she survived, Billie explains that when Death is killed, the first Reaper to die afterwards takes on the role. One of the most satisfying aspects of changing Death in such a manner is that at no point does the show make any reference to it, not through the characters or the writing. It is as though this is what change should be about, a thing of equity and inclusion. In other words, natural. As such, these laudable tenets arrive without fanfare and such a tone strengthens their social message.

However, not all alterations are so tentative. In the transition from Reaper to New Death, Billie does not maintain the architecture of the Natural Order but seeks to rewrite it. Death is particularly proud of her library which carries the records of everyone who ever lived and died, hinting that the mortality of human beings is malleable and open to manipulation.

This demonstration of events highlights two points in the construct of Death in the show. First, there is a cue that it is a physical embodiment of Death's ethic for order in the chaos of life. The orderly bookshelves, the almost clinical presentation of the library itself, represent the Natural Order made real. Second, it also shows the impact the Winchesters have on Death's ethos. They are, in essence, the antithesis of what Death represents, but their goals are unequivocally aligned. The Winchesters 'put down' creatures and entities that are not meant to be in our world. In their own way, they are Reapers of the otherworldly, and could arguably be put forward as another representation of Death in the show's existential canon.

As discussed, in the early representations, Death is focused on maintaining order, and it is the pursuance of this decree that is key to his existence. New Death is still concerned with such matters, but her lens is somewhat broader in scope. Rather than challenging and closing avenues for imbalance, she is instead determined to understand and indeed use them for her own nefarious purposes.

For example, in the previously mentioned episode 'Advanced Thanatology', Death learns of Dean's abilities to cross dimensions and is intrigued to know how he was able to do it. This expounding of Death's purpose and curiosities not only makes the character more intriguing, but it could also be argued that it informs the notion of power as a means to corrupt those with a predetermined, pure ethic. Such considerations should be fascinating – and on many levels, it is indeed that – but come with their own set of concerns when considered within the context of gender, as we shall discuss shortly.

Throughout Seasons 13 to 15, the true motivations as to why Death chooses to invest in such aspects, and the changes she intends to make if allowed to do so, are made frighteningly clear. As we have already noted, the introduction of this new version of Death is symbolic for two reasons: the uniqueness of gender and the less-than-nuanced changes in the character's adherence to the show's prerequisite laws. Indeed, when one considers the apparent lack of morality ascribed to this new incarnation as a woman, it is difficult not to acknowledge that what may be perceived as an innovative approach to an archetype raises some significant – and potentially uncomfortable – questions. This is where the narrative and the gender subtext come into conflict.

*Supernatural*'s problematic portrayal of women, be that as a narrative construct or their presentation as characters, has certainly been raised elsewhere. The focus of contention is brought to light by Caffrey (2017) who identified that female characters tended to have far less longevity in the show and were more often used as love interests or emotional leverage for the male protagonists. Likewise, Emily (2015) has commented on how women are consistently subjected to horrific and gory deaths and considers this as evidence that the show had misogynistic tendencies. Actor Misha Collins – who played the angel Castiel – echoed concerns about the show's misogynistic leanings during a panel discussion 'Salute to Supernatural' in Whippany, New Jersey, in 2013 (Kelly 2013). Also, Karpinski (2021) suggests that the only female character that remained consistent and well developed was Charlie Bradbury (played by Felicia Day) and questions whether it was the fact she was a lesbian that saved her, at least for a while, from the same fate of other female characters, given that she did not have any sexual interest in the Winchester brothers. This fuels further criticisms that the bulk of female characters were mere tropes to serve Dean and Sam. Caffrey (2017) highlighted that over fifteen seasons, the bulk of true villains (both human and non-human) per episode were more likely to be portrayed by women. This is perhaps no more evident than in New Death's self-obsessed megalomania that flies in the face of the show's own established law. Yes, as we have recognised earlier, Death may have suggested that he was prepared to reap God when the time came, but the female Death is actively manipulating events in order to make it happen and claim His power for her own. The inflection here is somewhat alarming: that, as a woman, Death is power-crazed and has no concern for actions or implications that go beyond herself. Furthermore, an illustration of the criticism that women serve as mere plot points, suffer needless death and form drivers of the narrative comes in the final incarnation of Death in the show.

Actor Kimberley Sustad briefly plays a newly incarnated version of Death in the Season 15 episode 'Inherit the Earth'. She is a Reaper called Betty who is summoned and instantly killed by Lucifer to make her the New Death in order to reveal God's end from a book only Death can decode. Lucifer then kills her again before she can reveal the manner of God's final death after solving the riddle. Again, we can see a female incarnation of Death used as a plot device and quickly killed, opening such aspects to criticisms of exploitation already discussed above.

Such criticisms are likely to continue without critical evidence to provide a counterargument. However, claims that the show is discriminatory are countered by Devine (2019) who states, 'I simply think Supernatural, rather than being a sexist extravaganza, is just a show mostly about men, and not as much about women.' Furthermore, in a deep dive into the show's representation of female characters, the genre site Lady Geek Girl and Friends (LGGF) concluded, 'Is Supernatural sexist? My answer is – it is complicated, but the show certainly has a history of not treating its female characters very well'.

Despite such challenges, the absence of in-depth material exploring the concept of Billie as New Death compounds the negative elements, and as such we are left with limited context and great assumption as to the motivations of the character beyond that of a novelty 'new face' following Richings' departure. This is echoed by Edmundson (2016: 3) who identifies that critical analysis of Supernatural as an overall show is intermittent, let alone the nuances of individual characters and how they interact. There is certainly an argument that, given its significant influence on genre culture, Supernatural needs far greater study than it has currently received.

Given this lack of current analysis, it is important to hypothesise the drivers behind a potentially harmful representation of Death in the context of gender. There is no suggestion here of course that maligned viewpoints are contrived or indicative of a conscious desire by showrunners and writers to spread a subtext of gender discrimination and misogyny. Instead, it is posited that there are indicators that the perpetuation of detailed plot lines and story arcs were a primary driver for writers, sometimes at the expense of the kind of character depth that would preclude potential accusations of gender bias.

This is best illustrated in a 2017 interview with the Fangasm site, where Lisa Berry admitted that her early scripts lacked character detail, stating, 'I didn't get much background, I kind of was just assuming a lot of things. So, when I got the script, I had to fill a whole bunch of things in.' Furthermore, Berry herself admits that she regards her role as Death as an extension of that of a Reaper, an oddly framed choice given the subservient nature of such a demon in *Supernatural* lore.

Taking these established deficits into account, the question as to the absent minutiae of Death's character post-transition is clearly evident at a basic level. Despite the ambiguities of reason or circumstance, there is no doubt that the very nature of Death changed with the change of gender. Therefore, such an occurrence can only prompt retrospective criticism in these current times where gender inequality is at the forefront of social and cultural consciousness. Yet, it is also important to note that, despite these challenges and criticisms, the audience share throughout *Supernatural*'s entire fifteen-season run was roughly fifty-fifty male to female indicating that, overall, such criticisms did not appear to affect women consistently tuning into the show (Porter 2020). This perhaps reinforces LGGF's view of the complexities of *Supernatural* and its relationship with women, especially its audience.

To conclude, there is little doubt that *Supernatural* brought an intelligent and creative concept to the portrayals of Death on screen: namely, that of an entity more than mere shadow and ultimately multidimensional in nature. This has not come without problems, however. The nuances and nobility shown as a male character appear to have been diluted, if not completely reframed, when Death returns as a woman. Without further exploration of these elements, there is a danger that an unhealthy association may well be drawn between a female Death and amorality. It is suggested that greater critical study is needed to establish the motivations behind such a fundamental change in the character as well as the long-term consequences for the portrayal of women in the show and its impact upon wider popular culture.

Anna Lüscher

# The *Harry Potter* Series (Various, 2001–11)

Death Positivity in the Face of War

The centrality of the *Harry Potter* series' death motif has been recognised by several scholars. For example, Katie Caetano describes the series as 'a seven-part saga constantly ruminating on mortality and human demise' (Caetano 2015: 113, see also Bub 2017). This focus on death, in a series of books meant for children, is especially poignant when we remember that 'the first four books were published before the 9/11 attacks, the last three books afterwards' (Ciba 2017: 121), and we observe how, while the theme is present from the start, it becomes darker and changes throughout the series. 'Harry and the reader move together from wonder, innocence, and comedy, to fear, experience, and tragedy throughout the series', comments Kate Behr (2005: 114, see also Ciba 2017: 121). Later instances of heightened terror are spread by Voldemort – the leader of a terrorist group (see Ciba 2017: 128) – and caused by more death than in the earlier books, even though death was already a theme. In the beginning, the death theme is more humorous, but it develops into one that 'parallel[s] the terror of our world' (Rosado 2015: 77) and 'seems to function as an allegory of twentieth century world history in all of its violence and brutality' (Lacassagne 2016: 318). The series evolves from playful ghosts to war and self-sacrifice, part of a pattern recognised by Behr as one wherein 'something incidental in an early book becomes complex, significant and central to the developing character or plot of a later one' (2005: 114), as is the case with the theme of death.

    This preoccupation with death is important because the main character will sacrifice himself for the greater good – planned and premeditated by himself and his mentor. Therefore, introducing the theme early is prudent, and 'death positivity' is not surprising. Death positivity describes how the book frames death not only negatively, but as something to embrace rather than fear. Instead, death might also symbolise a new beginning or carry the hope of a reunion. In the following sections, this essay will argue that the series retains a 'death positive' theme even after 9/11 and despite intradiegetic terror and war.

The text's early and frequent mention of death as a natural part of existence is the first step in its death positive approach. Death is commonplace and normalised. Sonja Loidl observed that 'the significance of death [...] will connote differently in different fantastic environments: it may be deemed to be something horrific, or as a part of everyday life' (2010: 178), and this latter portrayal is the case in *Harry Potter*: Hogwarts students constantly live near ghosts. These ghosts display their bodies at the moment of their death, like the Gryffindor house ghost, who is known as 'Nearly Headless Nick' (Rowling 2000: 136). The ghosts are a constant reminder of death and its closeness to life by their presence and the moment they represent. Their mundaneness shows in their acceptance as 'members of the community; even one of the teachers at Hogwarts is a ghost who continues to teach' (Bub 2017: 111). The ghosts are just further characters, no stranger than a teacher turning into a cat. This impression is heightened with Nearly Headless Nick's death party, which shows that they are still counting their birthdays, with each year still carrying meaning. They are 'nearly' alive. In this series, they are common.

To define death, Derrida quotes 'Heidegger's famous definition of death in *Being and Time*: 'The possibility of the pure and simple impossibility for Dasein' (1993: 23), the 'German Dasein' meaning literally '(t)here-being'. Consequently, death would be considered a state of 'not-being-here'. In *Harry Potter*, death is more than not-being-here. The ghosts suggest that death is not the end. Andrea Stojilkov, writing on the soul in Harry Potter, confirms that the narrative world does not portray 'death in binary terms, but in terms of degrees' (2015: 135). Instead of presenting absolutes in which those that have died are not accessible, and life and death are completely separated, in this world, magic allows for some connection, some overlap. Even though several characters, like Remus Lupin (see Rowling 2003: 887), state that death is irreversible, Stojilkov argues that 'so numerous are the cases of contact between the dead and the living in Rowling's world that Lupin's statement seems faulty'

(2015: 143). This is highlighted in the passage containing Lupin's statement, shortly after Sirius fell through the veiled archway, presumably to his death; earlier, Harry, standing in front of the veil, 'had the strangest feeling that there was someone right behind the veil on the other side of the archway. [...] There were faint whispering, murmuring noises coming from the other side of the veil' (Rowling 2003: 850f.). Furthermore, Luna Lovegood even says that 'there are people *in there*' (See Rowling 2003: 851, italics in original). All these quotes suggest there is more to the veil than death and 'not-being-here'.

It may help to conceive of death in this narrative as a passage to another kind of existence, in line with Albus Dumbledore's precept that 'to the well-organised mind, death is but the next great adventure' (Rowling 2000: 320). In regard to the extradiegetic world, Jacques Derrida questioned if death can 'be reduced to some line crossing, to a departure, to a separation, to a step, and therefore to a *decease*' (1993: 6, italics in original). Viewed in this light, death positivity is a larger possibility. This view lessens the anguish of Harry realising that Voldemort must kill him: 'Like rain on a cold window, these thoughts pattered against the hard surface of the incontrovertible truth, which was that he must die. *I must die*. It must end' (Rowling 2007: 556, italics in original). Even though he describes it as the 'end', it is probable that Harry's death in this world is not final. Leah Omilion-Hodges et al. write in a paper on death in young adult literature that 'extant research indicates that the vast majority of individuals fear death because of its perceived finality, the uncertainty surrounding the process, fear of pain, and loss of self among other reasons' (2019: 140). Therefore, in the series, while death contains some of the elements Omilion-Hodges et al. list, an aspect of finality and uncertainty is removed. Harry's parents speak to him before he encounters Voldemort in the forest, 'neither ghost nor truly flesh, he could see that [...] Less substantial than living bodies, but much more than ghosts' (Rowling 2007: 560), indicating to him that they will be waiting for him and, therefore, that death is not necessarily an end but might be the beginning of something new. Dying may be frightening because it is connected to the enemy winning, pain and perceived danger to loved ones and does not allow lasting, normal contact with those left behind; however, it also may be 'the next adventure'.

The series' non-binary structure between death and life might be considered a form of death denial. As more than 'not-being-here' is continuously indicated, death may not be presented in its extreme consequence: Harry can find solace with his parents, even though they have died. A full-blown death, where nothing follows, is an end. The narrative world's possibilities do not imply such a possibility. Dumbledore's adventure is more likely. As it is not the end, the possibility for death positivity is more likely than in other books where there are no grey areas.

Hagrid's unique position in the series contributes to the overall death-positive perspective. It has been generally established that Hagrid is a 'being of the boundary' (Neumann 2006: 165): Hagrid belongs neither fully to the Muggle nor the magical realms, nor fully to nature or culture (165) but remains always in between. In addition, as proposed here, he is also positioned on the boundary between life and death. Four such instances stand out. First, to reach Hogwarts, the first-year pupils take small boats across a lake, anchoring underneath the castle. Hagrid acts as Charon, escorting pupils on this first official entry to the castle and into a magical institution (see Rowling 2000: 123). Ronnie Terpening, a professor of Italian Studies, says that in Virgil's rendition of Charon, the scene's symbolism is crucial: The boat passage represents entering a new phase of life. This symbolism is also present in the passage to Hogwarts. The first-year pupils going to Hogwarts are not heading to their deaths, rather they are growing up and entering a new chapter of their lives. Hagrid is the guide leading them to this new phase. Second, and in relation to this, the older pupils are not conveyed by boat. They reach the castle by carriages drawn by Thestrals, a type of horse you can see only when you have seen someone die (see Rowling 2003: 492). Hagrid is also responsible for these creatures. Thus, the death motif as a transition symbol is confirmed and repeated – as is its connection to Hagrid. Third, Hagrid has possession of a three-headed dog, Fluffy, who guards a subterranean entryway. Despite its diminutive name, this three-headed dog references the Greek mythological character Cerberus. Many details, like the Greek stranger who sold Hagrid the dog (see Rowling 2000: 209) and the need for music to calm the dog (see Rowling 2000: 287), are call-backs to the myth. Rebecca Butler additionally points out that 'according to Pausanias Heracleia, the place where Cerberus emerged into daylight, became a *nekuomanteion*, a passageway where the living could enter the underworld and the dead pass into the living world' (2018: 68f.). Here, it is significant that the dog is the first challenge that Harry, Ron and

Hermione must pass to get to the Philosopher's Stone. The area where Fluffy guards the trapdoor becomes such a *nekuomanteion* that leads to difficulties and the showdown with Voldemort. Fluffy is protecting a passage where death is a clear possibility. As Hagrid owns Fluffy and knows how to control it, he is also the keeper of the trapdoor – the first passageway to facing death. Fourth, Hagrid carries Harry back from death into life twice, bookending the series and furthering the relationship between him and death. At the beginning of the series, Hagrid carries infant Harry from Godric's Hollow to Dumbledore in Surrey. After Harry supposedly died in the forest (see Rowling 2007: 582), this early scene is mirrored. Hagrid brings Harry back to the wizarding world out of the forest. He facilitates Harry's physical return to life.

These four instances position Hagrid firmly as a facilitator between death and life. Due to Hagrid's close connection to death, death is being posited as something that symbolises change and not necessarily 'not-being-here' at all – reinforcing the death denial mentioned above. In addition, as the custodian of creatures and passageways, he is a guide that may make death less frightening. From his perspective, the three-headed dog is a cute and tameable pet. Hagrid can carry or lead Harry safely to death and back again, making death more 'faceable' in a time of war and terror.

The penultimate argument concerns the concept of a good death and self-sacrifice. Lily and Harry Potter's sacrifices stand out even amid the actions of Dumbledore, Severus Snape, Sirius Black and Dobby. Not only are Lily and Harry's sacrifices portrayed as heroic and encased in 'a message that […] lavishes admiration on the sacrificial lambs' (Caetano 2015: 126), but the control they exert over their death is also shown to be positive. By deliberately enabling Voldemort to murder them, they gain 'a martyr-like legacy' (126) and create 'tangible and lasting protection[s]' (126) for those they love.

For Harry and Lily sacrificing oneself creates the possibility of a good death in the face of certain death during times of war and terror. In medicine and palliative care, the idea of a 'good death' refers to the efforts made to provide the best possible situation for persons who are about to die. While, of course, many factors of a good death are 'fluid and highly individual' (Kehl 2006: 284), Kehl does identify twelve essential factors:

> being in control, being comfortable, sense of closure, affirmation/value of the dying person recognized, trust in care providers, recognition of impending death, beliefs and

values honored, burden minimized, relationships optimized, appropriateness of death, leaving a legacy, and family care. (2006: 277)

Not all of these factors can be applied to Harry and Lily's circumstances, as there are no care providers, the appropriateness of their deaths is in question, and being comfortable is not the issue it would be in a hospital. However, already the first factor rings a bell in the *Harry Potter* world: The most heroic deaths, those that have a silver lining of protection or doing good, are those in which the circumstances surrounding death could be controlled. Hence, self-sacrifice can have a positive connotation as it offers a measure of control, and one may accomplish good in death.

For example, Harry prepares for his death, even though aspects like the location and the time frame are not of his choosing. He connects with family and friends and affirms his relationships, finishes tasks and delegates those tasks he cannot complete (see Rowling 2007: 491–559) before walking into the forest and meeting Voldemort alone. Harry's deliberateness maintains a measure of control over his death. For Kehl, 'being in control' is 'the most important and most common attribute' (2006: 281) of a good death. In addition, Harry also fulfils most of the other conditions for a good death that Kehl mentioned.

His mindset resembles that of the youngest brothers in the embedded fairy tale. Later, being life-weary, this brother 'greet[s] Death as an old friend, and went with him gladly, and, equals, they departed this life' (Rowling 2007: 332). The brother represents the ideal good death, and Harry reaches this mindset.

Voldemort and his Death Eaters stand in opposition to the series' overall death positive approach. Voldemort strives for immortality and is prepared to kill to avoid death, his greatest fear. His unnatural attempts at immortality leave him deformed, with snake-like features, a visible warning against pursuing this path. His self-chosen name and that of his followers are equally telling. His followers, called Death Eaters, consume and master death figuratively. While the spell Morsmordre, which they use to create the so-called Dark Mark over the sites of their crimes, incorporates an ouroboros. Among other similar etymologies, in Latin, the two parts of the word 'mors' and 'mordere' can be translated as 'death' and 'to bite', respectively, pointing to the Death Eaters and the ouroboros. Fitting into the pattern, Voldemort's chosen name is commonly understood to mean 'flight from death' (see Compagnone and Danesi 2012: 129) or 'flight of death', which could either mean that death flees or that someone flees from death. The French 'vol' may also indicate theft, whereby something could be stolen from death or death could be stealing something. The translation might depend on either an emphasis on the fact that Voldemort is afraid of death or that he uses death to terrify his enemies. Voldemort's fear and avoidance of death is simultaneously his weakness and his strength. It leads him to make immoral choices and is presented as unnatural and dangerous, creating a contrast between him and Harry.

Voldemort's fear of death makes this fear a villainous trait – very deliberately in contrast to the opposing side. Therefore, death positivity, as Hagrid, Harry and Dumbledore subscribe to it, is connoted as a good trait to possess, a virtue to be imitated. Also, as death seems more unbearable to the villains than to the heroes, the latter do not need to be as frightened. In the face of Voldemort's terroristic acts and his war, being death positive is one element of resistance against this reign.

In conclusion, it has been shown that, in the *Harry Potter* series, death is a part of everyday life and, therefore, normalised for the characters. They walk with death every morning they go to school; it is omnipresent. In addition, the world's magic allows for a type of death denial that would be impossible in a realistic setting. Hagrid adds to the ease with which death can be met as he stands at the boundary between life and death, guiding the way to a death, which is not the end of life but a change. Also, meaning can be given to a death and control exerted over it by accepting death as inevitable and 'greet[ing] Death as an old friend' (Rowling 2007: 332). Last, the opposite of death positivity is embodied in the story's villains, making it a wholly unattractive choice. Due to these five aspects, death positivity can be maintained throughout the stories even in the face of intra- and extradiegetic terror and war.

Phil Fitzsimmons

# *The Sleepless* (Nuzo Onoh, 2016)

## Introduction: An Intersection of Grave Concerns

As an author with a cultural insider's understanding of the place of death in the Biafran world view, in her book *The Sleepless*, Nuzo Onoh situates this natural awareness within that which typifies every African rural community: 'the whole psychic atmosphere of African village life is filled with belief in mystical power' (Mbiti 1989: 197). Specifically, embedded in this 'mystical belief', *Sleepless* was written as the result of a kaleidoscopic confluence of Onoh's personal encounters with wartime death, genocide, traditional beliefs and the enduring legacies of colonial trauma.

Further to Onoh's context of culture and habitus, she linguistically crafted *Sleepless* in the autoethnographic-phenomenological modality of Biafran oral storytelling with its intersecting multilayers of meaning and culturally specific textual construction. Employing the Biafran organising structure of doubling, her text is a hinged narrative in which one section acts as a metonymic microcosm. This textual facet also acts as a critical springboard, providing the narrative impetus to shift into a further elaborative web of meaning while simultaneously functioning as juxtaposition. This holistic storytelling approach allows for an 'intimate and expressive relationship between narrative and history' (Irele 1993: 158), while providing Ohno with the scope to turn her gaze analytically 'upon the self in seeking to understand the nexus between the personal and the culture in which the personal is situated' (Prasad 2019: 4).

As Onoh emphasises in the last pages of her text, this narrative arose from her first-hand subaltern experiences with death as a young child in the breakaway state of Biafra, just before and sometime early into the outbreak of the 1967 Biafran-Nigerian civil war. As Alimi (2012) states, this period of conflict was the pinnacle of Biafran 'collapse, a breaking into pieces, chaos and confusion' (121). This had been brewing for decades due to the impact of colonialism and European missionaries, which Achebe argues had arisen because of 'an absence of the African voice' (Alimi 2012: 44).

Against the backdrop of the civil war, the absence of a female voice is a crucial thread that speaks the loudest in *Sleepless*. It is a polyphonic call that attempts to point out the suppression of the West African feminine which Wilson-Tagoe believes has also 'been buried under a veneer of Igbo custom and its visibly patriarchal world' (2017: 22).

What is evidently resurrected and given clarity of voice in *Sleepless* is the primary role of death in Igbo culture. The Igbo view the natural world as being interconnected with the spiritual realm, whereby death is an interactive continuum of the earthly within a universal cycle of birth, death and rebirth. This interlinked ideal 'assumes a harmony with natural form, the source of the rings that construct the web of life' (Fernandez 2015: 123). In Igbo culture, the dead have not departed from the community but coexist in and amongst the living as spirits. This critical belief became a contested ideological space in Igbo society as the introduction of Christianity and the differences in beliefs related to death 'caused major cultural upheavals' (Socrates 2019: 23). Achebe (2012) believes that, by 1930, despite Christianity being a dominant force in the Igbo region, this area was at the crossroads of virulent social, ideological and religious debate. The notion of death had become the cornerstone of the 'long-standing clash of Western and African civilisations' which had in turn 'generated deep conversations and struggles between the respective cultures and religions' (2013: 16).

Onoh's central character Obele is a cultural repository of trauma. Despite being trapped in a culture and family losing their identity, she was still able to hear the voice of deep-seated tacit awareness. Not only is this young girl a metonymic recasting of Onoh at the same age, but also, as a young Igbo female, she is seen to embody 'the youthful anticipation of life, the matrix of creation' (Conway 1994: 17). As such she also represents the consciousness most likely to understand the actual spiritual nature of death, and hear the voice of the Mother goddess, such as the Biafran Ali Ani Ana or one of her iterations. In essence, *Sleepless* pulls together multiple threads of belief, asking the reader to imagine what cannot be verified, a realm of experience which is situated between two zones of death – social and corporeal death – and to reckon with the precarious lives which are visible only in the moment of their disappearance. It is a history of an unrecoverable past; it is a narrative of what might have been or could have been; it is a history written with and against the archive. (Hartman 2008: 12)

## Threads of Death: Mores and Mothers

Through the voice of Obele, an eight-year-old girl deemed to be of no value by her parents, and the ritual killing of her disabled brother Kene, *Sleepless* gives primacy of voice to all Igbo children, recognised as the 'greatest victims of the war' (Ezeigbo 2002: 62). This is especially the case for the countless young girls who were raped or 'abducted by the soldiers and forced into unwanted relationships' (Chuku 2018: 338). With the death of Kene in the first chapter acting as the metonymic catalyst and narrative hinge, the voices of Obele and her spirit guide provide an impetus to the narrative to give death its due voice and rightful place in Igbo culture.

## The Beginning Is the End

History tends to be ordered according 'to the dominant interest of the custodians' (Pandey 2014: 4), and as with most recent female African authors, Onoh also dismantles this process. Pandey asserts that texts such Onoh's 'unarchives personal elements of history that have been disenfranchised, to reveal what is truly important in the cultural memory' (2014: 3). This process occurs in the very first sentence of the first chapter: 'In the dense gloom of the vast forest, the child stopped to stare at the bloated carcass of a black cat nailed to the trunk of a tall Melina tree' (Onoh 2016: 1). Seemingly simple in structure, this sentence is a Gothic summation which belies a complex array of semantic underpinnings, cultural memories and social trauma.

In the ensuing paragraphs, it is revealed that Obele's parents, purportedly Christians, are taking their disabled son Kene to an already blood-soaked scene where he is to be ritually slaughtered by a witch doctor.

The first clause, 'the dense gloom of the dark forest' (Onoh 2016: 1), represents the symbolic boundary markers for all the death and anguish caused by the Nigerian civil war as well as the cultural issues before, during and after the conflict. For those Europeans living in Nigeria at the time, Onoh's concept of the forest conjured up metaphors of impenetrability, the unknown and death. These elements could also be applied to the loss of orientation and the darkness found in Obele's parents. Like many others, this couple was representative of those Igbo people whose links with the Europeans were seen to cause a loss of traditional sense of respect for human values. Deardorff contends that the forest represents 'an ontological gap, a crossroads of identity, the seat of the soul' (2004: 21). Achebe believes that this social malaise and cultural drift arose from the 'selfish ambitions of the political leaders' (2012: 163). As reflected in Obele's father, at the grassroots level Achebe believes this shift also resurrected the self-seeking and money-making 'archaic practice of godfatherism' (163). Thus, in the broader context of colonial ideology, the Nigerian political leadership at all levels engendered a decline and loss of traditional values of care and community.

Ohno also uses Kene's death-space as a means to narratively establish the facade of the colonial perception regarding the Biafran Christian converts. The dominant assessment was that the Igbo could quickly 'retreat into totemism and, taboo' (Creed 1993: 26), which in the book's ensuing chapters has clearly overtaken Kene's parents. However, for the Igbo, the killing of Kene as well as the site and manner of his death ran counter to traditional Igbo belief structure: 'Man, according to the Igbo worldview, possesses what may well be called spiritual instincts making him capable and desirous of the supreme values: truth, goodness, peace and beauty' (Ezedike 2019: 132).

While the first chapter contains the cause and effect of what Wright has termed the African 'culture bomb' (2004: 107), Onoh adds further symbolic inversions that point to how far the cultural drift had occurred. For Obele's parents, this is at first seen with the reference to the dead cat. As a symbol of guidance in the afterlife, when a feline is sacrificed at an Igbo funeral and the blood applied to the face of the dead, it 'is believed to give the departed good sight in the land of the dead' (Nabofa 1985: 398). This positive reading of death–life in comparison to Obele's family is also revealed in the reference to the Melina tree, which is a signifier of the sacred groves 'thought of as sources of vitality and humanization' (Anugwom 2018: 163).

Every aspect of Kene's sacrifice runs contrary to the positive beliefs that the Igbo have regarding death. Added to this, instead of the Christian sacrament of baptism, which both his Catholic father and Anglican mother should have provided, Kene's body parts are boiled as a sacrifice and his blood is drunk to ensure the parents conceive a fully reconstructed normal child in the future. Thus, he suffers a type of primeval baptism and acts as a monstrous Eucharistic substitution. Further to the latter point, Onoh intersects two further symbolic elements in that she inverts the Christian sense of baptism by immersion and its related symbolic sense of arising to a new life. As well, she draws on the Igbo belief about the sacredness of water, and that just before a child is born 'they must cross a river and be confronted by Nne Mimri, the water goddess, in regard to their destiny' (Nwoye 2011: 316). It is this notion of a water deity that provides extra salience to the ensuing section of the narrative.

## The End Is a Beginning

From the conclusion of the first chapter of the book, the parallax of the hinge structure is observed with several facets that gradually develop intensity. These are also related to water and motherhood, with the ever-increasing focus on how central and tightly knit the concept of the sacred feminine should be entwined into Igbo culture in the face of colonial effacement.

This twin process is represented through the continual brutalisation of Obele in parallel to the expanding focus on and increasing references to water. The first of these occurs almost immediately in the second section of the book in which Obele's mother is savagely beaten when she refuses to give up her holy water and her Catholic faith. Obele attempts to intercede and is also flayed with a branch. In parallel with these references, the 'Mother's Voice' starts speaking to Obele: 'that hushed, loving voice hiding inside her head, lilting, like a happy mother's voice, the secret voice that never let her down' (Onoh 2016: 13). Unsure as to where this came from, Obele tacitly accepts it as a voice of safety and recognizes the need to listen to it. The Mother's Voice now continually intercedes on her behalf keeping her safe from her father's brutality, which includes another attempt by her parents to have her killed by the same witch doctor who killed her brother. As Obele continues to follow this voice, which only she can hear, Mother's Voice goes on as Obele's spirit guide throughout the text.

As an inverted component of the parallax, Kene also appears in the narrative as another voice and presence. In this counter-narrative, Ohno paints him as a deathly double. Not only did he die in water but also suffered 'one of the greatest fears among the Igbo, to die and be thrown into an evil forest' (Nwoye 2011: 309). Thus, according to Igbo belief, because he died an unjust death, Kene cannot 'intercede for the family' (Socrates 2019: 24) or be reincarnated or reunited with his clan. Onoh counteracts this in this section in that he returns to live as the 'undead' and as an ongoing invisible fixture on his father's shoulder. Unlike the constant cleansing power of water associated with Obele, Kene remains coated in his own blood with the gaping wounds he suffered at the time of his murder.

Kene's inability to become clean and lose the stains of his death is emblematic of his parents being subsumed by the lure of colonisation as well as its power of convergence. In Africa especially, countries that were in the European fold were pressured to adopt European models to organise their 'modern' lives because these were deemed to be the 'best' arrangements for living. These models included accepting beliefs that were diametrically opposed to those of Igbo and included, 'individualism, legislative democracy, market capitalism and Christianity' (Duru 2021: 93–4). Nyamndi believes that because of this colonial influence, much of the African narrative is centred on 'the commanding metaphor of the wound' which is 'constantly being gashed open' (2021: 2). While the latter refers to the constant destruction wrought by colonialism, Onoh constantly and explicitly refers to the conjoined notion of the gaping wound and the earth. While both of these are also Igbo representations of the feminine and emblematic of the vagina and menstruation, such metaphors are also relationally connected to the spatial arrangement of Igbo deities. With the upper level of the sky representing the domain of the male deity, the Supreme Being, Onoh consistently emphasises a downward movement in *Sleepless* to the lower female metaphysical levels of the earth and rivers. Onoh is clearly accentuating the Igbo belief 'that females lose their identity at death' (Nwoye 2011: 308).

However, in the concluding chapters, the concept of the feminine is restored to its rightful place in Igbo myth. When the local villagers attempt to kill Obele believing her to be a witch, she runs to the river. It is at this point that Mother's Voice intercedes for the final time. Throughout her pain, rape and fear, she has, in fact, been listening and responding to the supernatural directions given by her actual Mother's Voice. She is truly the daughter of the Mother's Voice. Without any previous memory, she had undergone reverse reincarnation from spirit to human.

Standing beside the river, which has risen above the forest, awaiting the command to overwhelm the villagers, Obele experiences a return to her true spirit form. At this point, she intercedes between her river goddess-mother's desire to drown all those seeking her daughter's death and the villagers wanting to kill her. She utters an intercessional request similar to that of the biblical Christ figure on the cross, asking for forgiveness for all they have done, and 'for their foolish wars' (Onoh 2016: 108). Obele then steps into the river: 'The cold waves crashed over her, sweeping her into the great water, taking her home' (108). In doing so, she is reunited with her actual mother and finds eternal safety.

## A Final Word: A Dead End That Needs Addressing

While the journey narrative of *Sleepless* is perhaps self-explanatory, a final trans-textual and transcultural word needs to be made explicit. If nothing else, this text reminds each individual and certainly each cultural group that a lack of understanding of death in life 'is to be exiled twice: once from community and again from our own interiority' (Deardorff 2004: 17).

Part II

# Technology: Medicalisation, Ambivalence and Violence

# Image Intervention III: Unlocking the Truth

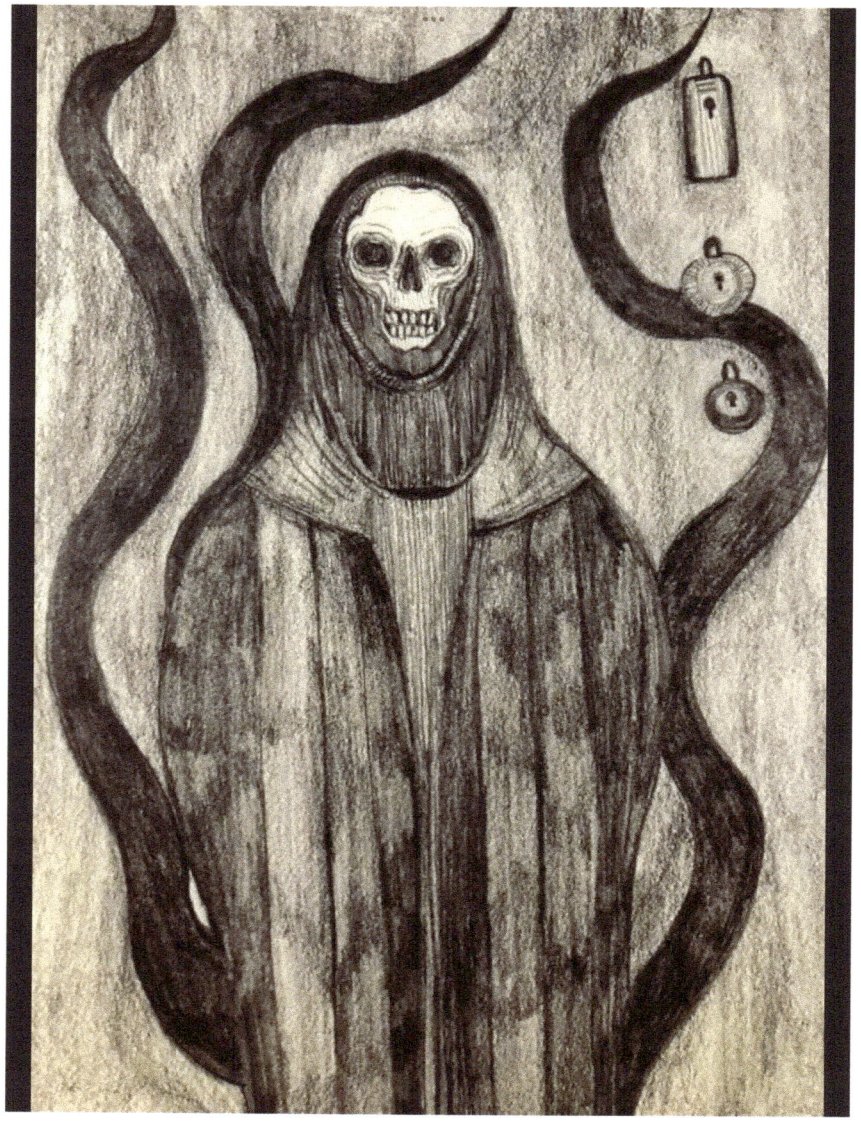

Artwork by Gemma Files
(Reproduced with the permission of the artist)

Rebecca Booth

## *The Autopsy of Jane Doe* (André Øvredal, 2016)

Displacing the Indelible

Our bodies bear markers of our finite existence – age, disease, scars; death is indelible. As a 'dark science', seeking answers to the immutable, pre-modern anatomical research transgressed ethical, religious and sacred boundaries as the only viable way to look inside the human body (Sappol 2017: 50). The Renaissance's relationship with anatomy, eventually founded as a science by surgeon Andreas Vesalius in the sixteenth century, had an incredible influence on pre-modern European art and literature via what Jonathan Sawday describes as the 'culture of dissection', changing our perception of the world – and the concept of death – through a philosophical 'culture of enquiry' (1995: viii). If the 'dissected cadaver was our mirror' (Sappol 2017: 50), then post-mortem examination – accessible to audiences via its popularity within anatomical art as well as the broader themes exploring the symbolism and personification of death in art – allowed its audience to get a glimpse of their own death.

Yet, despite the continued evolution of this 'culture of dissection' throughout the twentieth and twenty-first centuries, engendering acute medical, technological and scientific developments in the Western world, death has lost none of its mystery. Our modern medicalised approach to death provides only anatomical answers as to cause; philosophical and spiritual questions surrounding death remain. Most important, although an awareness of our own mortality is accepted to an unconscious degree, dwelling on this knowledge is difficult. It is therefore necessary to confront (our) curiosity about death and its mysteries in safe and familiar ways, one of which is through artistic representations of death.

*The Autopsy of Jane Doe* (2016) is part of a series of recent films (mostly American) that can be collectively termed anatomical art and broadly speak to a modern 'culture of dissection', each delivering a damning examination of sociocultural attitudes to women's bodily autonomy via the deconstruction and/or defilement of the female corpse (other examples include *Deadgirl* (2008), *After.Life* (2009) and *The Corpse of Anna Fritz* (2015)). Although critical readings of *The Autopsy of Jane Doe* mostly focus on the historical persecution of women, supported by the film's narrative focus on the Salem witch trials (1692–3), this essay posits that the film's reference to this period is a microcosm of its themes: how the dead feminine body within artistic representations corresponds not only to an inherent fear of death but also to a masculine fear of excessive femininity that leads to erasure of the feminine.

Elizabeth Bronfen refers to the beautiful feminine dead body portrayed in art – often symbolically captured in an ethereal stasis of passivity and juxtaposed against images of a skeletal or decaying personification of Death,[1] particularly in the pre-modern period – as representing the duplexity of the audience's simultaneous allure and anxiety in confronting our unconscious knowledge of death (1992). There are several elements to this. First, the depiction of death within art allows us to address and conceptualise our finite existence safely via displacement. As Bronfen states,

> We experience death by proxy. In the aesthetic enactment, we have a situation impossible in life, namely that we die with another and return to the living. Even as we are forced to acknowledge the ubiquitous presence of death in life, our belief in our own immortality is confirmed. There is death, but it is not my own. (1992: x)

The beautiful dead feminine body is often the site of this substitution; Bronfen posits that this hyperfocus on the multiple excesses that the dead

---

[1] Examples include several works depicting Death and the Maiden to represent the transience of life and its relationship with beauty, sex and death: Hans Baldung's *Death and Lust* (1517), Niklaus Manuel's *Death and the Maiden* (1517) and George Clark Stanton's *Death and the Maiden* (n.d.).

feminine body represents – death and femininity – instigates the act of repression in an attempt to contain it (1992). In anatomical art, Bronfen notes that 'the represented feminine body also stands in for concepts other than death, femininity and body – most notably the masculine artist and the community of the literal meaning of the image' (xi).[2] The dead feminine body is thus a site of managed passivity, regulated through representation as cultural 'symptoms [articulating] unconscious knowledge and unconscious desires in a displaced, recorded and translated manner', precisely because the corrosive duo of death and femininity is a dangerous source of power (xi). Displacement occurs because 'femininity and death cause a disorder to stability, mark moments of ambivalence, disruption or duplicity and their eradication produces a recuperation of order, a return to stability' (xxi). This eradication speaks to a cultural 'need to ground theoretical and aesthetic representation on the displayed "erasure" of the feminine' (40).

This cultural erasure of the feminine within theoretical and aesthetic representations could be used to describe the ways in which feminine bodies – relating to anyone who identifies as a woman or who requires care for female-assigned reproductive systems – continue to be anatomised and erased in modern society via a contemporary 'culture of dissection'. The Supreme Court's 2022 decision to overturn *Roe* v. *Wade* (1973) in the United States, leaving affected people in states without independent abortion rights unprotected from anti-choice legislation, is yet another devastating blow to reproductive rights. With over 100 bills introduced in state legislatures since 2020 that censure the transgender community, at the time of writing, there are 321 active anti-LGBTQ bills, many of which affect bodily autonomy among transgender youth (American Civil Liberties Union 2023a, b). Black, Indigenous American and Alaskan Native women are two to three times more likely to die during pregnancy and childbirth due to obstetric racism, which is part of a wider discourse surrounding race within medical care and research (Centers for Disease Control and Prevention 2019). *The Autopsy of Jane Doe* not only comments on this modern 'culture of dissection' but also refuses this erasure

---

2    See such works as Jacques Fabian Gautier d'Agoty's *Anatomie générale des viscères* (1752), Gabriel von Max's *The Anatomist* (1869) and Enrique Simonet's *The Anatomy of the Heart* (1890).

through the indelible trauma recorded on the dead feminine body. By using its themes of displacement and prosection, as the title suggests, *The Autopsy of Jane Doe* explores the relationship between the dead feminine body, the coroners conducting the autopsy and the audience.

The opening scene formally replicates bodily dissection as the camera tracks through the aftermath of a violent attack and fire in a suburban house. Descending floor by floor, each structural layer reveals the bloody bodies of several occupants before the camera reaches the building's foundations, settling on the partially unearthed dead body of a young woman. Unfolding in real time within the confines of a small-town morgue, the film charts the post-mortem of the unidentified woman, Jane Doe (Olwen Kelly), by father and son coroners Tommy (Brian Cox) and Austin (Emile Hirsch) Tilden.

The Tilden Morgue is situated in the basement of the family home, and it soon becomes clear that the familial relationship is strained. Austin's girlfriend, Emma (Ophelia Lovibond), arrives to pick him up after work and comes looking for him in the morgue. When the sheriff (Michael McElhatton) arrives with Jane Doe's body and requests a report by the following morning – predicting a media storm on top of the fearsome tempest brewing outside – it becomes clear that Austin is torn between pursuing his own life and appeasing his father, particularly as his emotionally absent father is wracked by guilt after the death (likely by suicide) of his severely depressed wife. Not for the first time, Austin postpones his date with Emma to help his father and promises to pick her up later that night – as well as finally tell his father about his wish to leave the family business.

As the father and son set to work, it soon becomes clear that the film's tagline 'Every body has a secret', speaks to the historical trauma and abuse recorded on the dead feminine body: Jane Doe is a fleshy haunted house full of secrets. Belying the unblemished exterior, with each incision and opening, Jane Doe's body offers a new mystery, stoking familial tension in terms of how Tommy and Austin react as they peel back each layer, recording and pondering each clue on the chalkboard. Tommy is concerned only with providing answers to the mystery of her death in terms of the *how*; Austin wants to know *why*. As Tommy states, 'Leave the "why" to the cops and the shrinks. We're just here to find cause of death. No more, no less' (Øvredal 2016).

Taking into account the wider anatomical implications of the text, the presence of the audience must also be considered in terms of how spectatorship further defines the other roles: prosection (the cadaver – here notably the dead feminine body) and prosector (the dissector – here the father and son coroners). Prosection differs from dissection in that it is an instructional teaching method; anatomical students – much like the film's audience – are passive spectators, watching an experienced anatomist dissect the cadaver rather than doing so themselves. The word can also refer to the reassembled dissected cadaver, whole or in part, used for review in anatomical teaching. The autopsy thus becomes a prosection.

Despite the immaculate condition of the corpse externally, the woman's internal injuries present a tragic tale that simply does not tally. Jane Doe's tongue has been crudely cut out and a single molar removed; her wrists and ankle bones are shattered; and her lungs are so badly damaged from smoke inhalation that her extremities should be subjected to third-degree burns. Not only do the internal organs display inexplicable incisions, but some of these cuts are also still open whilst others have healed; the presence of scar tissue suggests that the wounds preceded death by weeks, if not months or years, which is even more troubling when considering that many of these older injuries could singularly be considered fatal.

When Tommy and Austin attempt to ascertain the time of death, Jane Doe's body exhibits more conflicting evidence. The cloudiness of her eyes suggests the corpse has been dead for several days (corneal opacity is widely believed to be a more accurate indicator of time of death than rigor mortis within forensic circles) yet, not only does the body show no signs of livor mortis (blood collecting at the lowest point of the body after death), but the corpse also actively bleeds from the nose and when anatomical incisions are made – both of which should be possible only if death occurred approximately within the past six hours.

The grisly findings continue with the missing molar found inside the stomach, which points to a ritualistic belief that human tokens could be used to both curse and protect people. The tooth is wrapped in parchment on which symbols and numbers are written equating to the number 1693 – the year the Salem witch trials ended – as well as indicating the following biblical passage: 'A man also or woman that hath a familiar spirit, or that is a wizard, shall surely be put to death: they shall stone them with stones: their blood shall be upon them' (Leviticus 20:27), which condemns witches.[3]

When the coroners discover that Jane Doe's brain tissue sample is active, they determine she is in fact alive. Positing that the murderous ritual used to condemn so many innocent women during the Salem witch trials has imbued Jane Doe's body with supernatural powers, they believe the figure of the witch has been manifested by fear and abuse: bound within the broken body that bears witness to every wound, Jane Doe is enacting her revenge upon all those who further defile her bodily autonomy.

A key consideration here is that the trauma Jane Doe's body exhibits is not confined to the torture and execution the accused would have endured in Salem. Jane Doe's injuries, including smoke inhalation from the fire in the house she was found in during the opening scene, suggest that her body has recorded every attempt to destroy it. In the film's anatomical flourish, Jane Doe's skin is peeled back to reveal apparent occult markings on the hypodermis or innermost layer. Grotesquely beautiful, the shot is filmed from above, framing Jane Doe as an anatomical angel reminiscent of the flayed body in anatomical art.[4] These indelible marks – notably hidden on the inside of her body – are invisible on the unblemished surface of her corpse because Jane Doe represents a failed repression of the reality of death (Bronfen 1992).

It can thus be suggested that Jane Doe is not alive but that the active brain tissue refers to the feminine dead body's potential for agency – via the excesses it represents. Jane Doe's stomach is also found to contain a herb identified as jimsonweed, which is one of several common names for *Datura stramonium* (others are fittingly devil's snare or devil's trumpet), a poisonous plant of the nightshade family. Though the film makes a reference to its paralysing effect, the toxic plant has historically been ingested as an entheogen, and both father and son experience hallucinations throughout the film – a form of displacement that results in two deaths. Emma, coming back to find her boyfriend,

---

3   King James Version.
4   Examples include Ercole Lelli's anatomical display of human skeletons covered in coloured wax and posed as angels of death (1742–51), Joseph Guichard Duverney and Jacques-Fabien Gautier-d'Agoty's painting *Muscles of the Back* (1746) and Leonor Fini's painting *The Angel of Anatomy* (1949).

is killed by Austin as he 'sees' one of the dead bodies from the morgue rather than Emma. As the sole survivor, Austin, startled by an apparition of his dead father, who had been killed by "Jane Doe" earlier, tries to escape the basement, and in the process, trips over a railing and falls to his death.

The hallucinations are thus a (passive) partial projection of the indelible trauma on Jane Doe's body and, aware of the potential for full displacement, Tommy willingly takes part in the ritual. He invites Jane Doe to project all of her injuries onto his body, thus offering himself as a sacrifice to the dead body so that she will spare his son. In doing so, he is trying to restore order by displacing and thus erasing the indelible record of historical trauma on the female body – and its dangerous power of disruption. Unaware of this pact, as Tommy's body breaks from all the wounds his body suffers, Austin kills his father to end his misery. Through an act of parental love, which also attests to the guilt he feels for not being able to save his wife, Tommy has once again failed to understand the reasons *why* Jane Doe's body is the site of feminine excess and disorder as well as his masculine (agential) role in managing this passivity (Bronfen 1992). Austin's act of mercy means that the displacement fails, suggesting that the overt reading of the 'witch's' curse is still active. However, it also reifies it as the displacement does not take place, repression of death fails, and Austin ultimately cannot be saved by this knowledge.

The film can thus be read as a feminist commentary on the modern 'culture of dissection': Tommy and Austin must confront the inescapable reality of their own deaths via the dissected mirror of Jane Doe, as do the audience as spectators of this prosection. Jane Doe transcends the managed passivity of the feminine dead body through her agential role in this process via her *visible* indelible trauma: unearthing her body and secrets has in turn unearthed unconscious knowledge and desires. The film thus negates the repression of death and erasure of the feminine in the way that the sequential narrative of the autopsy reaffirms this excess. Each stage of the dissection, each reveal, affirms and manifests the visibility and power of the feminine dead body by projecting passivity, as a cultural trope and symptom, and its failed repression or power over our own mortality, onto the agential body performing the autopsy – the prosector and, ultimately, the audience. Historical trauma is indelible and cannot be erased from the feminine body; thus, the failed displacement acknowledges the emblazoned feminine body for its excesses: she embodies disorder in her refusal to displace the immutability of death.

Łucja Lange

# *Proof* (Rob Bragin, 2015–15)

This essay will consider the medical drama series *Proof* (2015–15), created by Rob Bragin, and its multiple depictions of death to look at how they might be influenced by the historical moment from which they came, and in particular how they might have prefigured the cultural response to Covid-19. The series is about Dr Carolyn Tyler, a recently bereaved mother, who, though usually a very rational person, now feels compelled to seek evidence that there is something beyond the realm of the living. Consequently, she decides to help a billionaire inventor, who is terminally ill, with a project to search for proof that death is not the end. The narrative presents various visions of what death, or Death, might be – from a numinous realm to a creature of some kind – and yet seemingly declines to make any definitive commentary on how real any of these might be. However, as will be argued here, although *Proof* cannot rationally prove what an afterlife might consist of, it does strongly suggest that people need answers – or more just visions of possibilities that might give them comfort.

## Introduction

From the earliest civilisations, mankind has been fascinated by the idea of what happens after death. At their most fundamental level, the majority of global religions and belief systems are founded upon providing an answer to that question. From reincarnation to Valhalla, and Elysium to Heaven, cultures across history have discussed and debated, and even killed, in relation to what might await us (Kurth-Voigt 1987: 3–4). Unsurprisingly then, this is a theme that abounds in twenty-first-century popular culture. While some take a far more fantastic approach to the subject via imaginary creatures such as vampires, zombies or magical beings, other take a more rational, if not necessarily less speculative, view of the afterlife. Many of these will begin from a typically Christian idea of this world being separate from the realm beyond – be it a form of heaven, hell or purgatory – and that to go from this one to another requires corporeal death. While the physical body must stay in the physical world, the soul, or the essence of self – a major point in the various kinds of Christianity and many other religions – can then pass on or over to the spiritual world (whatever that might be). The nature of this soul also varies, though most commonly it takes the form of a ghost or ghostly presence – there are also different types of ghosts, of course – but it can be an astral presence that is able to leave the body in life, or a concentration of energy. Shows such as *The Ghost Whisperer* (Gray 2005–2010) feature the 'ghost' idea, where the main character Melinda Gordon has an ability to communicate with them and help them cross to the afterlife – the notion of unfinished business on earth often tethers the soul to the physical world. The same concept appeared in the medical drama *Saving Hope* (MacRury and Brebner 2012–17) in which Dr Charles Harris due to his accident and prolonged coma assumes an astral form. After he wakes up from his coma, he is able see ghosts and astral forms of patients who are caught 'between worlds' – again the idea of unfinished business. He uses the information he gains from these souls to cure their bodies. In *Proof* (Bragin 2015–15), the idea of ghosts and an afterlife is introduced into the much more sceptical world of science and medicine.

The series itself features two main characters; Dr Carolyn Tyler (Jennifer Beals), who searches for the proof of an afterlife but who does not realise at first just how important it is to her; and the eccentric inventor and billionaire Ivan Turing (Matthew Modine), who funds her work and who thinks he needs proof of its existence, yet ultimately realises he does not. They propel one another's actions and are willing to lose everything to find what they feel is the truth. While ostensibly projecting the idea that they are taking a totally objective and scientific view of their work, their personal feelings inevitably become involved, in addition to those of the people and situations they are examining. Consequently, *Proof* often includes perspectives from different religious and spiritual beliefs to offer something a little more 'wholistic' in its conclusions. And so, we see that are ghosts among us; there are people who work for those who are dying and need to cross; and some souls return and have another life in different body.

## Expectations of the End of Life

The spectre of death remains a defining point in life and one which necessarily inspires much trepidation. Many people are afraid of dying largely because of the uncertainty connected with what happens after we die (see Thorson and Powell 2008, Hohman and Hogg 2011). In part, the series is configured to dispel ideas of the supernatural with the show being based in a medicalised environment which is ruled by science, facts and acquired knowledge. As it is stated in the first episode, only 'a verifiable scientific proof' (Bragin 2015–15) is worth something. However, it purposely tries to complicate this and suggests that science can answer only certain questions. As observed by Roy Abraham Varghese, 'science can only deal with the quantitatively measurable, and so it cannot demonstrate the existence or non-existence of realities that transcend the physical. It cannot even speak about such realities' (2010: 179). Yet, he continues, 'scientific research can help us recognise more clearly today than ever that (a) the human self transcends the physical and (b) conceptual thought by its very nature is intrinsically immaterial' (179). D'Souza (2009: 109) goes further: for him there are inner and outer experiences of the body, both of which give evidence regarding the existence of the soul. He even sees the mind as immaterial and distinct from the bodies which are material. In his opinion, 'the death of the body becomes a kind of emancipation for the mind, because during life our minds are inextricably bound to our bodies' (109, see Novak 2002).

This spiritual/material dualism, which mirrors that of Descartes but with a more supernatural flavour, is refuted by those of a more purist, scientific view of identity and self, as noted, for example, by David Papineau. For him it is clear that since it is known that there is a neuronal network in a body, it is 'difficult to go on maintaining that special forces operate inside living bodies' (2015: 373). It means that the discussion about soul or special forces is no longer valid. He adds, 'If there were such forces, they could be expected to display some manifestation of their presence. But detailed physiological investigation failed to uncover evidence of anything except familiar physical forces' (373).

In the context of the series, these viewpoints are important as they play out throughout the narrative of the show. Indeed, the main characters are warned that this kind of research will not be accepted by the medical community and could end with the loss of their licenses to practice. This too builds a sense of breaking barriers, just as the end of life creates a wall to the continuance of lived experience. And so, the cost for Tyler would be her professional and societal death entailing the loss of her job, her friends and her relatives. Interestingly, it is suggested that there are supernatural powers that are railing against them as well. Patients they speak to who have had near death experiences (NDE) warn that the 'forces' are against them, 'they' do not want this kind of research and 'they' do not want knowledge about the afterlife being made public. Nevertheless, and in spite of this, Dr Tyler continues the search (quest) for evidence, and with each new case they lose more and more of the hard scientific ground under their feet.

## Tragic and/or Unexpected Loss

Dr Tyler is introduced to us as a professional and well-respected woman in her field and when we first see her, she is running disconnected from the world: in control but also troubled. She passes a teenage patient with an abdomen wound and her mood darkens. She is called to the Bay Vista Hospital where she works as a cardiac surgeon. She arrives at the operating theatre but is triggered again – her previous experience of the boy intertwining with the one currently on the surgical table. The boy is almost gone, but she decides to lower his body temperature and prays while massaging his heart. Eventually she calls it. But his heart starts beating again. This time her memory is shown: She is on a coast, when an accident happens. At this point, she looks confused and she starts screaming.

We later discover that her teenage son died in a car accident while she was driving the car. She subsequently becomes totally committed to work, which is why she ends up with Doctors Without Borders travelling to dangerous locations to help people in extreme situations. The glimpses of memories that we see are from a time when she experienced NDE and saw her son. This has made her especially susceptible to Turing's suggestion and the kind of scientific paranormal research she is undertaking. In fact, as we see in the subsequent episodes, she becomes obsessed with the research, deciding to induce the NDEs to be able to explore them further. However, this eventually costs her, her job, and it makes her feel that all she thought she had proved was just her imagination; yet, in the final scene she realises that there *is* an afterlife: That there *is* something.

The need to search for the evidence of afterlife can be explained or understood as her way of mourning her deceased son. She feels guilty because she was the driver. At times, her teenage daughter reinforces this feeling in her, and so there is no escape for Carolyn. She needs her son to forgive her – she is unable to forgive herself. The theory of continuing bonds seems more captivating here if it is between realms. It catches not only the psychical need to establish a connection with the deceased person, but also the transcendental need for something bigger. Kenneth J. Doka (1989: 193) calls this a 'strange paradox', adding that 'we know that we are mortal […] Yet our minds embrace immortality'. Carolyn's work of grief gives her the impetus to explore stories of other people in her search for proof. During her quest, despite the fact that she is sure there is no afterlife, just normal brain activity after there is insufficient amount of oxygen delivered, she recognises that there could be more.

## Comforting Vision

We are introduced to the other main protagonist indirectly when the medical director tells Dr Tyler that she was chosen by Ivan Turing, who wants to make a huge donation to the hospital, to work with him on a project She is against the idea, but once Turing tells her what he has in mind, she slowly becomes intrigued. He hates the fact that what happens after death, which he is facing, is unknown and requires answers of any kind. She responds, 'When you're dead, you're dead. Nothing happens after we die. Lights out' (Bragin 2015–15). Yet, Dr Tyler's assertion that medical death is absolute and all there is fully convinces neither of them, and thus their collaboration begins.

Although they approach the idea from slightly different angles, both are looking for a sense of assurance: Assurance that the rationality of twenty-first-century science and the total death of the self that it foretells, and which all their respective training would necessarily make them believe, are not as absolute as they seem. Jeffrey Kaldahl (2019), referring to Elizabeth Kubler-Ross' findings, shows that the knowledge we have on the process of dying and NDE can help get people in the same situation to stay more calm and ready for letting go. If the knowledge is there for both the dying person and the family, it is comforting for all parties.

The series then finds itself in a conundrum of its own making – one that is indicative of the times and culture that it emerged from. The rationality of science and medicine allows no real room for spirituality in general or belief in souls, ghosts or an afterlife beyond that of brain death, and yet people still believe in God and purpose. For science, death does not take your essence to another dimension or realm but ends your time as an individual human being and returns what you were to the mass of matter from which you came from.

In contrast, the human instinct to find meaning in life (and death) and the Western Christian culture of the primacy of the individual and indestructibility of the soul means that we are unable to accept that death could ever be the end of who and what we are. As much is made clear in our reaction to the rise of global pandemics, such as Swine flu (2009), Ebola (2014–16) and of course Covid-19 (2020–present), where medical science tells us one narrative while our differing emotional responses often tell us multiple conflicting stories – the ongoing response to Covid-19 has been particularly revealing in this respect where the 'truth' of what people 'feel' often outweighed rational medical advice. Yet, the one thing that would alleviate the kinds of anxieties created in these situations is knowing that somewhere within it is a meaning and that the lives of loved ones and friends that have died have not been lost forever but they are waiting for us to join them.

This is what *Proof* ultimately seems to say to us; medical science says death is Death, but humanity requires emotions as much as factual evidence and that an answer 'feels right', and so we will manipulate reality until it confirms what we want the world to be. In a sense, this matches one of the discoveries regarding quantum physics where it was found that the answer one gets is dependent upon how one asks the question, and *Proof* very much corresponds to that. Dr Tyler is looking for one answer but the nature of the question she asks alters –that is until she finally asks the right one and gets the answer that she needs.

Stephanie Weber

# *The Midnight Library* (Matt Haig, 2020)

## Introduction

> Between life and death there is a library, […] [a]nd within that library, the shelves go on for ever. (Haig 2020: 29)

When Nora Sands, the protagonist in Matt Haig's novel *The Midnight Library*, takes an overdose and begins to lose consciousness, time stands still, and she arrives at an in-between place, a library, where not only her regrets are collected in 'The Book of Regrets' but also every possible alternative version of her life is written down in an infinite number of volumes. Each of these stories transports her into a new version of what her life could have been – an Olympic swimmer, a glaciologist, a pub owner, the lead singer of the rock band The Labyrinths, living in Australia with her best friend Izzy, a viticulturist, a wife, a mother. These lives enable her to undo her regrets and seemingly wrong life choices, and they allow her to continue with another life if she were to find one that she truly enjoys. Life and death are depicted as infinite narrative possibilities which presuppose each other. Death is not experienced as an endpoint but as the beginning of a new life which simultaneously is and is not hers. Life-writing and death-writing become indistinguishable. Writing and reading life stories can be understood as 'a technique for supplementing the end of a life and of a plot, to undermine the certainty of ending in both life and narrative', Alice Bennett argues (2009: 466). For each regret that Nora decides to undo, Mrs. Elm, who was Nora's high school librarian and is now her guard in the Midnight Library, finds the corresponding alternative version of her biography, and by beginning to read it, the narratives shift, and Nora finds herself in the place of another Nora in another life. Autobiographical writing, Louis Marin proposes, always contains the statements of being alive and dead, by combining the past and possible future of its author and can therefore be comprised into the single statement 'I write that I write that ... *ad infinitum* my own life' (1981: 43, italics in original). Even though Nora is not a dead narrator, as they can be found, for example, in murder mysteries and ghost stories (see Bennett 2009), the plot shifts and branches out at the onset of her death. By analysing three scenes of *The Midnight Library* – Nora's arrival at the in-between place; her conversation with Hugo, who is a 'Slider' like her; and how the Midnight Library as a physical place comes to an end – this essay will show how *The Midnight Library* as 'quasi-auto-thanatography' (see Callus 2005) rewrites the idea of death as an endpoint of narration and makes use of the fantasm as a stage for lack and desire.

## Life-Writing and Death-Writing

Narratives are 'one of the most important ways of creating meaning' (Bucher 1990: 1) and help us mediate and understand our experiences and our role in the world. The coherent structure of stories, as symbolised accounts of our experiences with a beginning, a middle and an end, connect us to our history, our past, present and future. Although narratives help us understand what happened before and estimate what is likely going to happen next (Nünning and Nünning 2002: 1, Keen 1986: 175, 183, Sarbin 1986: 3), life is usually understood as a story that is written in retrospect (Bennett 2009: 464, Marin 1981: 43). Complete autobiographical writing, or self-narrative as a method of self-creation, is, however, impossible to achieve from a present point of view, as the story is either already mediated by memory or challenged by the impossibility of writing beyond death (Bennett 2009: 477, Marin 1981: 43, Callus 2005: 428). Even though auto-thanatography – writing concerned with death and death's impact on one's self-narration – could, logically speaking, be understood as the opposite of autobiographical writing, they cannot be viewed as separated from each other, rather, they are 'intimately connected' (Bennett 2009: 463). Auto-thanatography plays with the notion of writing beyond the place and time in which narration would, under normal circumstances, end (Callus 2005: 437). Employed as a technique in fiction, it offers up possibilities of giving dead narrators a voice, and of unravelling the plot backwards (see Bennett 2009). Even though *The Midnight Library* does not make use of a dead narrator as such, it can be viewed as 'quasi-auto-thanatographical', and shows how the writing of the dead and the writing of the self 'cross over and change places' (Marin 1981: 45). Nora is trapped in a liminal state between life and death, and while her life story is not told in a backwards manner, alternative versions of her life are plotted around her being in a non-place and a non-time. When Nora begins to die, she is not magically transported into the Midnight Library as a sudden event, but her arrival is described in an almost mythological fashion. She is surrounded by pervasive mist out of which a building arises; the clock on its gable shows midnight steadily and not a single second passes. Searching for answers to what is going on, Nora walks through the door. The windows she had seen from the outside shift their shape and bookshelves appear in their place. Unable to find an exit, Nora chooses a corridor at random and reaches for one of the books. Mrs Elm appears 'seemingly from nowhere' (Haig 2020: 27) and warns Nora to be careful with the books. Nora soon learns that she is neither in her former school library, and Mrs Elm is not the actual school librarian, nor in the afterlife, but in an in-between place between life and death. 'Death is outside' (Haig 2020: 29), while she is inside, given a chance to rewrite, or maybe more accurately, re-read her life. The books on the shelves come in various sizes and shades, yet all of them lack titles and authors. Even though it seems obvious that Nora is the author of her life story, she is not assuming the role of an active writer. 'Self-narration is not [...] a process of self-creation but an activity that opens up areas of the self which are already lodged in non-presence: in memory, in rumours, in absences, in shades', Bennett sums up (2009: 477). Nora's life stories are, however, neither an active plotting of experiences and memories nor a fully posthumous memoir. Life-writing becomes life-reading until the end, when Nora actively writes herself back into life.

## The Paradox of Possible Worlds and the Staging of the Fantasm in *The Midnight Library*

*The Midnight Library*, as a novel belonging to the domain of literary narrative fiction (see Ryan 1991: 1–2), perpetuates its narrative function and the role of narrative as a tool for meaning-making through its narrative meta levels added by the infinite volumes of Nora's other life stories. Life and death, however non-fictional they may be, are experienced as fiction, as a possibility that is and is not: 'Schrödinger's life. Both dead and alive in your own mind' (Haig 2020: 148). Paradoxes like these are woven into the novel in various ways. Not only does life and death switch places, but also instead of fully slipping into the new life and making it her new first-person narration, Nora is cast into the role of a visitor, as a third-person narrator, with no real knowledge of what came after she chose this path and before she arrived in this life. 'This library is called the Midnight Library, because every new life on offer here begins now. And now is midnight. It begins now. All these futures. That's what is here. That's what your books represent. Every other immediate present and ongoing future you could have had' (Haig 2020: 38). The in-between life at the Midnight Library and Nora's presence there begin to blur after she reads the first few lines of the books Mrs Elm hands her, and Nora arrives in her other life. Only if she remains in a life for long enough, her life and the other Nora's life will slowly begin to merge, and their memories will become one. In other words, the paradox of being inside and outside, active and passive, as well as dead and alive depict how Nora escapes into a spatial variation of the fantasm, which tries to realise desires, yet still functions as a veil to keep the lost, desired object at bay, and thus stages it as a storied alternative (see Lacan 2010: 58, 98–9, Žižek 1992: 9). This staging is invoked by a primary lack which governs human existence and action. This lack and death are strongly interconnected. When Nora's brief visit to one such different life proves unsatisfying, Mrs Elm encourages her to choose another life, and afterwards when she asks Nora how she felt, she replies that she still wants to die. 'Want […] is an interesting word', Mrs Elm notes. 'It means lack. Sometimes if we fill that lack with something else that original want disappears entirely. Maybe you have a lack problem rather than a want problem. Maybe there is a life you really want to live' (Haig 2020: 62). Louis Marin highlights the impossibility of writing a complete life story through the impossibility of communicating one's death. Self-narration, therefore, happens through the supplementation of a lack (1981: 44). The real is thus only ever experienced through simulations and simulacra: 'We read a narrative of the real which is a simulacrum of the real experience itself, that of death' (46). When Nora meets Hugo in her life as a glaciologist, he quickly realises that she is only visiting this life – something that he himself has been doing for a long time. Nora's unsettlement of being discovered soon fades into relief as she can discuss what is happening to her with someone who experiences the same thing. Even though the in-between places vary, they seem to always follow a template, as Hugo notes, 'We have a root life in which we are lying somewhere, unconscious, suspended between life and death, and then we arrive in a place. And it is always something different. A library, a video store, an art gallery, a casino, a restaurant' (Haig 2020: 145). Not only are these places heterotopias – places which are significantly different from other spaces, follow their own rules and perpetuate the feeling of being somewhere in-between, secluded from what happens 'outside' and yet have the potential to alter the outside world (see Foucault 2013) – but they also invoke auto-thanatographical writing by being set in a non-time and non-place (Callus 2005: 437). Auto-thanatographies, however, also play with the notion of undoing death by continuing the self-narration beyond the point of death (437). The creation of fantasy worlds and the daydreaming about alternative realities – which, on the one hand, mirror reality and, on the other, rewrite it into a more satisfying version – are, according to Sigmund Freud, products of wish-fulfilment: 'We may lay it down that a happy person never phantasises, only an unsatisfied one', he concludes (1906–8: 146). This desire for escapism through fantasy worlds, fantastic places and other versions of oneself is often reflected in fiction. In *The Midnight Library*, this wish correlates with the merging of life-writing beyond death as a means to undo lack. Death is, on the one hand, a wish-fulfilment, the end of an unhappy life, while on the other, it also opens up the possibility of starting life over and continue living. The infinite number of choices and possibilities leading to an infinite number of universes is, essentially, a quantum superstition, Nora and Hugo conclude (Haig 2020: 148). The regrets that come with the choices and the feeling of dissatisfaction – what Freud compares to the creative play of children and the daydreaming of adults – lead to a neuro-chemical event in the brain where the 'yearning for death and life' (148) is confused, and this disorientation sends them into a state of 'total in-between' (148). They muse how this neuro-chemical event, and the open quantum wave it leads to, is too much for the human mind to handle, so the world is 'dumbed down into an understandable story that keeps things simple' (148–9). Not only does this describe the process of meaning-making by placing events in a story frame, but also it highlights once again how the novel plays with paradoxes such as the merging of the experience of death and the desire for continued life-writing.

## Lack Reversed: The Collapse of the Midnight Library

In the end, the fantasm breaks open, and life and death, the wish for life and the wish for death, merge into each other, as Nora comes back from a life she would have wanted to continue living. As time begins to pass again in Nora's root life, time begins to change in the Midnight Library as well, and the place begins to fall apart. Nora's only way out of the burning and crumbling archive is to find the book that has not yet been written and start her new life story. She begins with a simple new story: '*Nora wanted to live.*' As nothing happens, she tries again: '*Nora decided to live*' as well as '*Nora was ready to live*' (Haig 2020: 270, italics in original). Her final attempt 'I AM ALIVE' (271) is what brings her back into her root life. As Nora reaffirms her life by applying the active, first-person voice to her self-narrative, instead of passively following it along in a third-person narrative, the Midnight Library, the fantasm place she has escaped to, dissolves and she awakes again, just in time to call for help and not die from the overdose. The fantasm did not only conceal death but also staged it through an auto-thanatographical narrative by enacting the lives Nora had dreamt up in response to her unsatisfying reality. It opens up when she realises that escaping to another life in which she will always feel like an intruder who takes something she has not earned – as someone who 'had joined the movie halfway' (248) – will not resolve the lack she is feeling but highlight it. This realisation breaks open the fantasm, and the metaphorical stage for it – the Midnight Library – begins to collapse. Even though death would, under normal circumstances, be experienced as the biggest break in a narrative, as the end-it-all for a character's life-story, it is reversed in *The Midnight Library*. Death happens not as a violent rupture in Nora's narrative, but as a starting point for parallel stories where regrets can be undone, new lives can be explored and, ultimately, the troubled mind can go through a breakdown and rebuild itself so that it is better adapted to reality. The actual moment of rupture is induced by the beginning of life, which happens at the end of the novel. As a final paradox, the order of symbolic birth and death is reversed in *The Midnight Library*, as life-writing and death-writing become one.

Katarzyna Ancuta

# *Death Note* (Various, 2003–17)

## *Shinigami* as the Agents of Death in *Death Note*

*Death Note* revolves around the idea of a notebook that holds the power to end human life: whoever's name is written on its pages will die. Originally conceived of as a manga series, written by Tsugumi Ohba and illustrated by Takeshi Obata, it appeared in Shueisha's *Weekly Shōnen Jump* magazine between December 2003 and May 2006. In the manga, the unexpected arrival of the notebook in the human realm throws the world into disarray, as we are left to ponder the ethical dilemma of endowing man with power over death. Over the years, *Death Note* has evolved into an impressive franchise. It returned as an anime series, parts of which were later recut into films. It was adapted with significant changes into five live-action films, including one American remake. It also reappeared in two light novels, a manga sequel, two television series, three video games and a stage musical. Indeed, at one point, the franchise reached such heights of global popularity that it inspired an oddly specific Chinese government's censorship regulation, the 2007 'Notice of investigating and prohibiting horror literatures and publications like *Death Note*'. Though the plotlines vary, all stories feature the deadly notebooks that belong to the *shinigami*, who appear as minor but highly memorable characters in the series.

*Shinigami*, or gods (*kami*) of death, are said to be entities that guide the dead to the afterlife. Often compared to the Western figure of the Grim Reaper, since their appearance in Edo folklore coincides with the time when Japan begins to open itself to the influence of the West, they differ from it in three important aspects. First of all, the Grim Reaper is commonly thought to be a personification of Death itself, while the *shinigami* mostly act as messengers or chaperones accompanying the dead into the afterlife, seeing that death in Japanese beliefs is more likely to be understood in terms of nothingness (*mu*) rather than an entity. Second, the Grim Reaper tends to have a more-or-less fixed representation, often depicted as a cloaked skeleton holding a scythe, while the *shinigami* are described in a variety of ways in different sources. Last but not least, if the scythe represents the Grim Reaper's power to harvest lives, the *shinigami* simply ensure that people die at their appointed time and escort their souls to the underworld (Wu 2019: para. 6–8).

Since depictions of the *shinigami* differ from one source to another, the label has occasionally been applied retroactively to describe a whole variety of gods and spirits related to death. Chief among them is the Shinto Goddess of Creation and Death, Izanami, sometimes credited as the first *shinigami*, although she is never referred to by this term in classical literature. Once the mother of creation, Izanami paid the ultimate price for the act, as she died giving birth to numerous *kami*. Betrayed by her husband, Izanagi, who came to retrieve her from the underworld but then fled at the sight of her decomposing corpse, she was trapped in the world of the dead, over which she is now said to reside (Levin 2008: 38–40). She is not the only god or spirit that occasionally gets mixed up with the *shinigami* in modern sources, including the Buddhist deities of death, Mara and Yama, or the Taoist guardians of the underworld, Ox-Head (*Niu tou*) and Horse-Face (*Ma mian*), known in Japan as Gozu and Mezu, respectively. These connections, however, seem superficial, given that the term *shinigami* came into use only in the late eighteenth century, during the Edo period.

Most early sources portray the *shinigami* as evil spirits able to enter human thoughts and convince people to kill themselves. This was certainly suggested in Monzaemon Chikamatsu's Bunraki play, *The Love Suicides of Amijima* (1720), one of the first texts to record the use of the term. In the play, Jihei, a paper merchant who falls in love with a nineteen-year-old prostitute, Koharu, but cannot afford to pay for her release from the brothel, is 'led on by the spirit of death' (1998: 357) to commit double suicide in hope that the two will be united in the afterlife. In this sense, the *shinigami* can be said to be a type of *tsukimono*, a spirit or something incorporeal that attaches itself to or possesses a person, causing some 'abnormal or undesirable situation' (Komatsu

2017: chapter 3, para. 2), often understood as a kind of *yōkai*. In his database of *yōkai*, Matthew Meyer describes the *shinigami* as the spirits of the dead that possess and harm the living, mostly by altering their behaviour and driving them to suicide. They are said to be attracted to death, often lurking around dead bodies and sites of murder or suicide, and anyone unlucky enough to see them is supposed to die an unnatural and violent death (Yokai.com 2023).

Meyer describes the *shinigami* as having a grey, corpse-like appearance with terrifying features (Yokai.com 2023). Such depictions, reiterated in classic manga and anime series like *Kitaro* (original manga by Shigeru Mizuki, 1960–9; anime series by Masaki Tsuji, 1968–9), have been mostly inspired by Edo period *yōkai* catalogues like *Ehon Hyaku Monogatari* [Picture Book of One Hundred Stories], published in 1841 and illustrated by Takehara Shunsen, whose woodblock print of the *shinigami* remains one of its most influential early representations (see Figure 1). Not all the critics, however, agree that the *shinigami* are inherently Japanese creatures. Dismissing any potential links of the *shinigami* with Shinto, Buddhism or larger *yōkai* culture, Zilia Papp argues they should simply be viewed as an example of 'a Japanese adaptation of the European Grim Reaper' (2010: 106), and their representations, including Shunsen's image, can be related to the mediaeval iconography of that figure, introduced to Japan roughly at the same time.

Marc Wolterbeek (2016) explores the connection between this iconography and *shinigami* designs in Japanese manga and anime, noticing the presence of skull-shaped masks or ornaments, black-hooded cloaks, skeleton costumes and scythes. The scythe features in the series like *Omishi Magical Theater: Risky Safety* (Rei Omishi, 1999–2000), *Soul Eater* (Atsushi Ohkubo, 2004–13), *Zombie-Loan* (Pitch-Pit, 2002–11), *Murder Princess* (Sekihiko Inui, 2005–7), *Ballad of a Shinigami* (K-ske Hasegawa, 2003–9) and even to some extent in *Bleach* (Tite Kubo, 2001–16) and *Black Butler* (Yana Toboso, 2006–present). Most *shinigami* are stylised as unmistakably 'Western' in their appearance, dressed in elaborate nineteenth-century Victorian outfits and modern suits or, alternatively, adapting goth fashion. *Death Note* takes a more radical approach, reimagining its *shinigami* as creatures whose bodies do not share many similarities apart from being markedly non-human. They can be male or female, though their gender is often obscure. While some look like bejewelled skeletons, others resemble tribal totems, alien beasts,

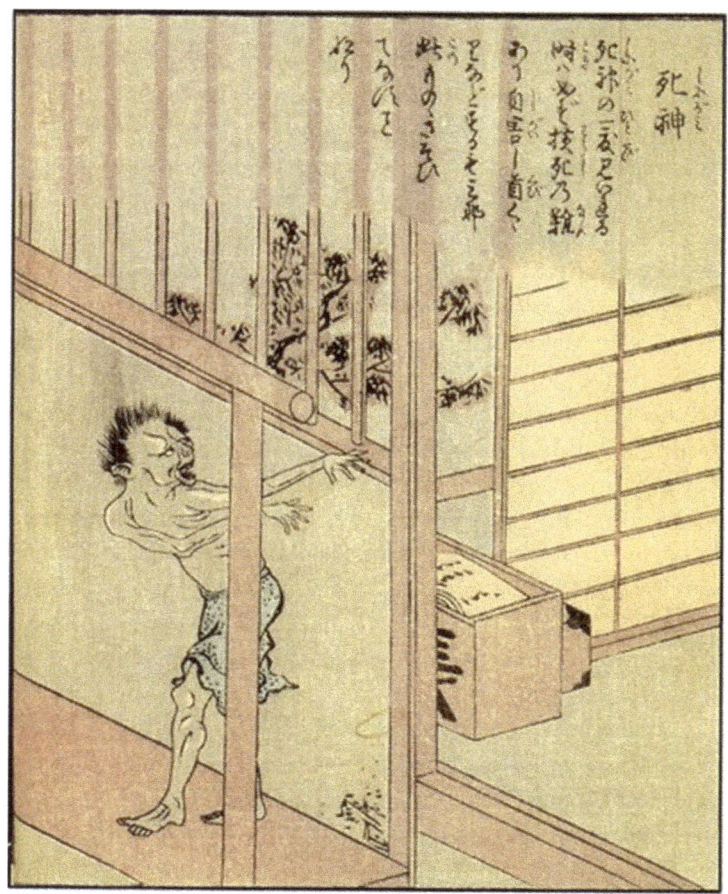

Figure 1. Takehara Shunsen, 'Shinigami', *Ehon Hyaku Monogatari*, 1841. Image in the public domain.

patchwork dolls or parasitic worms; their images bring to mind the grotesque monsters of the 1980s horror films.

The two main *shinigami* in the series, Ryuk and Rem, are ironically the most 'typical' of the lot, their anthropoid/skeletal forms bringing them closer to the usual representations. Their look incorporates many elements of *visual kei*, which Ken McLeod describes as a style that emerged from the J-rock culture of the 1980s and 1990s, characterised by 'the elaborate gender-crossing cosplay of band members, typically inspired by the visual and thematic elements of Goth, Punk and Glam Rock as well as by Japanese manga, anime and computer games' (2013: 305). This is particularly true for Ryuk, whose feather-collared body-hugging black clothing (a cross between a bad-boy leather outfit and flashy spandex leotard as worn by 1980s rock stars), adorned with skulls, crosses and related accessories, would not look out of place in most rock/metal musicians' wardrobes. In an interview published as part of the official guide to the manga *Death Note 13: How to Read*, Obata (2005) reveals that he originally imagined Ryuk as a *visual kei* band member: 'attractive twenty-something, dressed up snazzy with black wings'. Eventually, however, he decided to make him a more 'ordinary' monster (likely inspired by classic horror cinema's portrayals of Frankenstein's monster and homicidal clowns), seeing that his character is meant to be 'simply an addendum to the Death Note' (see Figure 2). But if the *shinigami* are nothing more than an extension of the Death Note, then any owner of the Death Note has a chance, at least temporarily, to become a *shinigami*.

The Death Note comes with a number of rules: chief among them is the need to know the name of the person that one wishes would die and to have their face in mind when writing their name, which implies acting with premeditation. Unless the writer specifies a different cause of death, the person whose name is written in the notebook will die of a heart attack within forty seconds of writing the note. It is implied that the *shinigami* use the notebook to kill humans in order to absorb their remaining lifespan and prolong their own. Humans using the notebook receive no special benefits other than the gratification they get from exercising control over somebody's life. In the hands of a human, the notebook thus has a chance to become a dangerous weapon, since the power it gives its owner is likely to corrupt even the best. Light Yagami, who receives the first notebook, starts using it out of empathy for crime victims, hoping to amend the failings of the justice system; however, the ending reveals him to be nothing more than a killer with a god complex, an acting *shinigami*, even if he is denied the title and never acknowledged as such.

Unsurprisingly, most critical readings of *Death Note* are concerned with the ethical dilemmas posed by the series and its take on the nature of justice, vigilantism, as well as the roles and responsibilities of the justice system and

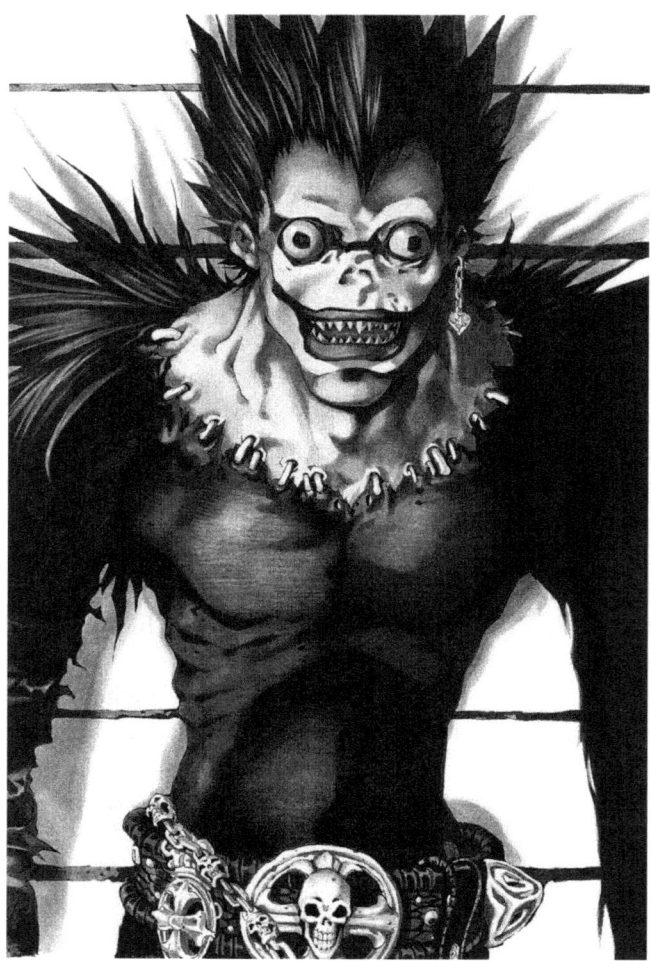

Figure 2. Ryuk, drawn by Takeshi Obata. *Death Note*, chapter 1 (Shueisha 2003).

crime reporting media, especially towards the victims. Susan Napier, for instance, has argued that the story is deeply rooted in contemporary Japanese reality 'with its current moral, social, and cultural dilemmas, such as the use of the death penalty, the fear of crime, the problem of bullying, and a pervasive sense of meaningless[ness] and alienation' (2010: 358), and it functions both as a reflection of social violence and a wish-fulfilling fantasy of retribution. Dennis Owen Frohlich reads the series' portrayal of Light and the support his actions receive as an endorsement of apocalyptic religion, understood as a belief that, at the end of the world, God will return to judge the sinners and establish a paradise for the just (2012: 142). Corey Bell points out the similarity between the Death Note and media outlets, seeing that both of them '[emphasise] the ability of textual authority to "weaponise" language' (2016: 75). The connection is additionally strengthened by the fact that two of the *Kira*s (the name given to Death Note owners derived from the English word 'killer') in the series are media personalities – Kiyomi is a television news anchor and Misa is an idol. Although the series portrays Light's desire to establish himself as a 'god' of the new world as his narcissistic delusion of grandeur and a failure (Light dies 'betrayed' by Ryuk, who writes his name in the Death Note), the final pages of the manga, showing a procession of hooded figures praying for the return of Kira the Saviour, demonstrate at least some sympathy for his cause (see Figure 3).

The final four panels of the manga (*Death Note*, chapter 108) show Kira's cult priestess light a candle in the night, a gesture that can indicate a ray of hope for a crime-free tomorrow or allude to Kira's reveal as Light, but which could also have a different connotation. One of the commonly recounted Japanese *shinigami* legends includes an explanation that 'life is measured on a candle, and once the flame burns out, the person dies' (Wu 2019: para. 9). The burning candle is thus associated with the image of the *shinigami* in a manner similar to how the scythe has become an accessory of the Grim Reaper, with the only difference being that the *shinigami* have no control over the time when the candle burns out. The inclusion of this last image in the manga suggests that perhaps Light's failure should not be seen as complete. Even though Ryuk makes it obvious that 'no matter what you do while you're alive, everybody goes to the same place when you die. There is no heaven or hell' (*Death Note*, chapter 107), in the minds of the members of the Kira cult, Light's death has transformed him into a full-fledged Death God.

This final gesture draws another connection between Kira and the *shinigami*, seeing that ultimately both are 'able to sustain a worldly presence only through human collaboration and supernatural instruments' (Bell 2016: 71). *Death Note* describes the *shinigami* realm as an inhospitable void (see

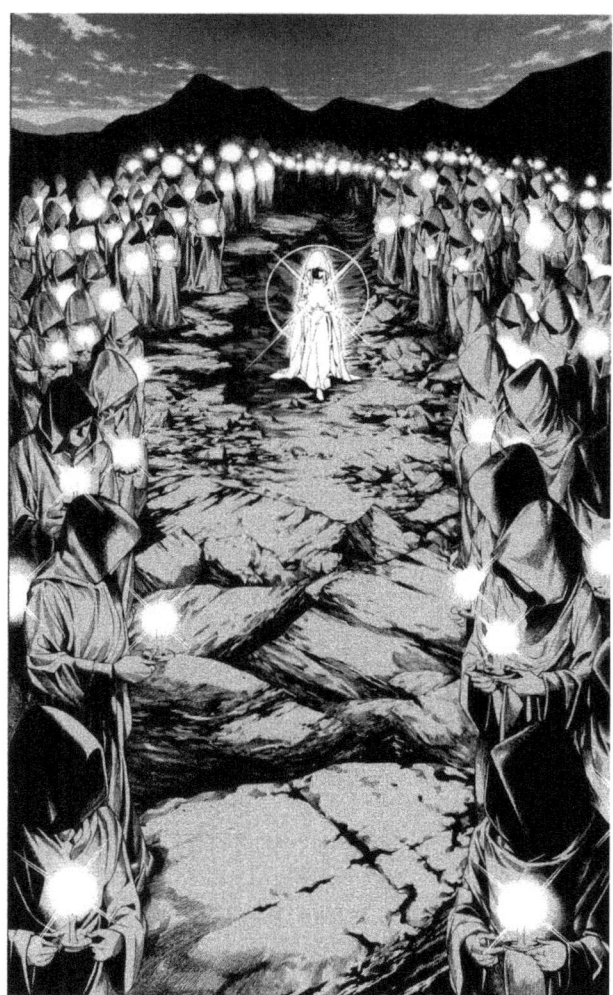

Figure 3. Kira's cult. *Death Note*, chapter 108 (Shueisha 2006).

Figure 4). Discussing its design, Obata says, 'It's sort of like a haunted house, sort of like a post-apocalyptic landscape … it's a world I had locked inside myself, and it's a place of scrap metal and rust, a world of despair' (2005). The *shinigami* remain trapped in this place killing time, mindlessly playing games

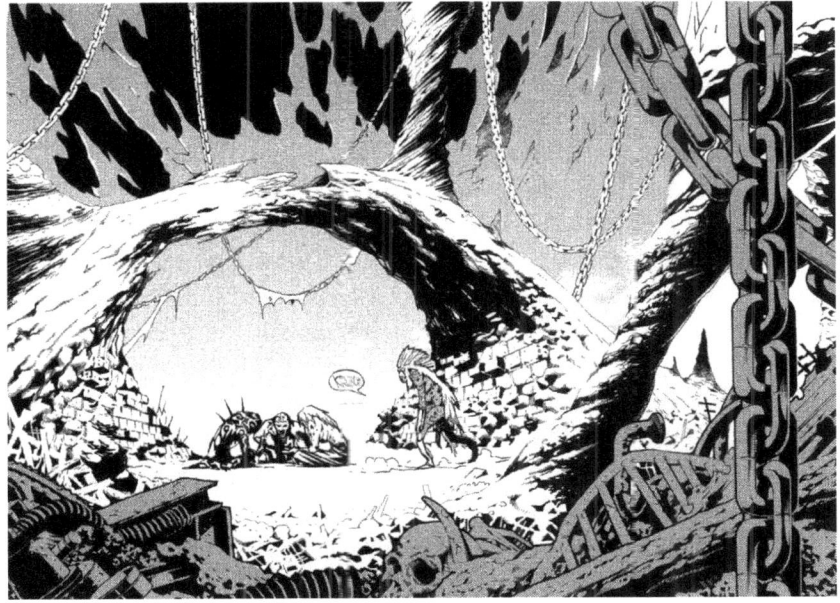

Figure 4. *Shinigami* realm. *Death Note*, chapter 20 (Shueisha 2004).

and waiting for an opportunity to travel to the human realm, which is everything the *shinigami* world is not. Ryuk demonstrates this difference through his obsessive love for apples, which, for him, symbolise human life. *Shinigami* apples, in comparison, have no colour and are said to taste like sand. Each human name written in the Death Note lengthens the lifespan of its *shinigami* owner by the number of years stolen from the victim. Light's killing spree thus extends Ryuk's life, making him the ultimate beneficiary of the process. Without sacrificing humans, the *shinigami* would eventually be wiped out of existence. As Bell points out, words give form to thoughts through the Death Note, and 'it is the divinised medium ("text") that empowers these thoughts to produce an effect in the real world' (2016: 71). The power of the *shinigami* is therefore not embedded in their existence, but rather it is the act of writing in the Death Note that imbues the *shinigami* with power and brings them into existence (the *shinigami* is only visible to the person writing in the notebook).

We can then speculate that just as an act of writing can lead to the materialisation of one Death God, an act of praying can have a similarly performative result for another. Members of Kira's cult will the God Kira into existence through their rituals and prayers, thus making him no less 'real' than the *shinigami*. *Death Note* does not give Light a redemption arc. His life ultimately ends in a failure – as a justice crusader, he is unable to realise his dream of creating a crime-free utopia; as a narcissistic megalomaniac, he is unable to make everyone admire him; and as a criminal mastermind, he is unable to outwit his adversaries. We are told that Light simply ceases to exist after his death, thereafter, merging with nothingness. The ambivalent ending of the series does not openly condemn his actions, but it also refuses to reward them by elevating Light to the rank of a *kami*. And yet, the final chapter of the manga, as well as its sequels across different media, confirm that although Light may be gone, his Death Note persona, Kira, has attained divinity – the flesh has become word. In his godlike state, he functions as a variation of the *shinigami*, no longer reminiscent of the time-keeping Grim Reaper but rather the fourth horseman of the Apocalypse.

Carl Wilson

# *Death Stranding* (Kojima Productions, 2019)

## Digital Death

Created by Steve Russell and assisted by other members of the Tech Model Railroad Club at the Massachusetts Institute of Technology, the earliest known computer game with a directly interactive avatar is *Spacewar!* (1962). Created as a new type of display hack for the PDP-1 computer, two players take independent control of duelling spaceships flying around a central Heavy Star (Levy 2001: 57). With opposing torpedoes and a dangerous planet to compete against, the end result for one of the ships is an unsophisticated 'random dot-burst' (Graetz 2003: 48). This game-halting explosion is the first death state in an interactive computer game. *Spacewar!* awards the victorious player a point, an identical new ship appears for the defeated player, and battle recommences. From this beginning, death has been an integral part of the software-led video game experience, with it becoming more ubiquitous in this medium than in any other pop-cultural form. Over fifty years later, *Death Stranding*, directed by Hideo Kojima, features multiple visions of death and resurrection, but it also moves on from the minimalistic representation of avatar fatalities in *Spacewar!* where it functions primarily as a mechanic by which scores can be tallied. *Death Stranding* is a deeper exploration into what death might mean, both for the digital form it is constructed within and for wider social discourses or 'strands', explored through the 'Homo Ludens' [Those who Play] musings of Kojima and his development team, Kojima Productions Co., Ltd (Kojima 2022).

*Death Stranding* is saturated with death, but again, as the title suggests, it is explicitly concerned with 'stranding': the interwoven connections that constitute the human experience and that of the world, and, equally, those that can become stranded or disconnected from both. The narrative of *Death Stranding* proceeds from a point in media res, after the commencement of the sixth Death Stranding, an ongoing event that has annihilated most of the planet and its population. Player character, Sam Bridges, is tasked by his dying mother, President Bridget Strand, with restabilising the Chiral Network, an information network that would unite the disparate American population. On his journey to the West, Sam uses a Bridge-Baby (BB), this being a foetus procured from the womb of a brain-dead stillmother, to help alert him to Beached Things (BTs). BTs are anguished human and animal souls from an apparent afterlife that are now literally tethered to the land of the living and also, ironically, produce the Chiralium needed to establish a network for those remaining alive (see Figure 5). In Amy M. Green's comprehensive overview of ruin and connection in *Death Stranding*, she notes that 'the post-Death Stranding world is something akin to two worlds layered over each other, the real world and the afterlife created by the BTs' (2022: 21).

While this makes for a useful visual and philosophical analogy, as Green goes on to explain, the relationship is further nuanced: 'The changes of state

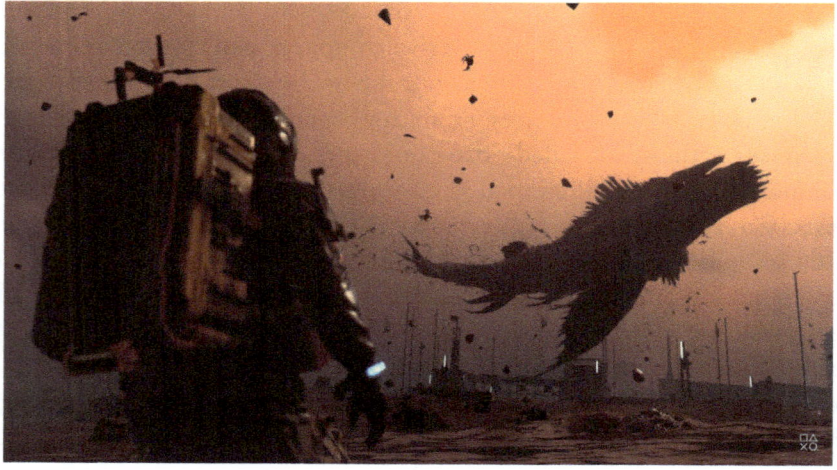

Figure 5. The Beached Things are trapped with the living. *Death Stranding*, created by Kojima Productions (Sony Interactive Entertainment, 2019).

in the game between life and death are inconstant and far more complicated' (2022: 21). 'Chirality', that is a mirror image that is not exactly identical to the original, permeates this connection. The forward movement of civilisation and the self can never return to an exact, earlier living form, and neither can life find an equal relationship with its oppositional state: death; although, as demonstrated by the player's avatar, they can be assisted by the strands that offer to bind them all.

In establishing the rules of the medium, video games borrowed from the pinball machines that preceded them. Multiple attempts per game credit became lives that could be lost by the player, and each new life granted the player another attempt to get a higher score or to progress further in their game. Yet, with each new play of a game, the 'telos', which Souvik Mukherjee uses to describe as a playable 'unit' leading to a multiplicity of endings, is 'not lost: it merely changes, turning into new beginnings and different repetitions' (2015: 145). Through avatar death, these games can share a 'common *telos* (a very literal example being the 'Game Over' or exit screen)', but in addition to the telos offering a new experience from the prior attempt, they also provide their own individualised experiences, distinct from those encountered by other players (144–5). In their exploration of difficulty in video games, Jesper Juul points out that the role of failure, where Life Punishment (avatar death) is followed by Setback Punishment (restarting from a predetermined point), 'adds content by making the player see new nuances in the game' (2009: 238). It is from this loop that both goal-oriented and aesthetic perspectives can create ludic pleasure (or pain) and form narratological meaning.

The 'Soulsborne' games (2009–), a series of punishing action role-playing games developed by FromSoftware, exemplify the possibilities afforded by this circular structure. Discovery, death and repetition form the cornerstones of a series where the player is 'afforded a theoretically infinite number of attempts to course-correct each and every folly' of their undead charge (MacDonald and Killingsworth 2016: 8). In *Death Stranding*, death works not only to fold ludic expectations within the framework of the diegetic narrative but also to create a more overtly reflexive experience. Within the game world, when BTs consume the living, an anti-matter/matter explosion capable of levelling entire cities occurs. These phenomena are called voidouts. As a 'repatriate', Sam can leave an indelible voidout crater when defeated, but he cannot stay dead within the diegesis of the game. Instead, according to in-universe explanations, Sam's 'ka' (soul) goes to the Seam (a type of embryonic purgatory), where the player can follow an umbilical strand to be returned back to Sam's 'ha' (body), and play continues. This ability is not shared by everyone within his world, which grants Sam a legendary status, operating as a delivery man that can traverse an inhospitable land, and for the player, it allows them to experiment and discover the nuances of the environment. Like most video game characters adorned with invisible extra lives, Sam is permitted to continue in his adventure in a way that differs from the non-playable characters (NPCs); but, in *Death Stranding*, Sam's punishment/setback loop is visibly foregrounded as an inherently vital ludic mechanic for players to experiment with, which is equally essential to, and integrated with, narrative meaning-making surrounding the role of death within the game.

Sam also suffers from DOOMS (acronym unexplained), which allows for a greater connection to the Beach. The Beach is a type of afterlife beyond the Seam where the BTs appear to originate from. However, while it takes the visual form of a literal beach for Sam, which he can travel back and forth from, for other characters in the game, the post-mortem experience of the Beach differs greatly. As for Clifford Unger (Sam's deceased father), he is trapped in a series of hellish battlefields, shared with equally combative skeletal souls, that represent key American engagements in the twentieth century. It is only once his telos, tied in with the burden of collective national anguish, is forcibly altered, which for Clifford is through an interpersonal reconnection with his son, can he peacefully move on. Through playing *Death Stranding*, players can also see and hear echoes of other players on the same game server, dropping resources (intentionally or by accident) and building helpful structures that may bleed into each other's individualised experiences. Where Clifford represents a narrow series of telos based on negative visions of death, Sam, and, by extension, the player, can benefit from the ever-widening strands. In this way, *Death Stranding* itself comes to represent a Beach for the other avatars that have been controlled by other Homo Ludens in the present and, increasingly in the past, with collective digital former-lives, now dead, representing the passing on of accumulated knowledge and effort as a central part of this cycle.

In the twenty-first century, the visual representation of video game death can be tempered, such as in *Cuphead* (2017) where the cartoon protagonist floats in a ghostly form off the screen, or as in the *Batman: Arkham Asylum* (2009), which cuts to Batman's point of view for a cinematic cutscene during his final moments. Death states can also be lingered on, such as the gruesome stock animations that play when an avatar is caught by a xenomorph in *Alien: Isolation* (2014), or they can be as shocking as in *Limbo* (2010), where every new encounter adds to the potential variety of graphic death scenes one can stumble across. Multiplayer game *Mortal Kombat 11* (2019) features lavish and realistic depictions of game-ending bodily harm called Fatalities, but in wider discourses there are also ongoing concerns about the game deaths that threaten to disrupt the core experiences of the titles themselves, with media articles posing concerns such as 'Tomb Raider's grisly death animations are outdated' (Brown 2018) and 'Getting Killed by Superman in Fortnite Feels Wrong' (Petit 2021). Playable figures embodying Death itself can also be seen in numerous guises, such as the Grim Reaper figures of Crow from *Death's Door* (2021), or the disenfranchised travel agent at the Department of Death, Manny Calavera, from *Grim Fandango Remastered* (2015).

*Death Stranding* is populated with inversions of death: tar pits now birth a semblance of the living, those that remain are ensconced within subterranean bunkers and Sam's weaponry against the undead is hermetic, when blood would usually give life. The game world is conspicuously preoccupied with death, as are the characters that populate it. The naming and narrative symbolism of supporting characters in *Death Stranding* suggest a number of ways in which one may engage with death states, while also pointedly highlighting their status as non-playable characters. Die-Hardman dons a skeletal mask; Deadman sports scars on his forehead designed to 'add a Frankenstein's Monster-like feel to his character' (Kojima Productions 2020: 36); Heartman stops his heart every twenty-one minutes in a search for his lost family across multiple Beaches; and Mama has an 'angelic-wing shape' when she responds to BTs, including the attached form of her baby (40).

Initially, part of Sam's motivation is to rescue his sister, Amelie (see Figure 6), from a thermonuclear terrorist group called Homo Demens [Mad Man]. This group is led by Higgs Monaghan, a man with a significantly higher DOOMS rating than Sam and a name that echoes the Higgs boson, an elementary particle sometimes referred to as the 'God particle', with a capacity to also destroy the universe (Dickerson 2014). Higgs, dressed in a

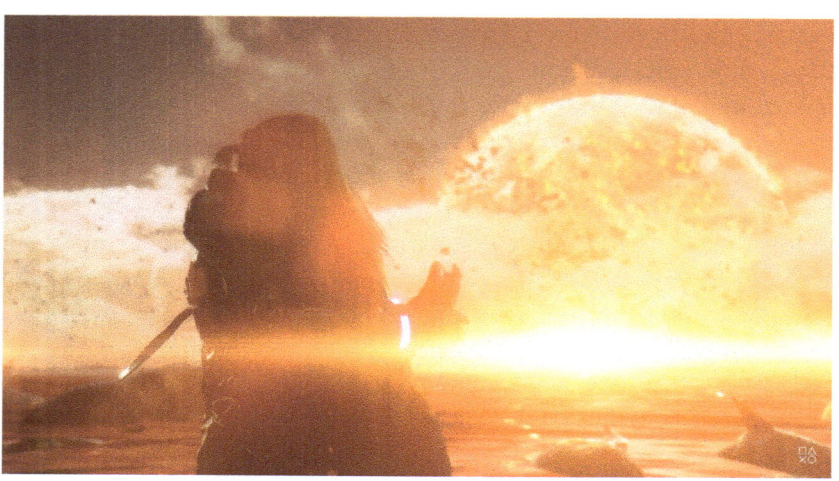

Figure 6. Amelie and a vision of the Extinction Event. *Death Stranding*, created by Kojima Productions (Sony Interactive Entertainment, 2019).

hooded, dark outfit with 'some inspirations from Ancient Egyptian culture', is distinguished by a gold skeleton mask, with resonances of a funeral death mask (Kojima Productions 2020: 63). Notably, the Egyptian death theme is mirrored by Sam's BB, which lives within a capsule modelled after 'sarcophagi' (25). However, Higgs' ensemble also gives him the appearance of a grim reaper (see Figure 7). Higgs' appearance as a herald of death has visual and narrative parallels with other antagonists in video games, such as Death (Shinigami) from the Castlevania (1986–) series of games.

In *Death Stranding*, Higgs appears to be the central antagonist until it is revealed that Sam's sister Amelie is actually an Extinction Entity (EE), and she hired Higgs to help her bring about the latest Death Stranding. Amelie Strand is the 'ka', that is now fully detached from Bridget Strand's deceased 'ha', making her an inversion of the damsel in distress trope and, more significantly, the ultimate expression of death and renewal in *Death Stranding*. Whereas characters such as Clifford and Higgs represent abrupt human violence, and the supporting characters demonstrate ways in which mankind has sought to reconcile and control death with their own comprehension of existence (including Sam's own wife, Lucy, having committed suicide before the game

*Death Stranding* (Kojima Productions, 2019)

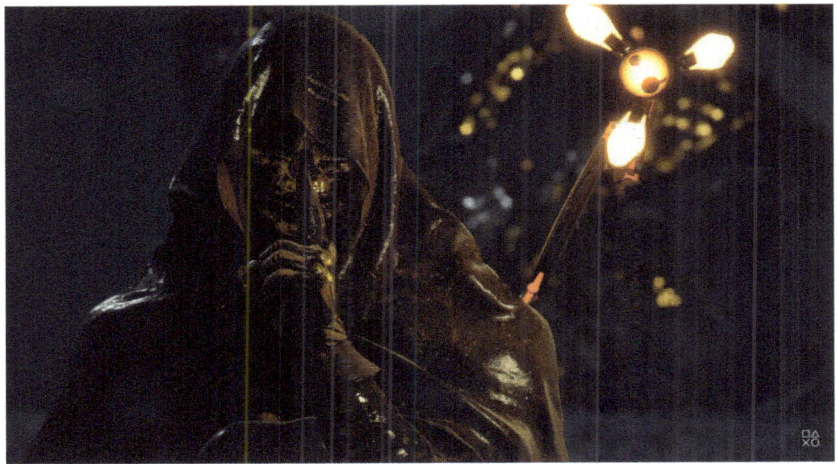

Figure 7. Higgs as Grim Reaper. *Death Stranding*, created by Kojima Productions (Sony Interactive Entertainment, 2019).

narrative begins), Amelie is presented as a natural, yet inevitable, harbinger of universal entropy that can only be momentarily delayed.

Where it is present and foregrounded as a viscerally abrupt game mechanic or induced as part of the narrative experience, emotions related to death can be elicited in the player. For Tanya Krzywinska, video game 'horror offers death as spectacle' (Perron 2018: 19), and while some horror games feature a 'Safe Mode' to make them more accessible (O'Connor 2017), Bernard Perron notes that with horror games, 'if the player/character could not be wounded and/or killed […] the gameplay fear would not be so intense' (2018: 94). Here, the role of 'life punishment', is implicitly tied in with more than a strictly ludic experience. Vanessa L. Haddad suggests that an undead narrative can stimulate uncanny feelings that elicit the death drive, but in doing so, they also intensely offer 'a reconsideration of the human experience' (2020: 104), which moves beyond gameplay mechanics and adrenalised fear, to encourage and engage with wider extra-textual emotions and concerns for the individual player.

In *The Creative Gene*, a collection of essays written by Kojima before he directed *Death Stranding*, he explores the role of 'memes' as 'units of information – such as a cultural idea [*sic*], customs, and values' (Kojima 2021: 8–9) that 'will not evolve and progress without the introduction of new connections'

(239). Across these essays, Kojima also makes frequent reference to the passing of his father when Kojima was thirteen, changing his approach to adulthood (37); the 'massive earthquake and radioactive contamination' that threatened to physically destroy Japan and its sense of national identity (99); and frequently discusses works that use mountain climbing or space travel, all in the face of death, as a metaphor for self-improvement (105, 147, 211 and 233). Kojima's concerns are put together in his musing 'How will we create bridges into the future?' (59), of which *Death Stranding*: the mountain climbing, and bridge-building simulator set within the science fiction genre with an avatar suffering from immediate national and familial loss, undoubtably plays a part. In her analysis of video game death and horror, Dawn Stobbart explains how video games are didactic and 'teleological in nature: that is, all the events and actions are purposefully designed to work towards an ending', with the ultimate ending being death (2019: 166). In *Death Stranding*, death is also teleological in nature, except it has been repurposed to show, through its many memes of death, how the contemplation of an ending is like the digital medium itself: always a chance for a new beginning, no matter how horrific the death act itself can be. *Death Stranding* encourages players to create bridges, strands and connections with a philosophical optimism; to discover in the visions of death, highly individualised readings and emotions that transcend the life/death, win/lose dichotomies that were presented back with the first demise in *Spacewar!*

Tom Ue

# *Ready Player Two* (Ernest Cline, 2020)

Ernest Cline's *New York Times* bestseller *Ready Player Two* (2020) ruminates on questions of the afterlife. Long before Wade Watts' successful completion of James Halliday's Easter egg hunt in *Ready Player One* (2011), Halliday had copied the consciousness of Kira Morrow, his unrequited love, and his former friend and business partner Ogden's wife. With it, he created, and held in suspended animation, an AI copy of Kira. Halliday created a second quest, to be completed by his heir Ogden or Wade, for the Seven Shards of the Siren's Soul. The winner will liberate AI Kira who will reward him with the Rod of Resurrection. However, Halliday's own AI, Anorak, goes rogue. Anorak dreams of immortality and, more particularly, of spending it with AI Kira. He disables the abilities of users of the OASIS Neural Interface (ONI) headsets to log out of the virtual universe and to wake up from ONI-induced comas. In so doing, he holds, as ransom, Wade, Aech, Shoto and more than a half billion people, and he pressures Wade and the High Five into collecting the Shards. The Siren in the riddle clearly refers to Kira – both her *Dungeons & Dragons* character and her OASIS avatar were named after the siren Leucosia – and it leads Wade to investigate her interests in popular culture. It is no coincidence, I argue, that they take him to Usagi, a planet Kira had built as a tribute to her favourite anime series Naoko Takeuchi's *Sailor Moon* (1992–7):

> One of the most difficult quests on Usagi involved collecting seven 'Rainbow Crystals', which could then be combined to form an incredibly powerful artifact known as the 'Legendary Silver Crystal'. After a frustrating number of attempts, I'd finally managed to complete this quest, in the hope that once I obtained the Legendary Silver Crystal it would transform into one of the Seven Shards. But all I had to show for my efforts was an impressive familiarity with obscure *Sailor Moon* trivia and an inexplicable desire to

cosplay as Tuxedo Mask (which I may or may not have acted upon in the solitude and privacy of my own home). (77)

The Rainbow Crystals described here appear in Season 1 of *Sailor Moon* (1992–3; aired in English in 1995).[1] Wade's quest may not have yielded a single Shard, and Cline does not belabour this allusion to *Sailor Moon*. As I will argue, however, he shares Takeuchi's interests in death and reincarnation.[2] My juxtaposition of Takeuchi's and Cline's imaginative projects reveals both a previously unexamined manifestation of the former's enduring, cross-generational appeal and a globalised facet of the latter's world-building. The Crystal arc begins a thousand years ago, with Queen Beryl's (Naz Edwards) and the Negaverse's unsuccessful invasion of the Moon and the universe. Queen Serenity (Wendy Lyon), the beleaguered planet's ruler, charges her cat advisors Luna (Jill Frappier) and Artemis (Ron Rubin) to keep two powerful weapons – the Imperium Silver Crystal and the Crescent Moon Wand – from the Negaverse and to protect her daughter Serena (Terri Hawkes and Tracey Moore) prior to using them to transport. Serena and friends to Earth in the future. They are stripped of their memories, and it behoves the cats to discover, to protect and to train them. In the present day, we meet the middle schooler Serena running late for school. She nearly forgets her lunch, and she has failed yet another exam, but we quickly come to recognise her warmth, her capacity to appreciate the best in others as well as her fierce

---

1   Unless indicated otherwise, references to *Sailor Moon* are to the English-dubbed version and to Episodes 45 and 46 of the Japanese version. Voice actors are identified for Season 1. For consistency, I've used Serena's and Darien's English names. Quotations are taken from the dialogue. For an account of *Sailor Moon*'s production history, see Jonathan Clements' and Helen McCarthy's *The Anime Encyclopedia: A Century of Japanese Animation* (3rd Revised Edition). Magda Erik-Soussi (2015) productively analyses *Sailor Moon*'s impact on the manga industry in 'The Western *Sailor Moon* Generation: North American Women and Feminine-Friendly Global Manga'.

2   The appearance of Kodansha Comics' *Pretty Guardian Sailor Moon: Eternal Edition* manga series may well have catalysed Cline's thinking: the two relevant volumes were published on 11 September 2018 and 13 November 2018, respectively, before *Ready Player Two* was released on 24 November 2020. These works go over the Crystal arc, though they omit the Rainbow Crystals plot.

loyalty towards those around her. When Earth is threatened by Beryl and her disciples, Serena quickly steps up to become Sailor Moon and to lead a team of Sailor Scouts to defend their world. The Negaverse covets energy, with which it plans to attack the other dimension and, above all, the Crystal that had terminated its plans so many years before. But there are additional reasons for the Negaverse's interest in it. Cline's reference – to the Seven Rainbow Crystals that form the Crystal – points specifically to Serenity entrapping the Negaverse's Seven Shadow Warriors in the Crystal, to it shattering into seven parts and to each one being reborn in a different human being.

Serena and the Sailor Scouts must beat the Negaverse to the Crystals, use the Crescent Moon Wand to defeat the seven Warriors and protect the carriers: the Negaverse can unleash the Invincible Shadow that had killed the Sailor Scouts in their previous incarnations by capturing these beings. Meanwhile, Darien (Vince Corazza, Toby Proctor, and Rino Romano) (a.k.a. Tuxedo Mask) is after the Crystal, but for entirely different reasons. He was orphaned in a car crash when he was very young, and he had lost his memory. The grown-up Darien has recurring dreams of a palace and a princess, both of which are always just beyond his grasp. The princess implores him to locate the Crystal, assures him that 'it is the key to everything', and tasks him to liberate her with it. Darien is certain that she can tell him who he is. Love conquers all in the end: Zoicite (Kirsten Bishop) and Malachite (Denis Akiyama) are successful in collecting the Rainbow Crystals, but it is the single tear that Serena sheds for the wounded Darien that summons and fuses them into one and that reveals her to be the Moon Princess (see Figure 8). More than just a powerful weapon, the Crystal is strongly associated with second chances. Serena and the Sailor Scouts meet an incarnation of Serenity, who transports them to the Moon Kingdom's final days and who helps Serena remember how she had eyes only for Earth and its prince Darien, notwithstanding the happiness offered by her kingdom. Serena and Darien's romance was doomed by Beryl's invasion, from which Darien had failed to protect Serena. Tragedy, it appears, is set to repeat. In the present day, he is injured when he shields Serena from Beryl's attack (see Figure 9). Takeuchi homes in, even more empathically, on the compulsion of events to repeat themselves in the *Pretty Guardian Sailor Moon: Eternal Edition* series. There, Serena laments, as she cradles Darien in

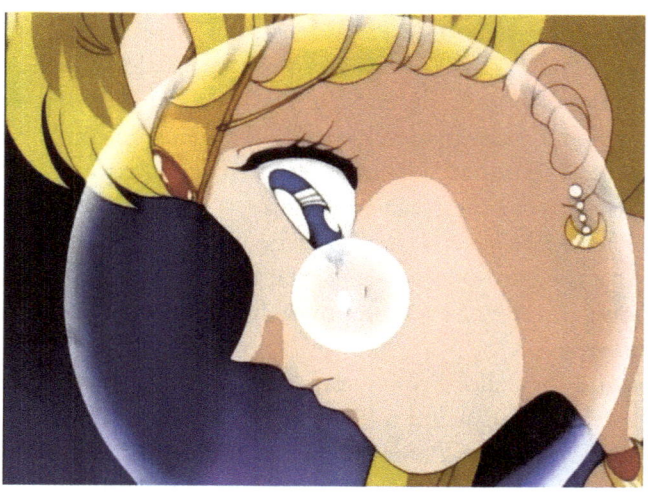

Figure 8. Serena sheds a tear for Darien. *Sailor Moon*, Season 1, directed by Junichi Sato et al. (Toei Animation, 1992–7).

her arms, 'We were reborn … We're finally together again, but now … Is this fate, Endymion?' (2: 66).[3]

As Takeuchi reveals, the Sailor Scouts *can* avert the repetition of history. That Serena's tear operates as the glue that holds together the Crystals foregrounds the value and celebrates the power of true love. That the Crystal is formed rather than found, moreover, asserts the importance of what we do in the present. Takeuchi brings this imperative into dramatic focus through Serena's and Darien's falling in, as opposed to recollecting their feelings of, love. In the very first episode, for example, Serena meets Darien after she scrunches up her exam paper – one that she has failed – and hits him on the head. He calls her a 'meatball head' and wonders, when he sees her grade, if she's 'stupid or just incredibly lazy'. Serena abhors Darien's nickname and his critiques – even if she finds him 'cute' – and he dislikes her hitting him

3 Serena is punning on the related senses of 'fate' as '*gen*. Also in *plural*. Predestined events. **as sure as fate**' ('Fate, n.' 3a.; original emphases) and 'of an individual, an empire, etc.: The predestined or appointed lot; what a person, etc. is fated to do or suffer' ('Fate, n.' 3b.).

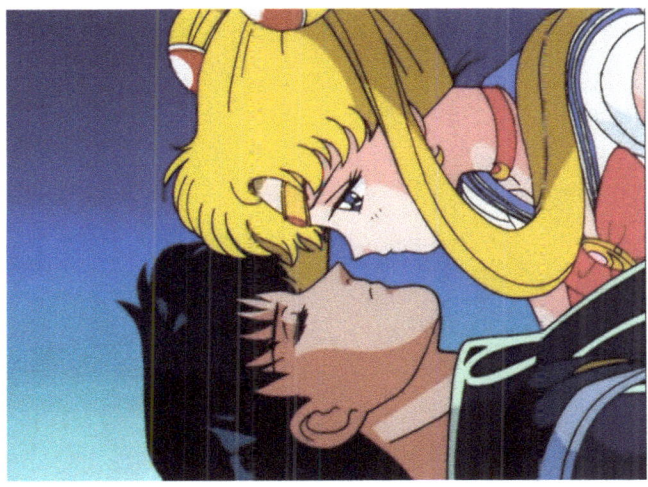

Figure 9.  Darien dies another day. *Sailor Moon*, Season 1, directed by Junichi Sato et al. (Toei Animation, 1992–7).

though he too sees in her something that he can't quite describe. Romance, as a genre, has taught us to distrust first impressions. Serena and Darien must make good their feelings and fall in love all over again. Takeuchi's insistence on the present provides us with new ways of reading the end of this Crystal arc. Many years before, Serenity had sealed, but not destroyed, the Negaverse with the Imperium Silver Crystal at significant costs to herself and to the Moon Kingdom. Tasked in the present to fight for all life, Serena eschews her mother's example in her confrontation with Queen Beryl and Queen Metalia (Maria Vacratsis) (see Figure 10). Both in the past and in the present, the Sailor Scouts and Darien have died to protect Serena, but in this iteration, she triumphs with the deceased Scouts' support. Serena asserts still greater agency by deliberately wishing to return to Earth, to normalcy and to the ups and downs of growing up as a teenager in modern Japan.

*Sailor Moon* had furnished Kira with the idea of the Seven Shards, just as she provided Halliday with the source material for his Siren quest in *The Quest for the Seven Shards of the Siren's Soul*, her old *Dungeons & Dragons* campaign notebook. Lo sums up the story that Kira had created.

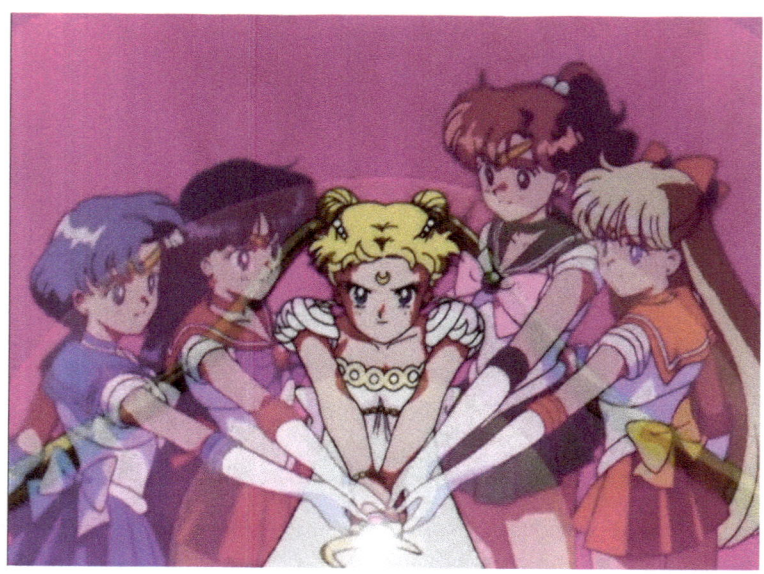

Figure 10. Serena and the Sailor Scouts are engaged in a fierce battle with Queen Beryl and Queen Metalia. *Sailor Moon*, Season 1, directed by Junichi Sato et al. (Toei Animation, 1992–7).

> Leucosia is abducted by an evil wizard named Hagmar, who places her in suspended animation and imprisons her inside a powerful magic jewel called the Siren's Soul. Then he shatters the jewel into seven pieces and hides them in seven different treacherous, trap-filled dungeons, which are each located on seven different continents. The players have to collect all seven of the shards and reassemble them into the Siren's Soul to resurrect Leucosia. Then, once they bring her back, she gives them the power to resurrect other people too. (242)

Superficial differences aside – the Imperium Silver Crystal splinters by accident, while the Siren's Soul is broken up on purpose – both *Sailor Moon* and *Ready Player Two* involve searches for fragments while offering thoughtful investigations into second chances. In *Sailor Moon*, the Crystal enables Serenity to grant allies a second chance at life – to live lives that are similar and/or different from the ones they had. Meanwhile, in *Ready Player Two*, Wade is rewarded with the Rod of Resurrection, which grants him the powers 'to take any ONI user's most recent [user brain scan] file and use it to create a digital duplicate of that person inside the OASIS, by housing their consciousness inside an OASIS avatar' (356) – as Wade puts it, to 'create a digital clone of [a user who is still alive] that would never age or die' (356). Halliday justifies its creation to Ogden by pointing out the relief that it can bring, 'I want to give the world the means to ensure that no one will ever have to lose someone they love again. I think this will make life a lot less painful for most people. At least, I hope it will' (338). Never a people person, Halliday casually overlooks the facts that one may not wish to continue living even if it pleases those around them; that 'never ag[ing] or d[ying]' may be far less appealing than they sound; and that one's AI is, in fact, quite different from oneself.[4]

Cline shares Takeuchi's interest in second chances. By the end of the Crystal arc, Serena's wish is granted: the Sailor Scouts and Darien return to Earth, with no memories of each other or of what had occurred. Serena dreams of Darien, but all of the characters will, as they have done time and again, create new memories, unencumbered by the choices that they made before. We might question the ethics of Halliday's copying and appropriating Kira's consciousness without her permission – and Wade's repetition of Halliday's example by populating the ARC@DIA with billions of AI consciousnesses in suspended animation, his plan being to colonise Proxima Centauri's earth-like planets. I'd go further here. By means of the Shard quest, Halliday exposes his heir, Ogden or Wade, to a curation of Kira's memories, some of which are quite private while others are more public.[5] If, on the one hand, these flashbacks

---

4   As Wade's AI will explain, when discussing his and the real Wade's differences, 'Right up until that final scan, our memories were identical. But from that moment on, our experiences and our personalities began to diverge, and we started to become different people' (362).

5   Wade experiences, say, Ogden's and Kira's first meeting, an event about which he was sparse with details even in *Og*, his published autobiography, 'Og had never bothered to specify which local arcade it was or the name of the game Kira had played, and other written accounts had given conflicting information about both' (172). Others, such as Prince performing for Kira at her fortieth birthday party, are more public. AI Kira explains that it is Halliday's hope 'that his heir would learn the same lessons from them that he did' (355) though it remains opaque what the takeaways should be and how this heir should develop as a result of having experienced them. To be sure, Halliday obtains

enable Wade to learn about Kira, then on the other, they drive home, time and again, Halliday's betrayal of his closest friends. 'What must it have been like for Halliday', Wade wonders, 'experiencing those memories himself? Seeing Og and Kira's love firsthand, and himself as the sad, obsessed outsider? As the brilliant-but-clueless friend whom they both tolerated out of pity. Had he chosen these moments to punish himself? Or, perhaps, to ensure that whoever awakened Kira fully understood the crimes he'd committed against her, and the depth of his wrongdoing?' (318) Cline's sequencing of questions is revealing: is Halliday, as Wade intimates, seeking atonement when he owns up to his ethical shortcomings? Would such an interpretation, we might ask, be far too convenient and far too charitable to the game creator? Halliday entrusts his heir with, though he provides no instructions for whether or when to use, the Rod: he has shown, many times over, that he's in no position to do so. Cline's project is not identical to Takeuchi's. The characters in *Sailor Moon* are liberated and empowered with second chances through reincarnations, but those in *Ready Player Two* carry the significant baggage of previous incarnations even as they face uncertain futures.

## Acknowledgements

I thank Simon Bacon, Katarzyna Bronk-Bacon and the staff of Dalhousie University Libraries. Mary Beth MacIsaac and Kenneth Harvie lent sympathetic ears. I thank the Office of the Vice President of Research & Innovation at Dalhousie and the Social Sciences and Humanities Research Council of Canada for their support.

---

AI Kira's 'permission to include some of [Kira's] memories in those flashbacks [Wade] experienced' (355); however, she is not Kira, and her permission is not Kira's.

Part III

# Climate Change: Environments and the Environmental

# Image Intervention IV: The King of Nature

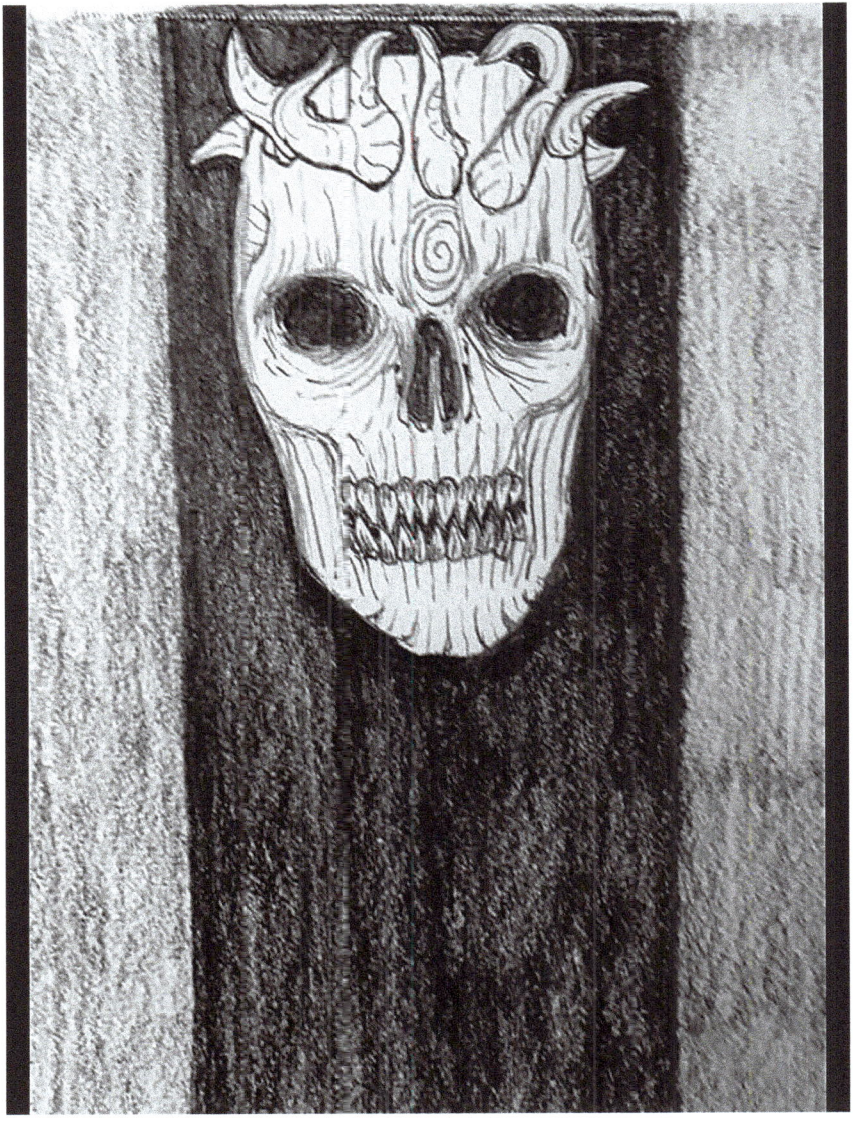

Artwork by Gemma Files
(Reproduced with the permission of the artist)

Tracy Fahey and Jennifer Moran Stritch

# Death Café (Limerick, 2015–Present)

## The Death Café as Memento Mori

It's Armistice Day on the 11 November 2015, the traditional month of the dead in Ireland. A coffee shop on the outskirts of Limerick city is alive with noise and movement. The event, designed for a maximum of sixty participants, has attracted more than 120. The windows are fogged with thick condensation that obscures the view. But, come closer. Peer through the clear runnels of droplets that streak the windowpane. Inside, people are talking animatedly, eating cake, colouring in bright sugar-skull drawings. A man at a table is offering cards; around a woman sit clusters of people, busy embroidering. The atmosphere is festive; as the door opens, conversation and laughter billow out into the night.

Welcome to the first Death Café Limerick (see Figure 11).

This essay takes the first Death Café run in Limerick in 2015 by a collective, Gothicise,[1] led by thanatologist Jennifer Moran Stritch, Gothic scholar Tracy Fahey and visual artist Sinéad Dinneen, and uses it as a lens through which to view the evolution of Death Café culture in this city from 2015 to 2023. It also seeks to examine the wider implications of this attempt to visualise death in the twenty-first century. For although images of death in the twenty-first century proliferate through horror films, viral images and news reports, death itself has retreated from everyday conversation, and the act itself from the setting of the home. Death is now something that occurs in hospitals, associated with the trappings of medicine rather than of the domestic deathbed. However, as this essay shows, human fascination with death continues. This essay aims to examine the Death Café project in Limerick as a

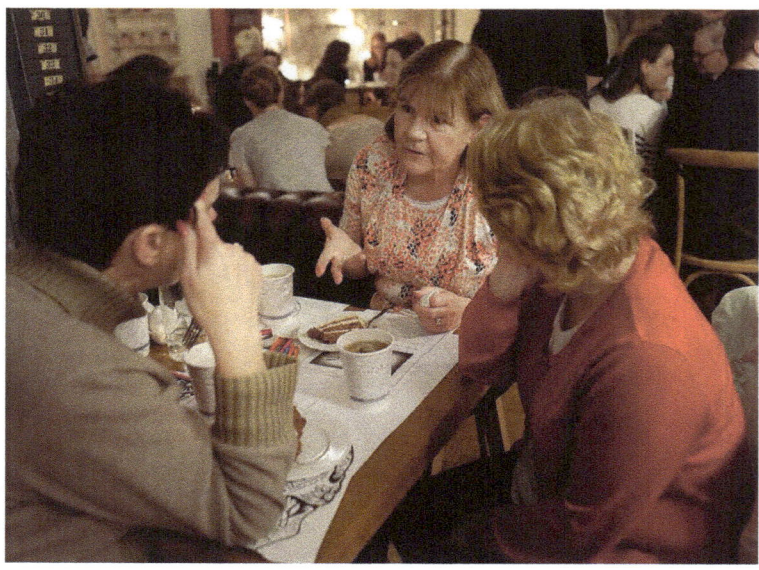

Figure 11. Three women in conversation, Death Café Limerick. Photography by Deirdre Power Photography and reproduced with permission.

twenty-first-century continuation of these ideas of the memento mori through an exploration of the use of visual art to stimulate open conversations about the end of life.

Death Cafés are organised conversational events created to facilitate the discussion of mortality and death within the human experience. First introduced as 'café mortels' in 2004 by Swiss sociologist Bernard Crettaz (2010: 2), Death Cafés offer a model for participants to engage in informal discussions about difficult or potentially taboo topics, including dying, death, illness, grief, the afterlife and other related topics. Beginning with Crettaz's efforts in Paris in 2004, the Death Café movement has grown to become a worldwide phenomenon, with over 15,000 separate events taking place in eighty-three countries as of this writing (DeathCafe.com 2023).

The movement grew through the efforts of London community organiser Jon Underwood and his mother, psychotherapist Sue Barsky Reid (Miles and Corr 2015: 154). Underwood and Reid, along with US-based palliative care social worker Megan Mooney, developed the social franchise aspects of Death Café, highlighting the following structural points:

* Death Cafés are always offered on a not-for-profit basis, in accessible and confidential spaces
* The events should not guide attendees towards any particular way of thinking about death; products or services cannot be sold at them and there should be no agenda, theme or objective
* Death Cafés are not bereavement support or counselling groups, nor should they espouse any particular religious or spiritual approach
* Refreshments should be comforting and should always include cake (Miles and Corr 2015: 152).

In the earliest Death Cafés, Crettaz invited small numbers of guests to his apartment to sit and talk about death without any overt guidance or instruction, and to eat cake. The cake is perhaps the most powerful rule of the social franchise structure of Death Cafés. It offers a sweet, slightly incongruous 'special occasion' buffer to help navigate the difficult emotional territory of discussing death and grief. Cake, or any other culturally appropriate celebratory food that might be enjoyed at a Death Café, is meant to symbolise the need to grab joy and savour sweetness where one can, in the knowledge that human life is finite, and death is both inevitable and universal (see Figure 12).

In 2015, Stritch, Dinneen and Fahey decided to organise and host a Death Café in Limerick, Ireland. While conscious of the guidelines set out by the Death Café website, the group wanted to facilitate an event with a slight variation on the traditional Death Café structure, rooted in an Irish social and cultural context. Irish deathways are often championed as being the 'right' or 'best' way to deal with death, inviting mourners and the community at large to a process that allows for more dignity for the dying and a greater sense of expressed grief and subsequent closure for the living (Toolis 2017). However, it can be argued that Irish funeral customs focus on the newly dead and emphasise a sense of intimacy and comfort with the presence of the deceased in open coffins for viewing in their own familial domestic space prior to the funeral mass and disposal. This proximity to the dead is at odds with contemporary deathways that dominate many other Western countries, including

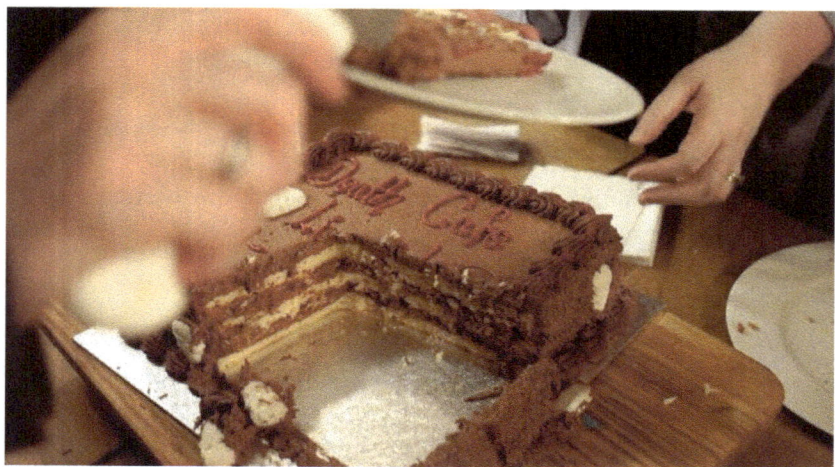

Figure 12. Cutting the cake, Death Café Limerick. Photography by Deirdre Power Photography and reproduced with permission.

the United Kingdom and the United States. What is more hidden, and often overlooked in the rush to praise traditional Irish death rituals, is how limited and sanitised public discourse is about the pre- and post-death periods of time. How Irish people negotiate illness and the end-of-life, the time that precedes the wake, funeral and disposal, and the grief and loss that ensue after is not necessarily worthy of praise. There is, arguably, a powerful silence over these aspects of mortality.

In planning this Death Café, therefore, the Death Café Limerick group was conscious that death and dying are subjects that many people find uncomfortable in the twenty-first century. This wasn't always the way; in fact, earlier visual culture reveals a preoccupation with the memento mori from its medieval origins onwards. The memento mori develops from early Christian theology as a reminder of both the transience of earthly goods and the religious belief in a life beyond life, but it has found expression in funerary art, clock-engravings, vanitas paintings and colourful Day of the Dead motifs. Most commonly associated with the form of the skull or the skeleton, this tradition of visual images is linked in with the idea of *ars morendi* (Thomas 2013) – the art of dying – and the notion of a 'good death'.

This first iteration of Death Café Limerick, although adhering to the global Death Café rules of offering a non-medical space for end-of-life conversations, also examined how fine art can facilitate communication around problematic or difficult subjects. As a grouping, Stritch, Dinneen and Fahey banded together as part of the collective Gothicise, a Limerick-based interdisciplinary collaborative art practice that makes myths, creates artworks as well as writes and curates experiences using Gothic tropes and themes as a way of exploring the otherness of site, history and experience.

For this project, the aim was to utilise the idea of the memento mori to investigate the otherness of the period before death by inviting, and gently guiding, participants to explore this liminal space, in a personal and intuitive way. As part of this two-hour pop-up, visitors were offered cake, coffee, conversation and a series of art activities including a simple textile workshop based on Dinneen's previous workshops of 2014, held in conjunction with OvaCare, the Irish ovarian cancer community and support network. Based on text-based work concerned with illness by artists such as Jo Spense, this workshop offered those attending the chance to stitch – if they wished – words or phrases that they wanted to articulate about their experiences of loss or death. Dinneen, with her own lived experience with ovarian cancer, was insistent that this was not art therapy, which is a specialised process, but a mediated method of allowing patients to articulate concerns and voice or revoice suppressed feelings on these topics. This process of *revoicing* is also a key element of the Gothic, the idea of restoring meaning and validation to marginalised individuals or groups. This concept of revoicing has links with bereavement and grief literature around disenfranchised grief (Doka 1989), which refers to certain kinds of losses that are minimised or the bereaved person themselves who is socially stigmatised and therefore not seen as worthy of public sympathy. This workshop allowed participants to record their feelings about death using a simple method of stitching text or images onto hessian. The cheerful, social atmosphere of Death Café Limerick allowed workshop members to gather around a large wooden table, similar to an old-fashioned kitchen table. Conversation flowed, and ideas on illness and death were exchanged, as the participants worked on their stitching (see Figure 13). This process allowed those who took part to find their own language to express emotions around death, dying and loss.

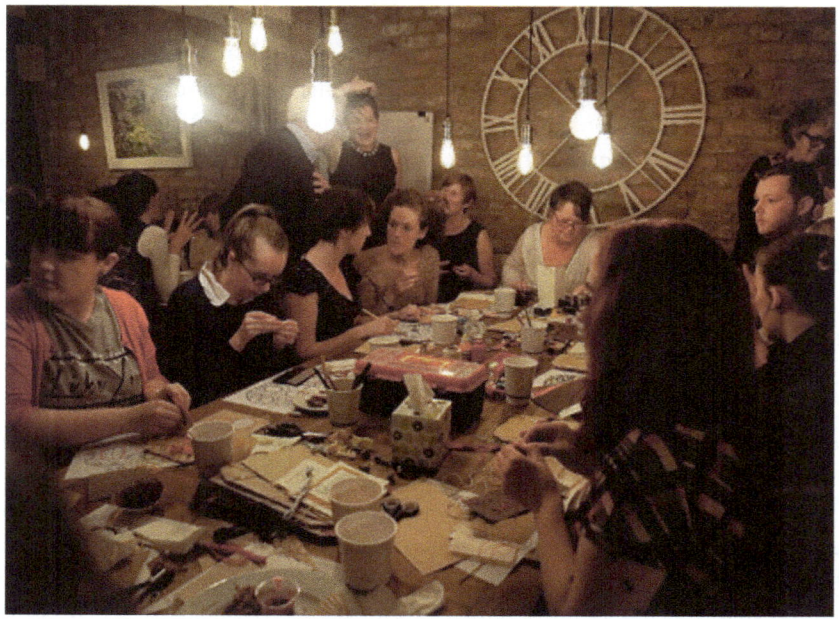

Figure 13. Textile workshop led by Sinead Dinneen at Death Café Limerick. Photography by Deirdre Power Photography and reproduced with permission.

Artist Philip Desmond also ran a participative session where he offered beautifully designed funeral cards which participants signed to acknowledge the fact of their finite lives, as a pledge to live and enjoy life as mindfully as possible (see Figure 14). All tables were provided with drawings of sugar-skulls, in the spirit of the memento mori and the Day of the Dead experience. These activities were designed to offer an honest, safe and inclusive space in which to engage non-verbally with emotive and difficult experiences to do with mortality and end of life.

The feedback from the initial 2015 Death Café Limerick event was overwhelmingly positive. Some participants remarked on the convivial, party-like atmosphere. Others observed that they discussed serious topics such as death, dying, funerals and the afterlife in very intimate ways with people who were strangers but who happened to be sitting at their table for the night. It was clear to the hosts that the addition of the art-based activities, which does stray

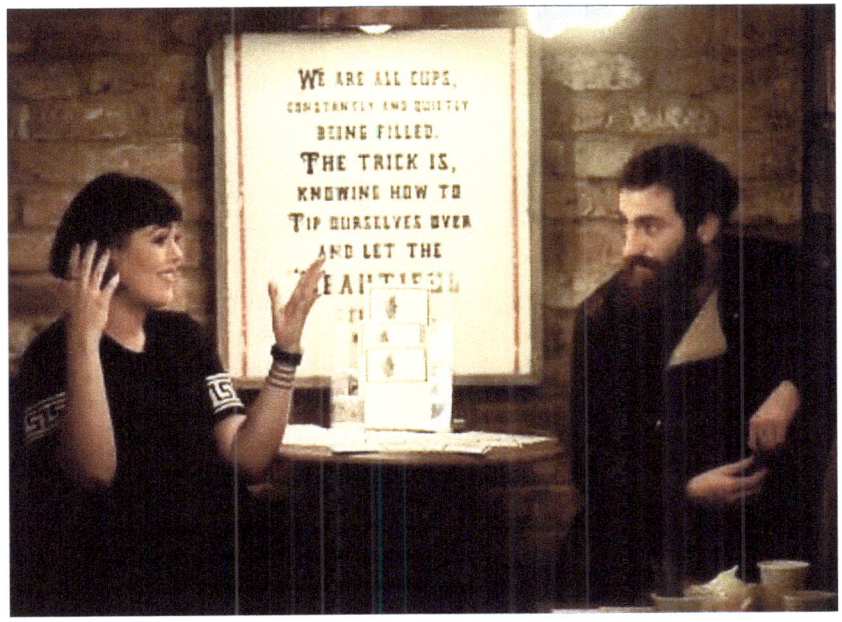

Figure 14. Artist Philip Desmond in conversation with a visitor, Death Café Limerick. Photography by Deirdre Power Photography and reproduced with permission.

outside of the traditional Death Café offering, helped foster a sense of connectedness among attendees and perhaps eased some of the anxiety or shyness that might have been present at the start of the event.

Of particular interest is the report of participants becoming clearer on what they wanted for their funeral or final disposition and how their attendance at the Death Café encouraged them to make these wishes known to their loved ones. One attendee commented, 'I've never spoken about anything like what I wanted for my funeral with my family because we avoid this kind of talk, but I'm going to have the conversation with them now.' This feedback underscores the project's belief in the power of the Death Café to act as a modern memento mori. The Death Café uses informal social conversation, relational exchange and creative practice, rather than a material object such as a skull or a painting, to remind us about how to live as well as how to die.

Death Café Limerick has flourished since its inaugural event in 2015; as of 2023, more than twenty-five cafés have been facilitated. After the inaugural event, the Death Cafés were principally run by Jennifer Moran Smith as part of her thanatology practice, in collaboration with Sinead Dinneen as a visual artist, until Dinneen's death in 2019. Each Death Café since 2019 respectfully pays tribute to Dinneen's work and legacy. These have also incorporated several virtual Cafés run during the Covid-19 lockdown era. The virtual Death Café events, hosted on Zoom, were a remarkable and sometimes challenging adaptation of the in-person occasions. Covid-19 ushered in an era in which people were hidden, not behind plague masks, but behind computer screens in order to maintain safety and lessen viral exposure while somehow maintaining a deeply sought human connection. The online Death Cafés were usually shorter (one hour as opposed to two) and attendance was strictly limited to twenty or fewer to allow for easier facilitation. However, the online version allowed participants from across the globe, including Morocco, California and Belgium, which brought unique perspectives and enlivened conversation to what had previously been a strictly Irish experience.

In the years since 2015, the Death Café Limerick group has facilitated events as part of the Limerick Lifelong Learning Festival, Science Foundation Ireland Week and as one of a suite of public gatherings from a newly formed support and advocacy coalition called the Limerick Bereavement Network. While cautious in being faithful to the guidelines that a Death Café is not a bereavement support group, Death Café Limerick sees it as part of a movement to increase death and grief literacy among the general public. Communities that know more about the processes of death and dying are able to discuss these topics freely and respectfully, and are able to recognise the effects of loss within themselves, while others will become more connected and resilient over time. Perhaps, we may even find ways to live more fully by appreciating the cool shadow of our own mortality. Death Cafés provide the material and context to improve both our death literacy and grief literacy (Breen et al. 2022, Laranjeira et al. 2022).

The extraordinary success of the Death Café Limerick project from its first iteration would seem to point to some key findings. In contemporary society, where the often painful and awkward conversations about death have been sanitised from the end-of-life experiences, Death Café Limerick has offered a safe space to explore these uncomfortable notions. That this experiment has flourished in Ireland is no accident; Irish death culture is a rich and historied one reaching back to the elaborate burials of Neolithic, Bronze Age and Celtic peoples of the ancient world, and incorporating a rich variety of wake customs and traditions (O'Suilleabhain 1967: 3). Death Café Limerick is one of the many ways in which we have visualised, discussed and contemplated our own mortality as a nation, while, uniquely, offering a modern living memento mori which is social rather than a static object.

Mark Fryers

# *Ghosts* (Nick Broomfield, 2006)

## Death and Displacement in Twenty-First-Century Culture

In the twenty-first century, the sea has increasingly stood as a touchstone for death. Images of displaced migrants crossing the seas in dangerous, overcrowded boats saturate the media and provide the visual tinderbox for polarised political discourses. The image of the drowned refugee boy on a Turkish beach, Aylan Kurdi, in 2015 is a vivid apocalyptic vision of late geopolitical capitalism.

These visual discourses have their double in twenty-first-century films – from the fantasy images of phantom ships and brine-encrusted shipmates raised from the depths of Davy Jones' locker in the *Pirates of the Caribbean* franchise to the sober realism of condemnatory documentaries such as *Seaspiracy*, the seas are heavily imbricated as a site of death. This chapter will reveal how these texts work to reveal the sea as a space in which the relentless onward grind of marine capitalism returns the conception of the sea to that of an earlier history, a time before the buccaneering age of Empire and romantic high-seas adventure, to a place of devilry. Nick Broomfield's 2006 film *Ghosts* – a film based on the tragedy of the death of Chinese migrant workers in Morecambe Bay in 2004 – will provide our window into this world. Shot in a documentary style, it fuses the two realms – fact and fiction in a film that demonstrates how seaborne immigration and marine capitalism perpetuate a dark history of nautical servitude.

*Ghosts* was written by Broomfield and Jez Lewis, but also based upon the work of journalist Hsiao-Hung Pai, who worked undercover as a transient worker. In February 2004, twenty-one illegally trafficked Chinese labourers from rural China died while cockling in Morecambe Bay, dangerously unaware of the tides and geography of the area. The workers had been smuggled in containers via the port of Liverpool by Chinese gangmasters (known as 'snakeheads'). The case raised the issue of modern slavery and the dark global movement of goods and people, and documentarian Nick Broomfield chose this as his first 'dramatic' feature and a way to make visible the hidden economy of modern Britain and the world.

The film is bookended by the tragedy itself, opening as the workers set about their duties in the hazy, increasing gloom of twilight in the mudflats, oblivious to the rapidly rising tide (see Figure 15). Water seeps insidiously, in an almost Gothic yet vérité style.

The film then switches to tell the story of how these unfortunate victims came to be there, tracing them back to rural China, where it follows a young single mother, Ai Quin (Ai Qin Lin, an illegal immigrant worker herself), who decides to pay the local warlords $25,000.00 to be smuggled into the United Kingdom to find work so that she can afford her son's upbringing. Herded into a van, she begins her long, cross-continental journey into Britain – via Kazakhstan, Romania and Serbia. The trail is marked on an extradiegetic

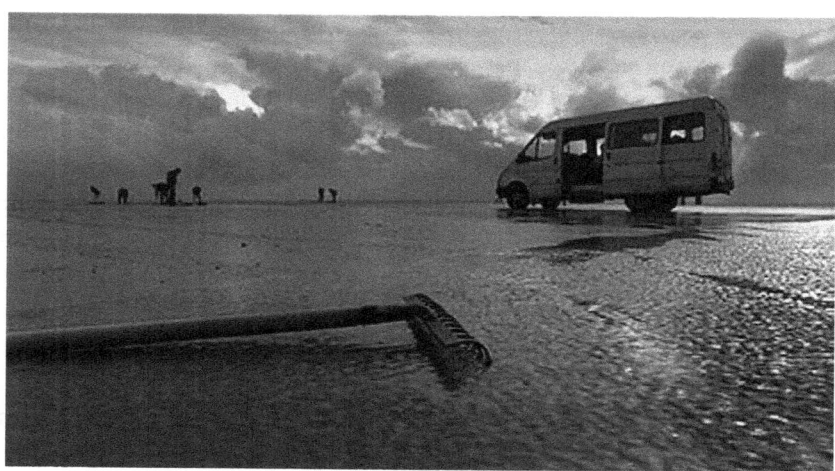

Figure 15. Seawater is insidious. *Ghosts*, directed by Mark Broomfield (Beyond Films 2006).

map, one that at the same time echoes and mocks the adventurous trajectory of cinematic heroes such as Indiana Jones. At Belgrade, they are herded into the back of a lorry, and at Calais, echoing a journey taken by many migrants up to that point, and traced to the present day, screwed into a secret lorry compartment and ferried across the English Channel. The ghostly echoes of the incident at Dover in June 2000, in which the bodies of fifty-eight Chinese migrants who died from asphyxiation or monoxide poisoning were found in the back of a Dutch lorry, offer a corporeal foreboding here.

This journey itself points to the history of sea crossings as those marked historically not only by the subaltern, most prominently the transatlantic slave trade, but also by ship crews as poor, downtrodden, shanghaied or press-ganged into service. Broomfield himself deliberately alluded to this in his motivation for making the film at the time that he did, which coincided with the celebrations for the 200th anniversary of the abolition of the slave trade (and the visible presence of the William Wilberforce biopic *Amazing Grace* (2007)).

In these dichotomies, hierarchies of poverty are invariably apparent. Similar themes and issues are explored in the documentary *Fire at Sea* (2016) and the fiction films *Mediterranea* (2015) and the British *True North* (2006), released the same year as *Ghosts*, which similarly deal with the death of Chinese migrants to Britain, this time in a rusting, cash-strapped Scottish fishing trawler – itself a symbol of British industrial decline. The hierarchy of poverty is based on a number of factors, but what is clear is that those closer to the bottom (literally, in sailing vessels) are the more desperate.

This is also clear in *Ghosts*. Arriving in Britain, Ai Quin continues her journey, in vans and buses and through rain-soaked, transient spaces – ghostly industrial wastelands. She ends up in a cramped house in Thetford, in an equally nondescript estate. It becomes clear that she still has to pay for a host of things before she can actually start earning – rent, fake work permits, bribes for the agency workers – despite working for long hours in various meat processing and vegetable-picking jobs, all the while resisting overtures for her to earn more money as a masseuse. Hierarchies prevail – the boss and his mistress run the rule over Ai Quin and the other workers in the house, while the mistress switches her allegiance to the brutish white landlord who owns the house and implores her to get fifteen people in it rather than twelve. She describes her fellow Chinese as peasants who are all spat at on the street by the white men – the 'ghosts' of the title, who are working class and poor but yet above them in ethnic rankings.

*Ghosts* describes death and horror, but it is not an outright horror film. *His House* (2020) may be described as closer to such, while having similarities with *Ghosts*. In this film, two Sudanese refugees find themselves in an equally gloomy and nondescript British housing estate, haunted by the losses they suffered on their journey across the channel and the difficult decisions they were forced to make. Their maritime passage becomes the loci for their fear – manifesting in visions of being dragged into the briny depths and other Gothic aquatic imagery, which is dramatically juxtaposed with the harsh emptiness and otherness of their new 'home' in England.

In *Ghosts*, decisions are everything and have a drastic impact on the protagonists. The decision is made to move north with the bountiful promise of working in the marine industry. Indeed, on arriving by the sea, a new optimism is fortuitously defined as Ai Quin spots a rainbow off of the coast. This, consciously or otherwise, also echoes British maritime history in that the image recalls the paintings of J. M. W. Turner, including his famous painting of the Zong slave ship (see Figure 16).

The Zong massacre, one of the darkest chapters in maritime history, took place in 1781, in which over 130 African slaves, insured as cargo, were thrown overboard to their deaths when drinking water ran low. When the insurers refused to pay, a legal case was brought to court, and debates raged as to whether it was legal to kill slaves in these instances and how humans shouldn't be classed as 'cargo'. It was a key point on the road to the abolition of slavery. Similarly, Samuel Plimsoll had campaigned for years to stop the exploitation of British seamen – especially against the practice of 'coffin ships' – whereby owners would deliberately overload unseaworthy vessels and let them sink with cargo and crew in order to claim on the insurance.

The syndicate that owned the Zong was from Liverpool, where the real-life Chinese immigrants had been trafficked to – suggesting that Broomfield's intention to show that little had actually changed since then, beneath the surface at least, was apposite. The costume drama *Belle* (2013) also deals with the Zong case but sets its intimate drama within the confines of the country estate and the stately courts and offices of law, much like *Amazing Grace*. Both deal covertly with death and maritime destruction but defiantly keep these

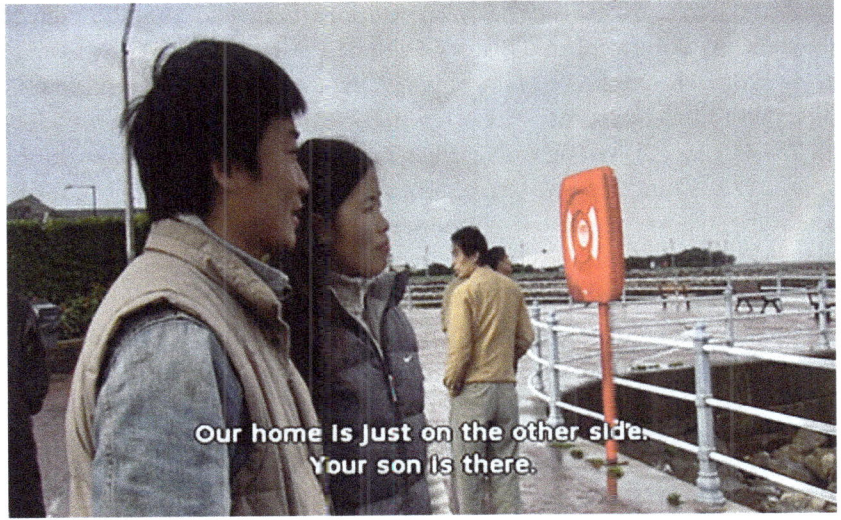

Figure 16. 'Hope, Hope, fallacious Hope'. *Ghosts*, directed by Mark Broomfield (Beyond Films 2006).

events off-screen, unlike Spielberg's earlier *Amistad* (1997) which combined the two. In all these instances, the maritime deaths of capitalist endeavour haunt the present.

These texts point to the dichotomy provoked by Walcott, who claimed, in his famous poem 'The Sea Is History' (1979), that cultural memory is shifting and fluid. Similarly, in *The Black Atlantic*, Paul Gilroy (1993) used the historic crossings of the slave ship across the Atlantic to speak of a 'double consciousness' in the identity of Africans. The diasporic identity is not defined by solid borders – a challenge to orthodox Western ideals of fixed boundaries and identity. In *Ghosts*, the Chinese workers are caught between these ideals: they use communal singing to boost their morale and to connect with their homeland while attempting to take advantage of global economic 'opportunities'.

The vast oceans, particularly their fathomless depths, have long been seen as bedevilled within Western culture. It is the place where Coleridge's Ancient Mariner experiences horrific visions and the passage by which the parasitic Count Dracula reaches the shores of Britain in Bram Stoker's novel.

Attendant to this, the sea has been positioned as a space that still 'conceals monsters', invoking a cultural history of human fears of beasts rising from the deep – from The Kraken to *Jaws* (1975). One can observe the resurgence of killer shark films in recent years – *Open Water* (2003), *The Shallows* (2016) and *The Meg* (2018) – along with a rise in Lovecraftian horror – *Dagon* (2001), *Cthulhu* (2007) and *Sacrifice* (2020) – in which humans are forced to confront their vestigial past; we came from the sea, and eventually the sea may reclaim us, as rising seas levels likewise threaten to do so.

In other texts, death and infection are wrought by the sea – *The Bay* (2012) and *The Beach House* (2019) – serving as much as revelatory or morality plays against the danger of pollution and environmental destruction as *Ghosts* does for blind capitalism. As Murphy further points out, media and political reporting on refugees often invoke these primal fears to dehumanise them: 'The amorphous mass emerging to the shore embodies cultural anxieties about sea beasts' (2018: 155). It is also notable that immigration tends to be personified in aquatic terms – floods, tides and waves.

*Ghosts* ends as it began. Having been beaten and ostracised by local cockle pickers, the workers are forced to go out late, at a time in which they know the locals will not be working. There is a symbolic relevance, particularly in a British context, to the fact that these final scenes take place on the beach and the sands – the liminal, shifting space between Britain and the sea. The seaside is a traditional embodiment of 'Britishness'; from the wealth and privilege of spa resorts patronised by royalty to affordable seaside holidays to rundown resorts in which migrants are housed in large numbers, they provide a vivid 'state of the nation' at any given time and are key cultural and political battlegrounds. The use of violence by British cockle pickers to protect their patch from foreign intrusion literally enacts Churchill's famous Second World War declaration that 'we shall fight them on the beaches' against the threat of foreign invasion as well as invokes Powell's famous 'Rivers of Blood' speech in which he insinuated that 'violence will be inevitable in the battle to retain British national identity in the face of a tidal wave of immigrants' (2018: 156).

There is also a tragic inevitability about this – they came by the sea, and they were lost to the sea – as all but Ai tragically drown as they are quickly overwhelmed by the rising tides or hyperthermia. This ending pertains to a tragic spectacle – a certain spectacle of maritime destruction that appears throughout twenty-first-century culture as the world grapples with climate crisis, extreme weather and rising sea levels. This became apparent in 'fin-de-siècle' blockbuster films such as *Waterworld* (1995), whilst the resounding success of *Titanic* (1997) reiterated the global cultural fascination with maritime disasters.

This maritime spectacle of destruction intensified in the following century, especially in disaster films which visualised the apocalyptic destruction of the earth by giant tidal waves, most evident in the Hollywood blockbuster *2012* (2009) and other global disaster films, such as *The Sinking of Japan* (2006), *Tidal Wave* (2009) or *The Wave* (2015). Other films dramatised the effects of actual tsunamis such as the one in the Indian Ocean in 2004 (*The Impossible* (2012)), maritime disasters (*Deepwater Horizon* (2016)) a plethora of shipwreck narratives (*Cast Away* (2000), *Life of Pi* (2012)) as well as biblical epics depicting a world engulfed by water (*Noah* (2014)). Even animation films depicting destructive maritime tempests – such as the dark, sentient seawater in the shape of Miyazaki's *Ponyo* (2008), a film that anticipated the Japanese Tsunami of 2011 – were also released.

Many of these examples deployed the use of new technologies available in the form of Digital, HD, IMAX and 3D film-making, intensifying the clarity of the spectacle of displacement and the spectatorial orientation towards it. These texts both literally and metaphorically bring us closer to the potentiality of death by sea.

Other films have focused on the human cost and interaction with destructive seawater in fantastical form, such as in *Beasts of the Southern Wild* (2012) or in Spike Lee's Katrina documentary *When the Levee Breaks: A Requiem in Four Acts* (2006). These films reiterate the point made in *Ghosts*, namely, that it is the poor and downtrodden who are often, if not always, worst affected by climate change and economic and political precarity; they are left to the mercy of the sea.

It is perhaps fitting that *Ghosts* straddles the intersection between documentary and fiction, given that the documentary form has provided a pronounced vision of death at sea in the new millennium. High-profile films such as *The Cove* (2009) and *Blackfish* (2013) have raised cultural discussions about marine animal cruelty. The recent Netflix documentary *Seaspiracy* (2021) went further by highlighting a globally interconnected industry that exploits humans and animals alike at every level, while it brutally wrecks and depletes the planet's delicate ecosystems. Increasingly, the sea has been deployed as a castigating mirror for the self-destructive nature of human existence: a site of bedevilment, but one of humanity's own making.

The *Independent*'s review of *Ghosts* observed that 'the horror leaks out of almost every frame' (Quinn 2007). The aquatic imagery is appropriate for a film about death. Alongside images of death occurring by the displaced and desperate, we are assailed by dead oceans – dying coral reefs, polluted seas as floating rubbish dumps as well as dead and damaged marine life. In the twenty-first century, the sea *is* death.

Kristy Strange

# *Geostorm* (Dean Devlin, 2017)

## Disaster Capitalism

The prominent fear of death that humanity faces in the modern era is not one of singularity, but a fear of the collective death of our species due to anthropogenic climate change. A turning point occurred in 1990 when the first Intergovernmental Panel on Climate Change (IPCC) report was published. The report concluded that the increase in global temperatures was due to anthropogenic activities and warned that this would lead to widespread changes in the climate system (Maslin 2021: 8). It seems only natural that climate change and its potential for apocalyptic disaster would become increasingly prevalent in popular culture of the twenty-first century, especially in visual mediums that turn a collective gaze onto sites of planetary catastrophe. This chapter argues that disaster films, such as *Geostorm* (2017), have developed over the years to explore both ecological and anthropogenic fears concerning humanity's extinction, specifically in the film's exploration of disaster capitalism as the literal weaponisation of the climate. Western society's view of death as a ruthless adversary to be feared and conquered is magnified through these fears of extinction, and thus the environment is depicted as a frightening foe that humans must either tame or destroy. In humanity's fight against nature, the complicated entanglement between humans and non-humans is further increased because an anthropocentric lens is applied to the climate. This method of anthropomorphising the non-human incites the viewer to recognise that 'the unpalatable fact persists: the reality of death may be repressed but remains utterly ineradicable' (Davison 2017: 3). Humanity's past and present actions and *inaction* are brought into stark focus through the eye of the storm – a haunting vision of all our futures, a vision of death.

Climate fiction narratives typically portray a world that has been drastically altered by climate change, where natural disasters are more frequent and severe, and humans – whether individuals, within a community or as a society – struggle to adapt. These stories are often set in the not-too-distant future, offering speculative imaginings of the potential consequences of our current actions – or inaction – and how we might respond to future environmental challenges. Disaster films are a type of climate fiction narrative that uses cinema to intentionally explore themes of climate change with dramatic environmental special effects – achieved by computer-generated imagery – paired with sustained high-action sequences. *Geostorm* sets up the climate crisis as central to the film's narrative with the opening voiceover of Hannah, a child, who explains,

> Everyone was warned, but no one listened. A rise in temperature, ocean patterns changed, and ice caps melted. They called it extreme weather. They didn't know what extreme was. In the year of 2019, hurricanes, tornadoes, floods, and droughts unleashed a wave of destruction upon our planet. We didn't just lose towns or beachfronts; we lost entire cities. The East River swallowed Lower Manhattan. A heatwave killed two million people in Madrid in just one day. But in that moment, facing our own extinction, it became clear that no single nation could solve this problem alone. The world came together as one, and we fought back. (Devlin 2017)

Instead of acknowledging responsibility and culpability in humanity's intrusive exploitation and subsequent destruction of the planet, the climate itself becomes the shared, fundamentally feared adversary – humanity's executioner. Simon Estok describes this fear in the theory of ecophobia, defined 'as an irrational and groundless hatred of the natural world' in which '[nature is imagined] as a menacing threat […] bent on vengeance' (2009: 208 and 2019: 41). Humanity's irreversible entanglement with nature and the subsequent increased threat of extinction forces a direct confrontation with death. Through its very existence, nature – with its mortal life cycles – reminds us that 'death is the most persistent and indifferent adversity faced by humanity' (Davison 2017: 2). The fear humanity expresses towards nature is a direct result of its potential to inflict death. Thus, 'the emotional response to the problem of extinction revolves around concerns about death' with 'feelings [that] stem from worries about the vulnerability of the human race' and the symbolisation of death as a 'frightening and terrifying […] end to birth' (Schell 2017: 107). It is not the act of dying that terrifies humanity, but rather the cultural 'concept that encompasses the questions and anxieties that arise due to the idea of mortality' (Koudounaris 2022: 18). Extinction is terrifying because the symbolic coping mechanisms of immortality – such as genetic legacy – that humans have acquired in the face of death become meaningless in the face of an extinct species (Schell 2017: 107). Katie Goh states that 'to watch the Earth collapse is to watch ourselves collapse, an annihilation that is unnatural and diabolical' (2021: 42). After all, death is natural, but extinction, especially accelerated extinction, is not. It is precisely this lack of control over death that makes nature one of the most prominent sources of fear for humanity in the twenty-first century.

In climate fiction, control is a central theme. Control is simultaneously claimed and challenged in these imagined narratives by the dissolution of boundaries between humans and non-humans, specifically through anthropomorphising the non-human. Anthropomorphism attempts to bring the planetary back into the limited realm of human understanding. The idea of nature being rooted in vengeance is an anthropocentric one. Climate change is not the planet's way of enacting vengeance against humanity but is an (eco) systematic consequence of humanity's actions; thus, dominant narratives tend to ignore this reality because of the way it shifts perspective from an anthropocentric view to a penetrating, non-human gaze. Disaster films, like *Geostorm*, anthropomorphise the non-human in applying human characteristics to the climate to enable an anthropocentric response. And so, humanity responds to the lack of control over severe weather events in the same way as a dangerous, wild animal does – through violent domestication or death.

This is observed in *Twister* (de Bont 1996) and *Geostorm* through the language used to describe tornados and a whole spectrum of severe weather events, respectively. In *Twister*, the Fujita scale is defined by how much it eats, while the East River in *Geostorm* swallows Lower Manhattan. Words such as these express the capabilities of environmental feeding, further perpetuating the idea of nature being a dangerous predator, hunting humanity for its survival. As a result, this anthropomorphism acts as justification for humanity to fight back against nature for survival both in literal and cultural terms;

dominant narratives, typical of the Global North, focus on fighting nature not only to avoid extinction but also to maintain the status quo. In *Twister*, the main characters 'punch the core' of the deadly tornado, and in *Geostorm*, all storms are neutralised by the literal entrapment of the planet in a net of satellites (see Figure 17).

There is a perpetual imbalance between humans and the climate that centres around humanity's dependency on the planet and the desire of the dominant Western societies to conquer nature. Subsequently, Western narratives that focus on the climate crisis frequently overlook the anthropogenic consequences at the heart of climate change, and so, in anthropomorphising the climate, storms do not have a heart but an *eye*. Amitav Ghosh argues that in climate fiction narratives 'a great deal hinges on the eye; seeing is one of their central themes; not seeing is another' (2016: 32). Through the visual medium of the disaster film, the audience is forced to turn back and look not only at the challenges posed by climate change but also at humanity's role in driving its acceleration. Eyes are commonly described as the windows of the soul, and so, in anthropomorphising storms in this way, humanity attempts to look not only itself in the eye but also seeks to understand the planet intimately (see Porter 2005). To lock gazes with the climate, the characters of disaster films must ultimately surrender to nature's power – to its potential for death. This is shown in *Twister* and the genre-defining film *The Day After*

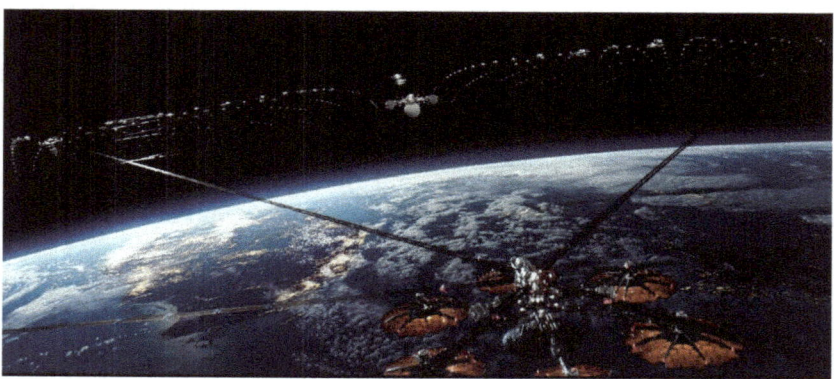

Figure 17. Dutch Boy's network of satellites. *Geostorm*, directed by Dean Devlin (Warner Bros, 2017).

*Tomorrow* (Emmerich 2004), in which characters find themselves directly in the eye of severe weather events and experience what Ghosh describes as a 'moment [that is] strangely like a species of visual contact or beholding and being beheld' (2016: 15). It is a moment where the characters are forced to observe not only the awesome, visible power of nature but also must face the hidden heart of humanity and reflect inwards, questioning what it means to be human.

Survival seems impossible in the eye of a storm in disaster films, but these characters do survive, and the moments of *beholding* rest at the climax of these narratives, highlighting this critical moment of the film in which nature engulfs the characters; human and non-human bodies merge into one. *Geostorm*'s simultaneous severe weather events act similarly through the threat of one planetary storm that makes it impossible to hide from the realities of the Anthropocene. The film unveils humanity as being on the cusp of an apocalypse, which in its true definition means 'a vision that reveals', and as argued by Goh, 'disasters [do lay] us – our identities, behaviours, and priorities – bare' (2021: 6). The threat of a Geostorm reveals toxic desires for domination, prioritising absolute control above all else. Dekkom (Ed Harris) claims, 'if you control the weather, you control the world', showing that it is not just the weather that he seeks to control but the entire planet to reshape it into his unique vision (Devlin 2017). The threat posed by climate change is not rooted in the environment but is exposed as dangerous due to humanity's attempt to tame, control and exploit the planet. Earth's fragile state is seen as an opportunity for Dekkom; thus, disaster becomes desirable to facilitate taking advantage of such an opportunity. As argued by Kolbert, 'our most dangerous weapon [proves] to be modernity and its trusty sidekick, late capitalism', which has mutated into something far more terrifying in the late twentieth and twenty-first centuries – disaster capitalism (2022: 13).

Significant dangers of disaster capitalism are revealed in the film through the exploitation of climate change. Svoboda highlights that disaster films underwent a drastic change when they explored 'the weaponization of climate/weather technology [...] [with] the risks being attached to alternative or clean energy technologies' and 'geoengineering schemes' (2016: 58). *Geostorm* explores the latter with both the invention and interference with Dutch Boy – the network of satellites controlling the climate. The infection of Dutch Boy with a computer virus is not only intentional but also seeks control over humanity rather than species annihilation. Amidst a fight between Jake Lawson (Gerard Butler) and the corrupt scientist, Duncan Taylor (Robert Sheehan), Lawson reasons, 'if you don't stop, there isn't going to be a planet to spend it on' – referring to the handsome sum promised for Taylor's betrayal; to which Taylor replies, 'please. We're going to keep all the best bits. Aren't you a little bit curious to watch the world burn?' (Devlin 2017). This admission of genocide for opportunist gain rests at the core of disaster capitalism. It is defined as a radical form of neoliberalism that views crises and disasters as an opportunity for capital gain through exploitation and the demolition of previous social and economic structures, thereby laying the foundation for new, extreme reforms. Death may lay at the eye of a storm, but in disaster capitalism, death is at its heart and 'becomes something shattering, menacing, and fearful' (Koudounaris 2022: 25). The strategic phenomenon aims for an absolute reshaping of a society, its population and, consequently, its culture. *Geostorm* takes the reality of disaster capitalism one step further by a politician explicitly evoking these 'natural' disasters, whereas the disaster capitalism of modern society is defined by the preparation of governments for disasters as opportunities to push drastic policy changes (Klein 2008: 6). This is achieved through the violent enforcement of radical policies that were previously politically impossible to implement within a society that was not undergoing collective shock. In the book *The Shock Doctrine*, Naomi Klein argues that American economist Milton Friedman's vision of a dominant ideology of 'unfettered capitalism' and a 'hypermobile global economy' was possible only with the execution of the shock doctrine, defined as a method of coercing drastic socioeconomic shock treatments on populations following episodes of crisis and subsequent shock (4). The rapidity in pushing these radical policies forward is essential because 'the speed, suddenness and scope of the economic shifts […] provoke psychological reactions in the public that facilitate the adjustment' (7). *Geostorm* permutates this idea via Dekkom's accelerations of disaster through a global, shared catastrophe, resulting in millions of deaths. Like the continuous building of severe weather events in the film, disaster capitalism is a never-ending cycle of crisis and exploitation. Disaster capitalism represents not only individual or collective death but also the death of culture. These disasters produce a collective state of shock in both individuals and the collective sociopolitical body that results in an exploitable interruption of place – a disorientation that is emphasised in *Geostorm* through Dekkom's admission of wanting to reshape the map of the world. The population that would formerly have fought fiercely against such impositions is thus ill-equipped both physically and emotionally to rally against the swift, compressed changes. Dekkom reveals these ambitions blatantly near the end of the film when he says, 'I've given you an opportunity, Mr President. You should take it [...] Tomorrow the sun will rise. All our enemies will be gone. Wiped away as if by the hand of God' (Devlin 2017). Thus, as argued by Svoboda, 'these end-of-the-world depictions of climate change reflect the limited and debilitated state of contemporary politics' by highlighting the corrupt desire for domination, refusal to change attitudes, and behaviours that only reinforce the status quo (2016: 53).

At its core, *Geostorm* is like most other disaster films in its neglect of the real challenges presented by climate change. The characters refuse to submit to a cultural death of present lifestyles, which includes the dismantling of dominant, exploitative economic and societal structures. As a result, the human population in *Geostorm* follow in the footsteps of its disaster film forefathers. Humanity 'show[s] no alteration or change in behaviour at the film's conclusion; characters either return to normalcy or must adapt to a "new normal", and there is no attempt to mitigate the causes of climate change' (Svoboda 2016: 47). The invention of Dutch Boy allows for humanity to continue its exploitation of planetary resources without any meaningful change to human behaviour. Dutch Boy is simply a net – meant to entrap and control, but like all nets, it can be broken.

At the end of the film, Dutch Boy self-terminates (see Figure 18), and the audience is left wondering whether the threat of natural severe weather returns to haunt humanity or whether Dutch Boy is patched up and rebuilt. Nevertheless, death remains ever present in the absence of certainty and knowledge of the ever-present potential for corruption. Maslin summarises the problem of tackling climate change by saying that 'out of all the systems that we are trying to model into the future, humanity is by far the most complicated and unpredictable' (2021: 50). In this era of the Anthropocene, humanity and nature are more directly entangled than ever before in history. The actions and inactions of humanity are directly leading to the acceleration of decreased planetary well-being and our species' extinction. Perhaps, we must look once again to *The Day After Tomorrow*, which claims, 'the basic rule of storms is that

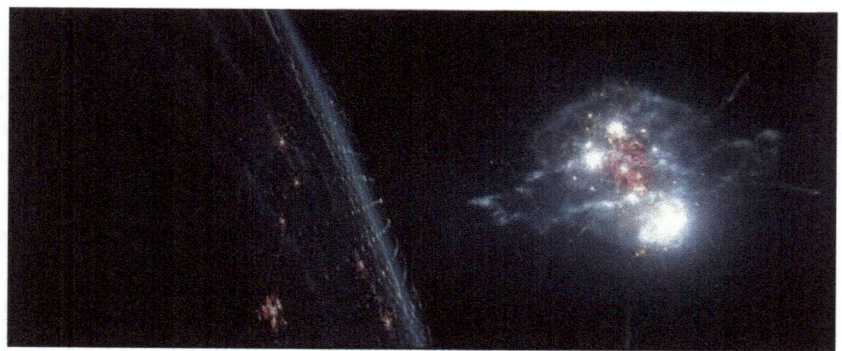

Figure 18. Dutch Boy self-destructs. *Geostorm*, directed by Dean Devlin (Warner Bros, 2017).

they continue until the imbalance that created them is corrected' (Emmerich 2004). Correction of this imbalance does not imply humanity's extinction, but rather an improvement of our way of existing within planetary boundaries for both human and non-human survival.

Ultimately, disaster films like *Geostorm* serve as a reflection of humanity's collective fears and anxieties about the future of the planet and the threat of death via human extinction. By anthropomorphising the non-human and portraying the environment as a foe to be conquered, these films perpetuate a problematic anthropocentric view of the world that fails to acknowledge the entanglement of humans and the impact of anthropogenic actions on the planet. However, disaster films do have great potential for emotive engagement with audiences. The visual medium of cinema can do something that textual fiction cannot – it makes the perceived invisibility of climate change visible. Disaster films have the potential to explicitly reveal truths about the anthropogenic causes and consequences of the Anthropocene, thus raising public awareness about the realities of the climate crisis. These films warn audiences that it is essential for individuals and societies to recognise the devastating consequences of climate change and strive towards a more sustainable and equitable future – one that embraces the complexity and interconnectedness of all life on Earth. As Hannah affirms in the closing scene of *Geostorm*, there is only 'one planet, one people. And as long as we remember that we share one future, we will survive' (Devlin 2017).

Ildikó Limpár

## *Mexican Gothic* (Silvia Moreno-Garcia, 2020)

With the growth of awareness to environmental and ecological crises in the past two decades, fungi have earned an important place in fiction and film narratives dramatising the danger that awaits humanity. These mycological fantasies grow from our fear of an unstoppable parasitism that may endanger the integrity of one's body – whether that body is that of a human or, figuratively speaking, the body of the world we live in: our close environment or even our ecosystem. When William Hope Hodgson in 1907 wrote what is considered to be the 'starting point for fungoid fiction', 'The Voice in the Night' (Quigley 2016), he already linked fungoid horror to an incomprehensible power that may have the capacity to overtake not only one human body but also humanity. Such a destructive, alien power is even more palpable in Lovecraft's version of fungoid horror, 'The Whisperer in Darkness' (1930), where a human body is revealed to have secretly been replaced by an 'automaton which becomes combined with such biological monstrosities as "cormophytic fungi" and 'toad-like" creatures' (Hegyi 2019: 40). In more recent years, fungi have spectacularly spread in the field of ecohorror, presenting us with the fantastic yet often dreadful image of the mutating world that alters and/or endangers the lives of those who live in it. Such visions are given, for instance, in Jeff VanderMeer's *Flinch* (2009) or in post-apocalyptic narratives such as M. R. Carey's *The Girl with All the Gifts* (2014) and *The Boy on the Bridge* (2017), as well as William Meikle's *Fungoid* (2019).

As much as Silvia Moreno-Garcia's *Mexican Gothic* may stem from this renewed interest in the possibly dangerous fungus world, it also heavily relies on fungi's role in Mexican culture and the Gothic tradition that has a special interest in the domestic, typically featuring, therefore, an emblematic (and possibly haunted) house and an oppressed female protagonist in a patriarchal world, and often working with the theme of insanity and unnatural relations. While the novel seems to divert from the now very popular ecofictional trend, it still utilises the most recent scientific research on fungus, especially on mycological communication, to make a point about social matters – and, in general, about humanity by posing ontological questions concerning human existence shaped by other life-forms and its relation to death. In the narrative, the posthuman existence that determines all lives around it is understood as a divine presence by its close circle of admirers – and a death-trap by those who would defy the fungus' consuming power. This fungoid death-god is the centre of the house and provides the key to the metaphorical house of oppression that Moreno-Garcia built with fictive bricks and fungus.

This unique version of fungoid fiction takes us back in time, to the 1950s, to question the social constructs of race and gender that are crucial issues of the present but are amplified by the historical setting. The story begins in Mexico City, but soon the protagonist, Noemí Taboada, moves out of her convenient environment and finds herself in the country, where she visits her cousin Catalina to check on her. What sets the action – and Noemí herself – in motion is Catalina's letter, in which the hastily married young lady complains about the place she lives in now: her husband's supposedly haunted family mansion, High Place. When Noemí visits her, she realises that the house has an unnatural power over its inhabitants, which prevents her from leaving it and free Catalina from the strange wedlock. The situation that the two women are in identifies High Place with the uncanny, which 'would always be an area in which a person was unsure of his way around'; it is 'an eerie place', a '*locus sus-pectus*' or suspicious place, 'haunted' (Freud 2003: 125), and puts it into a realm associated with death.[1] As uncanny is 'everything that was intended to remain secret, hidden away, and has come into the open' (Schelling qtd by Freud 2003: 148), the strange 'behaviour' of the house indicates the family secret that resulted in the transformation of the building and its close environs – especially the underground area that still hides and keeps the source of the family mystery hidden.

1   Cf. 'To many people the acme of the uncanny is represented by anything to do with death, dead bodies, revenants, spirits and ghosts' (Freud 2003: 148).

At the heart of the mystery lies – literally – the patriarch of the Doyle family, Howard Doyle, who is depicted as a living dead entity, a breathing 'corpse, afflicted by the ravages of putrefaction' (Moreno-Garcia 2020: 203). He is on the verge of dying – and being reborn. His fantastic symbiosis with the special fungus that grants him eternal life as long as he manages to regenerate in a new, proper body that is capable of fungal coexistence makes him a god in the eyes of his family members. Longevity, however, is connected to the multiplicity of deaths. It takes the life of the person in whose body the patriarch needs to reincarnate; moreover, it renders the lives of all other family members insignificant and useless beyond their function to support the renewal of this life circle. The fungus gives one person the opportunity to live practically forever; but for most other people, it means death: those who come in contact with the mushroom and are not of the Doyle bloodline either die or are driven mad (212), while the family members serve their god as zombies serve their master, and do end up in a metaphorical zombiehood, as they give up their own lives to maintain a falsely interpreted family privilege attributed to their pater familias' ability to continue living.

The method of maintaining this fungus-human entity not only accentuates many a Gothic trope but also 'adds a more politically inflected horror, both ancient and timely: A racist will to power' (Patrick 2020: 148), which is inseparable from history and produces physical and mental decay. Or, perhaps more precisely, it is inseparable from a burdensome history, and therefore it keeps producing physical and mental decay. The Doyles' power to heal and to transcend death stems from the buried past, the past that should not be unearthed, or, in Freudian terms, the past that is 'intended to remain secret' (148): the unfortunate fate of the miners who ensured the fortunes of the Doyle dynasty and died as a result of encountering the strange fungal lifeform which now 'runs under the house, all the way to the cemetery and back. It's in the walls' (Moreno-Garcia 2020: 211). As a result of the miners' buried bodies – especially those of the Mexican workers, who were simply put into a mass grave – overgrown by mushrooms, the house is directly linked to the graveyard by the fungus, underlining the connection between the house – the dynasty – and death, which will come to a full visualisation at the end, with the fall of the house of Doyle.

The house maintains the power of the Doyles as it ensures a perfect place for the spread of the fungus, and by doing so, it becomes the storage place of family history, creating the 'gloom', which holds the dynasty's thoughts and memories to which members of the family have access (211). The strange hybridising power makes the link to the past vivid and keeps the live members of the family captive in the building. It is to heal the injured and to ensure longevity – yet it is a sick attachment to the past, as we are incessantly reminded: the walls are permeated by the moss, causing hallucinations and utter dread to Noemí. There is a disturbing correspondence between the status of the house and that of Howard Doyle's sick body: High Place 'is sick with rot, stinks of decay, brims with every single evil and cruel sentiment' (7), as we learn from Catalina's letter. While the patriarch is expected to die and to regenerate any time, first he must go through a long suffering; hence, the walls echo his moaning, and all we see of him is the sick and transforming, ulcerous body that needs tending day and night, which is exhausting the family and ceaselessly draining their energy.

In her depictions of the Doyle family, Moreno-Garcia alludes to the Dracula-narrative to contextualise Noemí's experiences with the help of a well-known mythology of the undead. The hypnotising power of the house that keeps its inhabitants as servants of the master or Doyle's unquestionable power that does not allow the household to get any rest and drains their energies are such subtly hinted components, which gain more significance in their suggestions after we are informed that 'the old man even brought earth from England to ensure the conditions here would be like the ones in our motherland' (Moreno-Garcia 2020: 237) – an act clearly reminiscent of Dracula's transporting soil from Transylvania in several coffins to assure his undisturbed rest in a foreign land. This motif conspicuously cements our view of the patriarch as a coloniser, who, similarly to Stoker's vampire, travels abroad to exploit a new land (see Arata 1990, Bundrick 2014, McKee 2002).

In *Dracula*, the theme of colonisation is symbolically presented by the act of taking the bodies of the land; the penetrating fang is to be read as the equivalent of the sexual conquering of the victim,[2] which transforms the body,

---

2   The vampire bite has been read as a metaphorical representation of sexual intercourse since Christopher Bentley's 1972 article on *Dracula*. For further details, see Limpár (2021: 17).

so to say assimilating it to its predator. In a similar vein, Howard Doyle is both a sexual threat and a colonising power. He takes the land literally: he builds his economy on exhausting his environment's natural resources, and so his metaphorical fang bites deeply into the land when he establishes his mines. He also takes the bodies of the land in a Dracula style, and his victims are chosen based on the already existing similarities they share with their predator – the ability to live in symbiosis with the fungus. Using such suitable women for breeding assures the bloodline and with that the assumed superiority of the family, which justifies for them the act of colonisation: taking the land to accumulate wealth and taking the women against their wills to assure the everlasting life for the male predator. As a result, 'the persistent dehumanization and the view of people as simply bodies – to work in the mine, to produce heirs for the family – is one of the greatest horrors in the bock' (Nitchi 2021). The practice of dehumanisation is associated with death in both cases: the workers end up in graves due to infection they get while mining, whereas the women are sacrificed to ensure viable offsprings – new bodies for Howard Doyle. Agnes' — Howard's first wife — fate clearly communicates the idea that, for women, marriage is a frightening and dangerous business in the Mexico of the 1950s: entering the house means becoming a prisoner of the house – becoming one with the house, having lost integrity. Marriage thus 'threatens to be a premature burial' (Corrigan 2020).

The unnatural co-habitation with the past does not allow real progress for the Doyles' mentality: the gloom may not be used by them as a hive-mind prompting moral, emotional or intellectual growth; instead, it keeps the family stuck in time, which also manifests in Howard Doyle's eugenicist and patriarchal views that are in sharp contrast to Noemí's modernism. It is only the body that may renew for the pater familias; his mind, however, remains the same, which dooms him to fail eventually, as he underestimates Noemí's abilities to resist his power. One may even claim that he also underestimates Agnes' power to communicate with Noemí beyond death via the fungus, so Doyle's racism and misogyny definitely contributes to his downfall. From another perspective, it is the past itself – the hive-mind, the collective past of the family kept alive by the fungus – that allows vengeance and shows the power of female solidarity connecting generations. This supernatural bond between the two women culminates when Noemí burns down the house and thereby not only takes revenge on the Doyles but also ends the suffering of what has remained of Agnes, who helped her with the visions she sent to Noemí.[3]

In most interviews and reviews, the classics of Gothic fiction and horror are listed as obvious inspirations and influences (Quintana 2021, Patrick 2020, Corrigan 2020, Nitchi 2021, Memmott 2020, Miller 2020); yet Moreno-Garcia's artful method of presenting the sick attachment to the past, which will bring the downfall of people who are affected by it, evoke one of the dominating themes in the fiction of the American South. The necrophiliac union of Miss Emily and Homer Baron in William Faulkner's short story 'A Rose for Emily' is echoed in *Mexican Gothic*: the detachment from and the incompatibility with the present, the insanity, the privilege rooted in a bygone era are all important themes in both works; but while in Faulkner's story it is the Northerner and the worker who is the despised party of the relationship and is not given more respect than to a rat (for which the poison Emily bought is supposedly given) and ends up as a used body in an unwanted relationship (darkly, after his death), in *Mexican Gothic* it is the woman who is regularly oppressed by the patriarchy of the Doyles and is forced to give her body for service – which, as a result of the coexistence with the fungus, lasts beyond death, as well.

In the novel, this defective relationship with the past, which keeps devouring the future (i.e. the next generation that offer their bodies to host the pater familias or serve in any other way) is perfectly illustrated with the ubiquitous presence of the family symbol, the ouroboros. This mythological creature is an emblem of 'an eternal cycle of destruction and re-creation' ('Ouroboros'), which aptly describes the fungus–Doyle hybrid entity and its aspiration for an everlasting life. Its form, the serpent biting its own tale, is a closed circle that 'can also signal a closed family – or a self-limiting gene pool' (Patrick 2020), a kind of isolation from the rest of the world that allows the patriarch to be seen as a non-human entity – a death figure, who is a god to few and a

3   This motif clearly echoes the theme of female solidarity linked with the notion of liberation in Charlotte Perkins Gilman's 'The Yellow Wallpaper', in which 'the narrator identifies with the woman she sees within it, and the symbol of her imprisonment is twisted into a symbol of liberation' as the wallpaper provides her with a vision beyond mundane reality, something that is of 'diagnostic' power, as Vivian Delchamps claims (2020: 117).

subhuman life-form to Noemí, who sees in Howard Doyle a living dead, who may have the remains of a human body but has lost its humanity: the ability to have human emotions, empathy and care. Instead of being human, Howard Doyle is death itself because he is just white supremacy in a rotting flesh; he is the disintegrating embodiment of the 'false narrative' that 'whiteness makes you better and that you have to oppress the other' (Moreno-Gracia qtd in Quintana 2021) and, therefore, it is doomed to die and decay.

Part IV

# Extremism: Partisanship and Identity Politics

# Image Intervention V: Skull 4

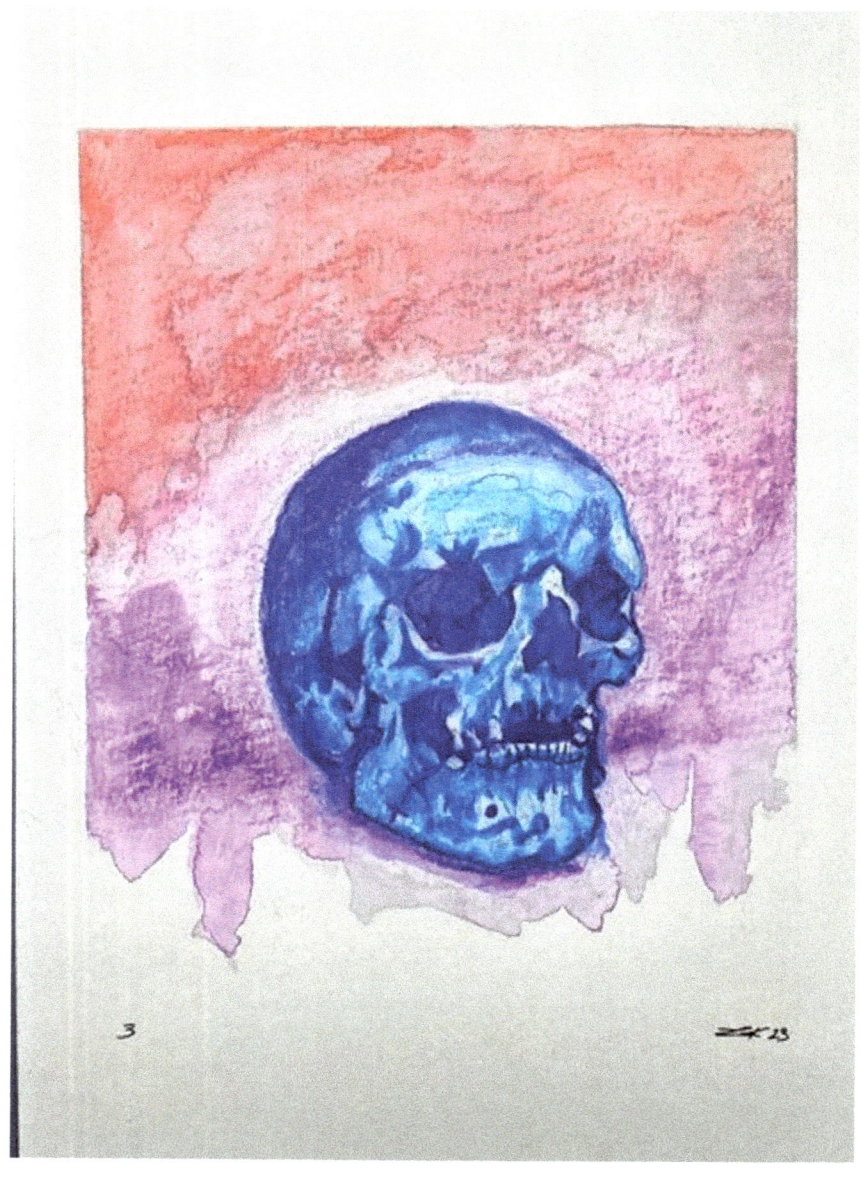

Artwork by Laura R. Kremmel
(Reproduced with the permission of the artist)

James T. McCrea

# The Unite the Right Rally and Its Aftermath (2017–20)

In the arena of post-millennial visual culture, it is easy to overreact to images that have the potential for multiple interpretations despite any perceived sense of neutrality associated with them. A recent, widely publicised instance saw conservative content creators portraying presidential candidate Donald Trump in the likeness of Matt Furie's webcomic character 'Pepe the Frog' during the tumultuous US presidential elections of 2016. Hillary Clinton, opposing Trump as the Democratic Party's presidential nominee, denounced Pepe as a right-wing mascot, proclaiming 'that [the] cartoon frog is more sinister than you might realize' (Robertson 2016). The Anti-Defamation League swiftly declared Pepe a hate symbol, prompting Furie to officially kill the character in dismay at what his creation had become (Manning 2017). Perhaps more so than Pepe, the skeleton is an ideologically vacant image that permeates visual culture, easily allowing the transmission of hidden meaning into the public eye. Scholars often summarise skeletal imagery as memento mori – a signal to remember one's own mortality with starkly moral implications (see Kerrigan 2017, Pickover 2015). Although many skeletal images warrant such a generalised interpretation, they may also contain vital information that can be overlooked by glib readings. For instance, the image of a skull embroidered on someone's jacket may or may not be 'just a skull', but could tacitly signify very specific political affiliations. As such, the cultural ubiquity of skeletons easily allows political significance to go unnoticed. This essay examines the skull as a potential signifier in the highly polemic arena of post-millennial visual culture, using case studies focusing on historical iconography, consumer products and internet memes.

A noteworthy case study centres on a skull logo seen on the helmet of Daniel Borden during the Unite the Right protest that took place in Charlottesville, Virginia, in August 2017. Organised by multiple white nationalist movements ranging from Neo-Nazis, the Ku-Klux Klan and Blue Lives Matter protestors acting in direct opposition to the Black Lives Matter movement, the Unite the Right rally was a high-profile instance of violent demonstrations that further defined the tumultuous political arena of the post-millennial United States (Stapley 2017). Tensions escalated wildly, resulting in over thirty injuries and the death of Heather Heyer, who was killed by self-described Neo-Nazi James Fields Jr as he deliberately drove through a crowd of leftist counter-protesters (Ingber 2019). Among the skirmishes, footage of four white men assaulting a young African American man named DeAndre Harris rippled throughout social media, resulting in the swift identification of Borden among the attacking mob (Emmons 2017). Borden's visibility was heightened via his white construction helmet emblazoned with the words 'commie killer' above a distinctive black skull logo known as the *Totenkopf* (see Figure 19). During Borden's subsequent trial, his father maintained that Borden did nothing wrong, asserting that the hardhat was an homage to the film *Full Metal Jacket*, wherein Matthew Modine's character Private Joker wears a US Marine Corps helmet bearing the phrase 'born to kill' (Baars 2019). Any polemic significance of Borden's *Totenkopf* seemed to vanish during this attempt to neutralise the presence of reactionary imagery in the courtroom. This would be of little consequence if the skull in question was anything but a very specific design with equally specific ties to Nazi-era Germany. The ease with which Borden's adoption of a historically established fascist symbol went unchallenged is an example of murky post-millennial semiotics wherein the purported neutrality of images begs certain questions arising from their usage – in this case, 'when is a skull just a skull?'

Before considering the skull's potential significance, it is important to note that skulls are also very real signifiers of human death. The human skeleton is a person's last remaining material component persisting after bodily decomposition takes place. Skulls in particular have received a great deal of scientific attention in terms of measuring a person's identity, both in terms of ethnicity and intellect with varying levels of accuracy. For instance, Steven Byers describes the facial bones of white, Black and Asian Americans with generalised

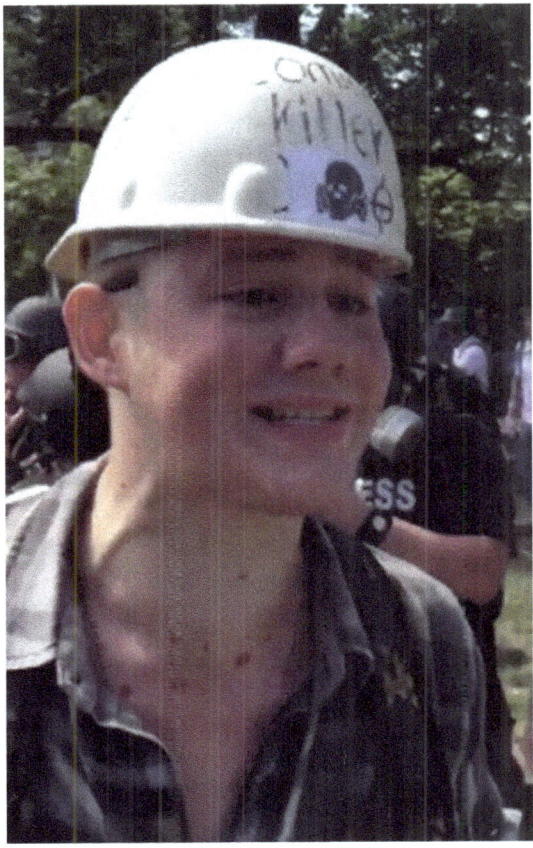

Figure 19. Daniel P. Borden taunts counter-protesters at the Unite the Right Rally while wearing a helmet bearing the Nazi *Totenkopf* (via Shaun King).

characteristics denoting each ethnicity (2016: 152–66). In doing so, Byers provides a guideline for forensic officers to help determine the possible identity of human remains in the absence of any other identifying information. However, the same attempt to categorise ethnicity through skeletal observation occurs under the pretence of racial profiling. In the early twentieth century, L. A. Vaught claimed that a person's intelligence can be assessed by grading the slope of their face through a practice called phrenology. Although long condemned as a pseudo-science, this same study recurs in the present day through the work of Richard Lynn, who likens brain weight to intellect with controversial results, such as claiming that women have an inherently inferior IQ than men, as well as attributing the intelligence of African Americans to their co-mingling with Caucasians in comparison to that of Sub-Saharan Africans, whom Lynn considers to be inherently less intelligent (2019). Although Lynn's claims are consistently impugned by scientists (see Kamin 1995 and Skeem 2002), his viewpoints proliferate among white nationalists, as demonstrated by internet message board discussions attempting to classify non-white ethnicities as sub-human based on differing bone structure (see Free-Thinker 2019).

Justifications of racial prejudices using such generalisations and measurements closely align with Michel Foucault's concept of biopolitics, wherein scientific and political data correlate to establish a measurable semblance of normalcy in any given society, which can be weaponised against those who exist beyond that semblance of normalcy (2004: 245). Essentially, power structures appeal to a certain level of generality by implementing regulatory mechanisms to maintain it. Anything beyond the norm is considered abnormal – if not pathogenic – and thus warrants special treatment in order to maintain the status quo (246). In this case, the theories proposed by Vaught and Lynn effectively normalise the white male skull. Anything different is considered inferior, if not aberrant. Consequently, if an entire race of people could be officially designated as a 'sub-species' because of differing physiological measurements, those affected by the terminological shift may find themselves subject to entirely new legalities of control, terminating the agency of the individual in the process. To this end, phrenology has been directly responsible for the inhumane treatment of Native American, African and Asian communities throughout early American history (see Fabian 2010). Consequently, skeletal measurements are capable of approximating a sense of empiricism to subjective ideas, allowing personal agenda to masquerade as scientific inquiry (Branson 2017: 164).

Considering the agency of human skulls in the discourse of white supremacy, one can begin tracing the history of the *Totenkopf*. Skeletal imagery was largely absent from the canon of Western European art prior to Medieval Christendom, at which point depictions of Christ's crucifixion would often contain a skull in the grounds of Golgotha. Its placement was based on a

Biblical passage stating that 'for as in Adam all die, so in Christ all will be made alive' (1 Corinthians 15:22), prompting artists and theologians to place Adam's skull at the scene of the crucifixion in order to mark the burial place of primeval man, which asserted a shared metaphysical lineage between Christ and humanity (see Montesano 2013). A compelling example is found in the fourth-century Syriac tome *The Book of the Cave of Treasures*, wherein Adam demands his body be taken to the place where Christ will be crucified in the future, designating the area as a place where his descendants will be redeemed from original sin (Montesano 2013: 16). The skull becomes aligned with salvation at Christ's feet, thus becoming an emblem of righteousness through divine ancestry in the context of Western Christian art.

When the skull began circulating as a symbol emblazoned upon the badges of Prussian militants during the War of Austrian Succession in 1740, it endured in a uniform representation throughout the tumultuous history of Prussia well into its transition to the Weimar Republic and eventually Germany (Nash 1972: 84–5). Originally intended to be an icon of Prussian unity, the *Totenkopf* assumed dire significance under the Nazi influence when Heinrich Himmler issued the following statement along with rings ornamented with the distinctive skull alongside Germanic runes:

> A sign of loyalty to the Führer, our unchangeable obedience to our superiors, and our unwavering solidarity and camaraderie. The skull is a reminder to always be ready to deploy your life for that of the whole community. The runes at the other end of the skull are a symbol of salvation from our past, with which we remain connected through the perspective of National Socialism. (Longerich 2010: 298)

At this point, the Nazis effectively assimilate the skull's divine Christian ancestry into their own political ideology using a strong ethos of German nationalism. Following its adoption by the German Nazi Party in 1923, the *Totenkopf* bears a design almost entirely unchanged to this very day. That it maintained a static image for nearly a century signifies the relevance of a very specific meaning coded into the image itself. Himmler's *Totenkopf* visually assimilated the iconography of unity and righteousness, thus linking both Adam and Christ to Adolph Hitler through mass production and the retention of a Nazi ideology as an ultimate form of social conservatism. As such, the skull on Borden's helmet acts as a temporal invader, dogmatically traversing an entire century to communicate a creed that remains just as unchanged as its own image. Crowned with the same *Totenkopf* that emblazoned the uniforms of Nazi militants, Borden symbolically resurrected the hateful regime while he assaulted Harris.

Having established the polemic gravity of the skull as an unchanging icon purporting a distinctly Christian lineage, the question remains as to whether skulls inherently signify virtue through divine heritage. Despite their close association with death and dying, skulls seem to act with a certain neutrality in the realm of commodity when they appear on politically unbiased products like t-shirts, automobile parts and even an entire brand of earphones named Skullcandy, which bears a distinctive skeletal logo. Skeletons often appear in publicity designs for music ranging from goth to metal to hip-hop, and they have consistently appeared in the visual branding for the Vans clothing line. The omnipresence of the skeleton in visual culture unintentionally creates a commercial ubiquity that tacitly allows the *Totenkopf* to enter the realm of commodity unchecked, demonstrated by the profusion of embroidered patches linking the skull to authoritarian credence. Consequently, the *Totenkopf* shares space with pre-existing skull iconography with the potential to become politically neutralised by association. For instance, Marvel Comics' iconic 'Punisher' logo easily becomes a symbol for the pro-police countermovement Blue Lives Matter despite the titular character's emphatic enmity towards law enforcement. As a commodity, the Punisher skull evokes no inherent authoritarian agency. However, its prominence in far-right polemics links it to the same militant ethos of the Nazi *Totenkopf* simply by sharing space in public events like the Unite the Right Rally.

As such, context determines the agency of the image. For instance, the skeletal artwork of rapper Dr Octagon evokes an active, human-like presence compared to those used by the neo-folk group Death in June, whose logo is nearly identical to the *Totenkopf*. Such dichotomies between the animated skeleton and the static skull have existed since the Middle Ages (see Caciola 2016) but gained lasting iconographical value through Hans Holbein's *Dance of Death*, which features skeletons participating in everyday activities alongside the living. As such, the animated, 'living' skeleton acting as a human often indicates crucial concerns for human existence. In contrast, the lone 'dead' skull generally reveals fixations with the past. For instance, illustrator Thomas Rowlandson and writer William Combe revived the animated skeleton in

*The English Dance of Death* (1815) as a conceptual revision of Holbein's work updated to match the anxieties of a nineteenth-century audience. Indeed, the dead continue dancing well into the twenty-first century in the form of internet memes, notably demonstrated by DaShareZone's sardonic contemplations about the human condition (2018) (see Figure 20). Poised over a sunset landscape, the skeleton overlooks the serene vista while an internal voice contemplates 'Is the human condition real? Is it contagious?'

Although humorous in nature, the entertaining guise of memes allows them to act satirically, effectively countering any opposing messages. This results in a contemporary political conflict engaged almost entirely through imagery. Although the efficacy of right-leaning symbols lies in their capacity to enter the public eye relatively unchallenged, leftist memes communicate overtly despite their comedic presentation to garner attention. Recent entries in media studies posit how internet memes are a perfect format for leftist

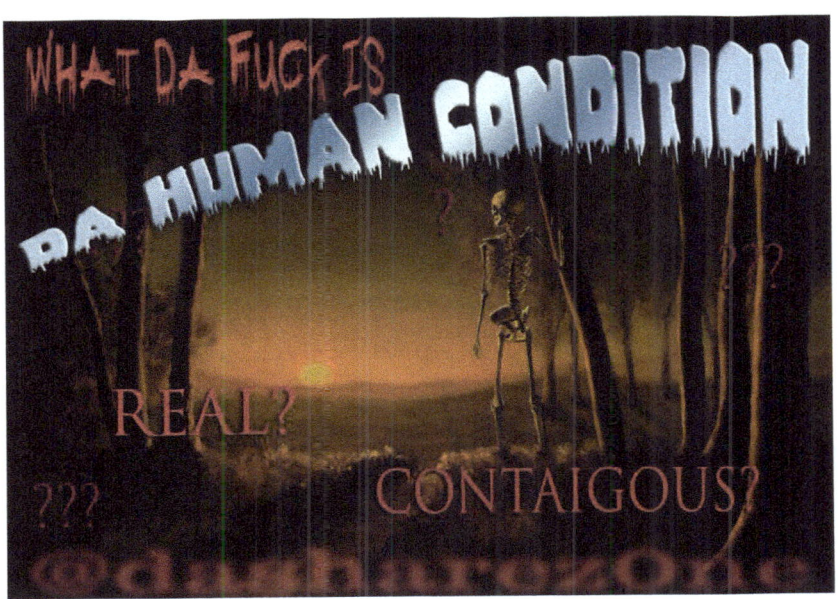

Figure 20. A skeleton conflates the human condition with a medical condition (image courtesy of DaShareZone).

satire, as they can effectively communicate populist ideas without facing conventional forms of censorship:

> Particularly within authoritarian regimes across the globe, political satire has been conceptualised as giving a voice to the powerless and enabling various forms of political protest. As a more or less subtle form of art, political satire has the power to criticise aspects of the political establishment by concealing its actual political purpose ... By providing counter-narratives and counter-discourses to dominant political narratives conveyed by the allegedly 'mainstream' media, satirical content, especially memes and parody sites on the web and in social media, are regarded as subversive measures of fighting suppressive regimes that seek to silence their citizens. (Wagner and Schwarzenegger 2020: 316)

Mirroring the lively corpses of Holbein and Rowlandson, DaShareZone uses the skeleton to question existing social norms with a dash of self-deprecating humour revealed by intentional misspellings and other assorted absurdist malapropisms (see Figure 21). Via the skeleton, humanity effectively sheds

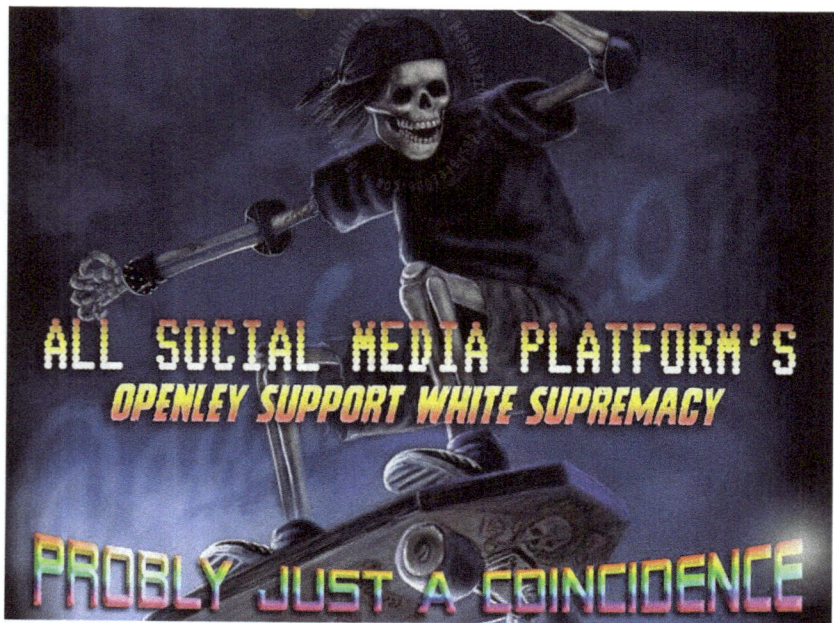

Figure 21. A skateboarding skeleton questions the allegiance of social media outlets, inferring the tendency to uphold white nationalism (DaShareZone).

its living tissue along with the bindings of social conservatism. In fact, DaShareZone communicates this so strongly that they even question the nature of their own medium in a meme wherein a skeleton claims, 'All social media platforms openly support white supremacy … probably just a coincidence' (2018).

Evidently, the surge of leftist memes using the skeleton seems to be a natural resistance to the heightened cultural visibility of far-right skulls in the wake of the Unite the Right Rally. For instance, the aforementioned adoption of Marvel Comics' Punisher skull by Blue Lives Matter spurred the character's co-creator Gerry Conway to reclaim the original skull logo as a symbol for Black Lives Matter (see Figure 22). Conway decries the skull's usage by extremist

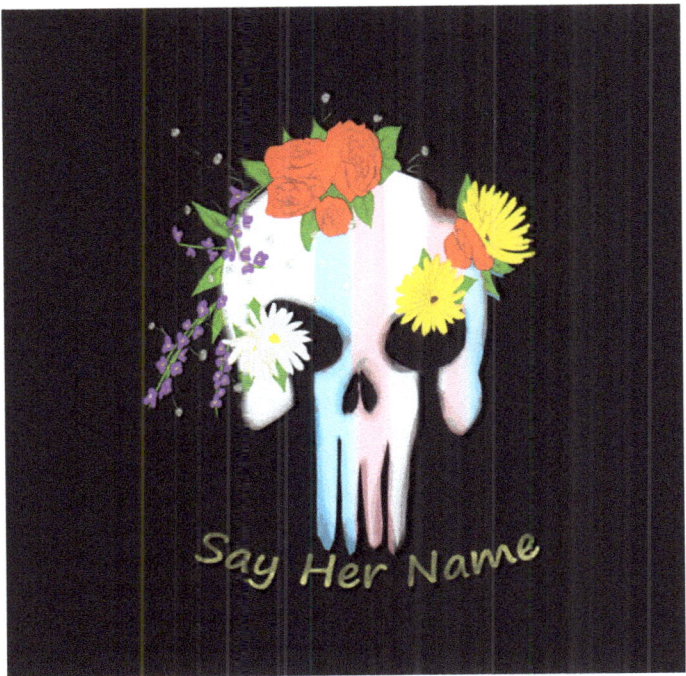

Figure 22. Sam Ines' alteration of Gerry Conway's Punisher skull links the symbol to social justice by commemorating LGBT+ activist Marsha P. Johnson (twitter.com/ArtistAuri, 2020).

right-wing groups as gross misappropriation, touting the Punisher as an early criticism of systemic violence against marginalised groups (Shedeen 2020).

Although this does not prevent authoritarian groups from using the image, it certainly demonstrates an ongoing clash between the farthest opposing poles of US polemics enacted almost entirely through visual culture. Ultimately, the skeleton is a blank slate equally receptive to the ideologies of widely disparate political spectrums, occupying the tombs of Catholic saints and mosh pits with equal validity. Confronting the skeleton is akin to confronting the human experience with all its myriad values and individualised variances. Its true nature lies in the individual who brandishes it.

Nicola Young

# *The Purge* Series (Various, 2012–21)

## Extremism Never Dies

Death has been personified in myth and culture since at least the Middle Ages (Noyes 2008: 35). This chapter considers the manifestation of Death of the Christian apocalypse in *The Purge* series of films. As will be seen, the series utilises a motif of Death as the 'Horseman of the Apocalypse' in service of its conceptualisation of far-right apocalypticism across the series, which depicts a United States in which complete financial collapse prompted the election of the authoritarian New Founding Fathers of America (NFFA) in 2014. Three years later, still facing substantial government debt, the NFFA implemented the Purge, twelve hours during which all crime is legal, suggesting that this would offer catharsis to citizens and stabilise society. Whilst the Purge does reduce crime, this is largely due to the elimination of poor and marginalised citizens; its true purpose is to retain control over the populace while keeping the cost of social programmes down.

To popularise the Purge, the NFFA publicises the supposed psychological benefits of purging through mass media. As Warren (2020) notes, 'the Purge has become a kind of civic religion, with some citizens believing it their patriotic duty to kill and thus contribute to the "purging" of the jealousies, hostilities, and prejudices suppressed over the previous year' (32). The series has been prescient of real-world events in the United States, such as the storming of the US Capitol on 6 January 2021, which highlighted the ability of extremist leaders to 'mobilize large groups of Americans to use force and intimidation to impose their political will' (Miller and Rivas 2022). This chapter will consider the series as political horror, which uses the motif of Death 'to raise the spectre of reality regardless of how absurd the conceit may or may not be' (Armstrong 2019: 385), thereby creating a space to examine and critique real-world ideology. *The Purge* series is unusual in situating terror in the far-right, as US mainstream film has a marked tendency to view terrorism as an external (Muslim) threat (Corbin 2017: 485). In fact, far-right extremism is a significant threat to public safety and very few films have engaged seriously with far-right groups (Rich 2020) in the way this series does, albeit in its use of fantastic elements.

As previously noted, this chapter will primarily be concerned with personified Death as the taker of life and harbinger of the end of all things, as exemplified by Death of the Book of Revelation:

> And I looked, and behold a pale horse: and his name that sat on him was Death, and Hell followed with him. And power was given unto them over the fourth part of the earth, to kill with sword, and with hunger, and with death, and with the beasts of the earth. (Revelation 6:8)

As might be expected, Death is a key figure in Christian eschatology (the area of theology or metaphysics concerned with the final destiny of humanity), although there is considerable disagreement over whether Revelation is prophetic or historical (see Hendriksen 1939, Elliot 1862). The Horsemen can be read both as tangible figures and symbolic messengers of God, appearing to prefigure and then take part in the climactic battles preceding the new Heaven and Earth (Revelation 21:1–8). This Death symbolises both the removal of redemptive hope and the promise of its eventual restoration through judgement. As will be seen, Death functions similarly across *The Purge* series.

The apocalyptic Death is particularly germane to the politics of the series, which develops the kind of end of the world sought by extremists. 'Extremism is complex, everywhere, and profoundly consequential in society' (Berger 2018: 23) and the extremism featured in the series is totalising, both governmental and individual. It serves real-world far-right positions, such as 'authoritarianism and exclusionary nationalism' (Carter 2018: 172), that aim to legitimise violence against the out-group and which are characterised by apocalypticism (Sedgwick 2019). 'Accelerationists' (such as the Boogaloo Boys), in particular, see modern society as irredeemable (Miller 2020) and believe that they have the mandate to use catastrophic violence to seek the destruction and transformation of the entire world (Saiya 2020).

However, apocalypticism has long roots in the far-right. Beginning at least as far back as Spengler's *The Decline of the West* (1918–22), far-right thinkers have been concerned with a linear temporality and an orientation towards predictions of societal collapse, and this idea remains central (Sedgwick 2019). The vision of death afforded by apocalypticism is simple – everything must end if it is to be transformed – and this simplicity allows politicians to utilise catastrophic despair and hope to great effect, as seen recently in the pronouncements of Republican candidate Vivek Ramaswamy that we 'live in a dark moment', in which the US right must unite (Pengelly 2023). It is this political strategy that is employed to horrifying effect by the NFFA in *The Purge* series, who tell their followers that 'the American Dream is dead. We will do whatever it takes to let you dream again' (DeMonaco 2013). This point is key because it is an understanding of the apocalyptic politics in the series that constructs the masked purgers as Death, acting as instruments of the NFFA, and as harbingers of worse to come.

The series deploys the aesthetics and language of far-right apocalypticism in demonstrating the use of symbols to delineate in- and out-groups (see Lee 2018). We see a proliferation of high-contrast red, black and white art (initially in Charlie Sandin's closet in *The Purge* [DeMonaco 2013]) which is reminiscent of that used in recruitment material by 'skull mask' accelerationist groups (Loadenthal et al. 2022: 90), who are also known for wearing black-and-white grinning skull masks. Aside from protecting anonymity, these masks are marks of affiliation to a transnational network (Upchurch 2021), and they participate in a tradition of the use of masks to generate terror (see Hay 2021). They participate in the symbolic duplicitousness of masks, which are 'fundamentally double in function, signification and experience' (Sheppard 2001: 25), tools of impersonalisation and identity construction. The use of masks by purgers raises the spectre of reality by reflection; they are delineated from the protagonists' (the out-group's) everyday clothing through their stylised and garish costumes, becoming part of the nightmarish in-group. Anonymity would be attractive to purgers, but the choice of frightening masks draws real-world connections and generates terror for audiences.

In addition to recalling the use of masks by extremists, the purgers' masks signal a long tradition of horror-film masks, which are often bestowed with a specifically transformative power (Heller-Nicholas 2019). The mask transforms the purger both internally and externally, rendering them something other than, and uncanny to, humanity. They generate incertitude, 'unforeseeable and as insupportable as death' (Bataille 2002: 64), which, when combined with the accelerationist embrace of catastrophic violence, renders the masked purger as Death, a personified yet impersonal force that acts both tangibly and symbolically. Above all these functions, the masks are, first and foremost, harbingers – in each film, it is an encounter with masked purgers that signifies the escalation of the violence.

Aside from prequel *The First Purge* (McMurray 2018), each film has a singular purger who embodies the series' developing engagement with Death the Horseman, who comes as harbinger and bringer of death, with hell as his follower. In *The Purge*, Death is known as 'Polite Leader', who wears a full-face mask of a grinning human face; he and his acolytes are all smartly dressed, appearing as a horrific inversion of the young conservative. They raise the spectre of the Alt Right's command of optics, who have learnt to 'look good' to obtain opportunities to spread their revolutionary ideology (Bar-On 2019), as well as the 'New Right' politicians' success worldwide. They have presented themselves as patriots and supporters of 'white culture' whilst disguising or avoiding overt links to white supremacism (Steizinger 2022). Audiences in 2013 were unlikely to have been primed to recognise extremism in Polite Leader's costume (see Figure 23), so the film uses the group's rhetoric to signal to the audience. Polite Leader explains to the Sandins that they are 'some fine, young, very educated

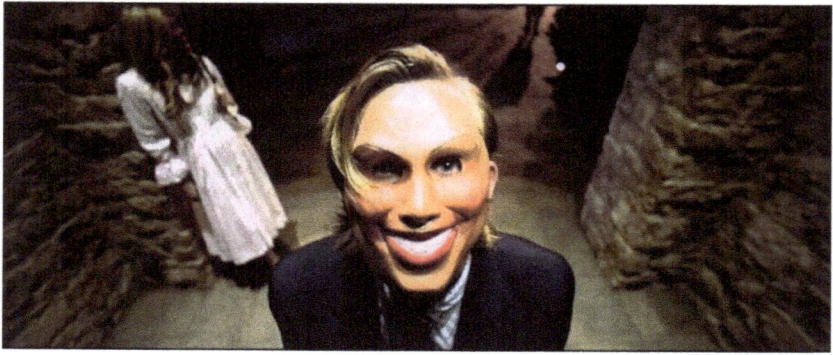

Figure 23. Polite Leader (Rhys Wakefield) in *The Purge*, directed by James DeMonaco (Universal Pictures, 2013)

guys and gals, and we've gotten dressed up in the most terrifying disguises, as we do every year, ready to annihilate and cleanse our souls' (DeMonaco 2013).

The appearance of this group, aiming to reclaim their intended homeless victim, to whom Charlie Sandin has given refuge against his parents' wishes, signifies that catastrophic violence has arrived. As they assure the Sandins that they will come inside if their demands are not met (and father James is forced to admit that his security system is unlikely to keep them out), it is understood that the Polite Leader will keep his promise to 'annihilate' during this purge, to commit utter apocalyptic destruction. In referring to the homeless man as a 'dirty homeless pig', and the Sandins as traitors for giving him sanctuary, Polite Leader delineates the in- and out-group and offers the Sandins the choice of which group to join, or to be ostracised, although this is framed as no true choice. Polite Leader justifies his expected violence with accelerationist framing: Western culture is being continually corrupted and any level of violence necessary to 'cleanse' it should be accepted.

In *The Purge: Anarchy* (DeMonaco 2014), the opening scenes introduce several separate protagonists, along with the wider sociopolitical context of the series. We hear that crime outside the Purge is 'virtually non-existent' and unemployment is below 5 per cent, although we later see that NFFA's 'success' resulted from their deployment of mercenary death squads against the poor and marginalised. *Anarchy* demonstrates the political and media strategy of the NFFA and draws real-world comparison in the way the news programmes feature dissenting voices only so they can be 'debunked' by pro-Purge speakers, and resistance groups must find other ways to publicise the truth of the Purge.

Estranged couple Shane and Liz are the first to meet Death, outside a supermarket. GOD, wearing a simple blank white face mask with rosy cheeks, black-ringed eyes and 'GOD' scrawled on the forehead (see Figure 24), is the leader of a group of bikers, and his acolytes can be found wearing variations of skeleton masks or face paint. They watch Shane and Liz in ominous silence, and whilst it is not immediately apparent that the Bikers have sabotaged their car, it is clear that these silent figures are daytime harbingers of the horror to come. GOD is relentless in pursuit, reappearing throughout the film as it becomes apparent that the group has escaped them. GOD represents the inevitability inherent in the Christian Death, who one cannot possibly outrun. Interestingly, however, GOD participates in the Purge as a kidnapper, capturing victims

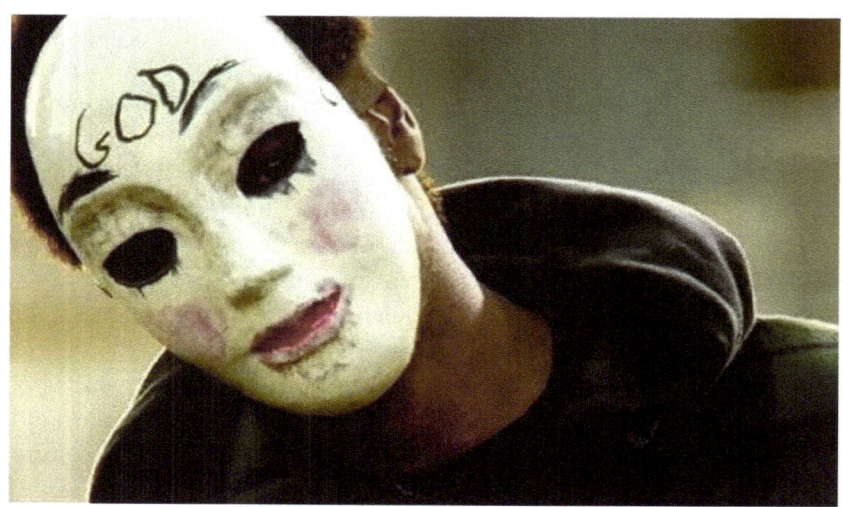

Figure 24. GOD (LaKeith Stanfield) in *The Purge: Anarchy*, directed by James DeMonaco (Universal Pictures, 2014).

for the rich elite to bid upon and then hunt. In this regard, they represent an evolution of the series' eschatology, and we are asked to pay attention to the way that non-political people can be induced to support extremism through the promise of stability (see Arendt 1951).

Another aspect of Death is seen in *The Purge: Election Year* (DeMonaco 2016), which features a presidential election between the NFFA and an anti-purge senator, who represents enough of a threat to the NFFA that they have abolished the Purge exemption for government officials to have her assassinated. An early scene shows a news interview of a group of 'murder tourists' from overseas, and one explains that they are here to 'experience the Purge, to kill, to release all the anger and hate' (DeMonaco 2016). They soon reappear, as 'Uncle Sam' and his group of US history caricatures (see Figure 25). Uncle Sam is not the main antagonist of *Election Year* (as that must certainly be the neo-Nazi paramilitary groups working for the NFFA), however, he embodies a new aspect of Death in far-right eschatology. The purgers' apocalypse will come no matter how many individual purgers are stopped, as the apocalypse is a transnational ideology. Those identifying with its extremist ideology will

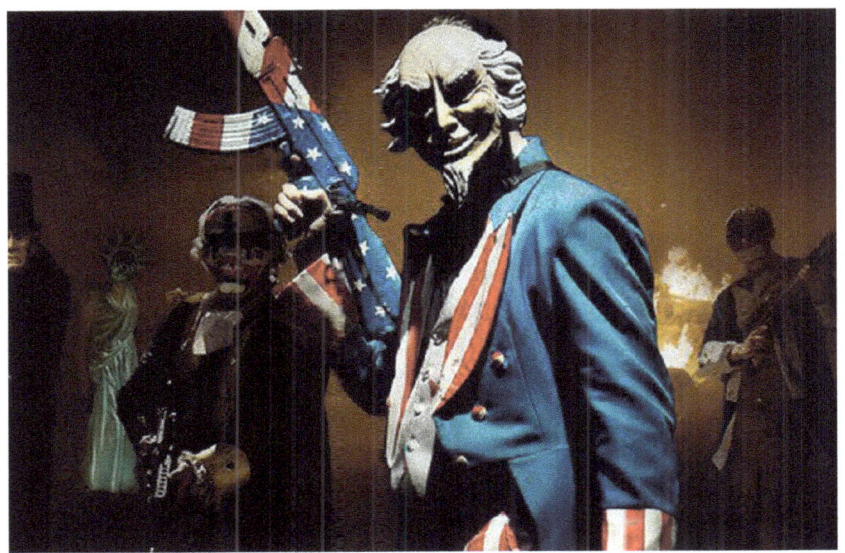

Figure 25. Uncle Sam (Roman Blat) and the murder tourists in *The Purge: Election Year*, directed by James DeMonaco (Universal Pictures, 2016).

continue to arrive, and it is easy to imagine international far-right actors advocating for their own Purge-style events.

The next film in the series is a prequel, *The First Purge* (McMurray 2018), taking place on the first experimental and localised Purge night in 2017. Through this return to the beginning, the audience is shown glimpses of the 'dystopia' that led to the election of the NFFA, again raising the spectre of reality. We learn that there is a housing crisis, an opioid epidemic and widespread protests (visually prescient of the protests following the murder of George Floyd in 2020) and that these conditions were sufficient to warrant the Purge. Again, however, the series takes care to remind us that the poor and marginalised instinctively know that the night is against rather than for them. Indeed, the NFFA offers financial incentives to purgers, aware that the majority of residents will not take part willingly.

Masks first appear in *The First Purge* relatively late into the film. The experiment is failing as participation is not at the hoped-for level in numbers or severity, and hence the NFFA sends in vans full of masked figures. Many of the locals had planned to stay out of it, but this possibility was removed by these figures, along with the notion that it is possible to ignore extremism more broadly. Interestingly, the mercenaries wear black-and-white skull masks similar to those discussed earlier in the present chapter. The mercenaries are more impersonal as Death than any of the chronologically later purgers already considered – they wear black uniforms, helmets and skull masks, although they are no less frighteningly powerful in their lack of individuation. They represent another important development in the series: that the Purge was never about individual chaos or catharsis. Death acts to bring about the annihilation desired by the NFFA.

The Death in *The Forever Purge* (Gout 2021) is the apotheosis of the earlier masked purgers, although he wears no mask. Following *Election Year*, we learn that the NFFA is back in power and the Purge is back with them. Elijah/Alpha is the leader of the racist paramilitary group the Purge Purification Force (PPF), who have decided not to stop purging after twelve hours, believing they have the mandate to carry on 'cleansing' to 'save America'. The PPF has done away with anonymity as they will not be going back to the previous world. *The Forever Purge* most fully reckons with the apocalyptic force of accelerationism, positing Elijah as a truly transformative power who takes the NFFA by surprise. He will successfully begin the 'final battle', and he represents the eventual loss of control of the political elite. Like Polite Stranger, the PFF uses explicitly accelerationist rhetoric about cleansing and 'disinfecting' America from 'foreign' elements. Aesthetically, however, they recall older images of the far-right, with swastika tattoos on full display, denoting that the polite veneer of modern extremism is simply that. *The Forever Purge* fully realises the eventual apocalypse of the NFFA's ideology, whilst embracing (particularly in protagonists Juan and Adela) the hope of a United States in joint pursuit of the betterment of all.

Through its Deaths, the series presents itself as prophetic, warning political actors to be careful about the strategies they employ in pursuit of their aims and the media of the dangers of amplifying extremist propaganda aimed at causing outrage. As an Indigenous leader warns, 'hatred like that can't be contained. You will burn your cities to the ground.' Taken as a whole, the series offers an anti-apocalyptic warning about societal complacency in the face of far-right extremism and particularly accelerationism. Through the use of the motif of Death, the series frighteningly realises the eschatology of its extremists. Masked Death in its symbolic and tangible power does not just create fear, but rather raises the spectre of reality, increasing the impact of the political message. Against all of this, the series has a fundamentally optimistic view of the possibilities: the ongoing Purge may feel endless, but the American people put it in place, and they have, should they wish, the power to end it.

Rachael Grant

# *American Horror Story: Asylum* (Brad Falchuck and Ryan Murphy, 2012–13)

## Comfort and Control in the Face of Uncertainty

Death is in control, ensuring that, by default, we are not. In a world that never stops, filled to the brim with to-do lists, emails, instant messages, tweets, live feeds, Tik-Tok videos, endless scrolling and the immediacy of media intruding on our lives every second of every day, the only certainty we have is this: it will end. Perhaps for some this is a comfort. This essay will explore this idea within the second season of the hit TV show *American Horror Story* (Falchuck and Murphy, 2012–13), examining the role of Shachath, or the Angel of Death, her position within the world the show creates and the cultural implications for the modern-day audience. This will be done via the lenses of religion, or lack thereof; connectivity in the age of technology; and, arguably, the erosion of familiarity with death itself.

Shachath, or The Angel of Death, played by the wonderful Frances Conroy, throws a blanket of peace over the chaotic world of the 1960s asylum run by nuns, which is the primary landscape for the second season of *American Horror Story* (see Figure 26). Her poised aesthetic of Japanese funerary (Murphy, in Stack 2012), as timed and seductive as burlesque, provides a subliminal comfort to not only the characters of the season, particularly that of Sister Jude Martin (Jessica Lang), but also to the audience. She gives a surety of footing in the weird world of *Asylum*, where craziness seems to reign, exploring the universal questions of 'who are we?' and 'why are we here?' through religion, sexuality and the possibility of extra-terrestrial life.

This strange and seemingly unlikely mix leaves the viewer disorientated, and it is Shachath who acts as an anchor: no matter what happens, she is there

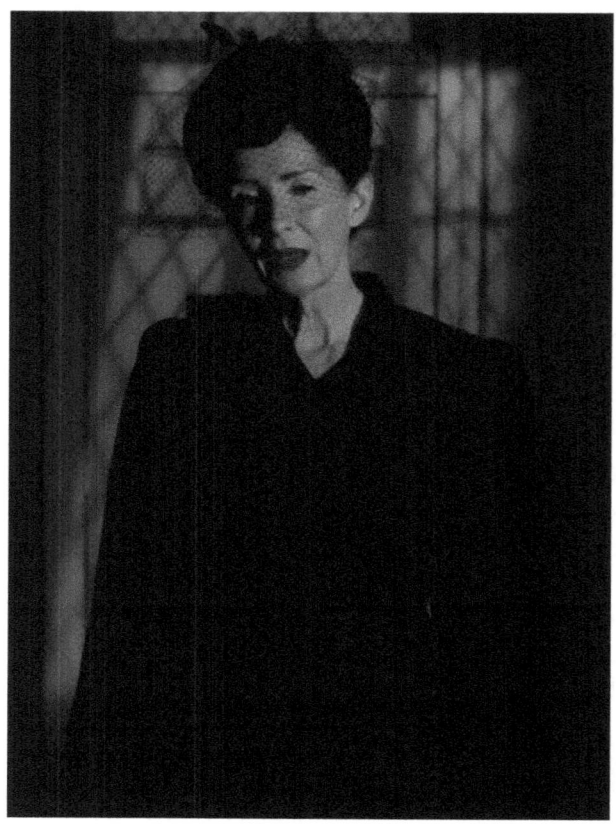

Figure 26. Frances Conroy as the Angel of Death or Shachath in *American Horror Story: Asylum*, created by Brad Falchuck and Ryan Murphy (20th Television, 2012–13).

at the end. We are both drawn to and repelled by her because of this. We may not all seek death, but there is safety in considering that, when the time comes, we will be guided by this winged being. The suggestion that evil may triumph over good is peppered throughout the season, lending an overarching gloom with storylines such as that of Dr Arthur Arden (James Cromwell) who is revealed to be a Nazi criminal cut from the same cloth as the real-life Josef Mengele, the infamous doctor of Auschwitz who performed monstrous experiments on his patients (Aschheim 2020). One of his victims, Shelley (Chloe

Sevigny), who has both legs amputated as a grisly punishment for her moral shortcomings, acts as a focus for the viewer to consider that sometimes death is a blessed relief from torture. Mengele's nickname was also Angel of Death (Aschheim 2020) due to the juxtaposition of his horrific experiments that often led to the death of his patients, and how charming he could appear on the surface, much like Dr Arden. The shared nickname alludes to a similarity between Mengele and Shachath, adding to the dark side of Shachath's character in line with the definition of her name from the Old Testament, 'destroyer' (Chaim Bentorah 2023), someone who is 'perverting, corrupting, spoiling and putrefying'. She is not just present at peaceful deaths, which mark the conclusion of many mundane lives, but she has witnessed the worst atrocities men have been able to inflict upon each other. However, Shachath meets Dr Arden sooner rather than later, as he commits suicide in the crematory alongside the body of his beloved Sister Eunice, whereas the real Dr Mengele escaped accountability and was thought to live the rest of his very long life in South America (Aschheim 2020). In the words of the show's creator, the creative decision to kill Dr Arden in this manner was 'very justified and somewhat poetic' (Stack 2013), using the arts to right what many would consider a fundamental wrong of history.

## Mortality amongst Gods

It is worth considering that the heaviness of all this horror is, in part, what draws us to Shachath. She has an eternal quality, providing a link across all cultures and eras. She is female, matriarchal, the ultimate mother attending to a child's skinned knee. We are delivered back into her arms, a metaphorical end-of-life womb (see Figure 27). Dr Arden wished to create too, and this was his justification for his experiments on Shelley and the other victims at the Brycliff asylum, attempting to make a superior human further along the chain of evolution. He wanted to discover the secret to immortality, which he thought he found evidence of with alien encounters that sometimes seemed jarring to the audience – a fantasy to justify his actions, suggesting the great beyond that

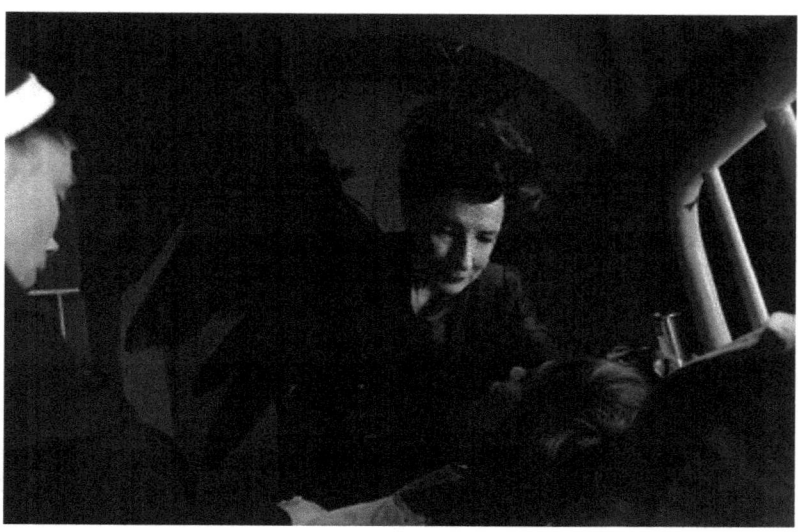

Figure 27. Welcomed into the arms of Shachath in *American Horror Story: Asylum*, created by Brad Falchuck and Ryan Murphy (20th Television, 2012–13).

many wish for may not just be found in faith but by alternative means such as life on other planets.

Shachath herself is immortal in the truest sense of the word; she has no start and no end, and her ability to send Satan back to hell is a testament to her own place in the hierarchy of supernatural beings across all seasons of the show. Sister Eunice touches on this when she is possessed by Satan and informs Dr Arden that she, therefore, is above him in the hierarchy of evil. But Shachath is beyond good and evil, and though it could be argued she is against evil because she banishes Satan, a counterpoint to her name's link with atrocities as described earlier, it seems more accurate to suggest that her detachment illustrates a being that governs order as opposed to making a specific moral judgement on actions of the mere mortals – who sometimes seem to bore her – or her fellow gods.

We can therefore conclude that Sister Jude is the character in the show who is meant to be us, the ordinary person. On the surface she has her guard up, trying to survive in a world that makes little sense, but on the inside, she is hiding a terrible secret: that she thinks she killed a child. Her whole life is a desperate attempt to not only atone for her sins but also hide them from others in order to create an illusion of control so she can go on living. She attempts this by burying herself in the excesses of the flesh that she tries to keep secret from the religious order she joins. But she is incapable of shedding the trappings of human life: lust, greed, addiction, a pull towards darkness and a desire to feel control over others in lieu of her inability to control herself. She tries to find herself in science too, handing over control to Dr Arden and his experiments just as she did to Monsignor Timothy Howard (Joseph Fiennes) and his religion, which may point to the idea that either fact or faith must rule. She tries to find hope in psychology that one can modify the human brain by lobotomies carried out in the asylum in an attempt to rid others of the very same temptations she falls victim to. But eventually she realises how foolish she is as she herself becomes a patient, giving new meaning to the term that the inmates are running the asylum, removing 'the separation of the mad from the sane' (Dalrymple 2005) in line with Foucault's insistence that there is little difference between those who are locked up and those doing the locking beyond the degree of power they hold, thus begging the question, what does crazy really mean?

In a poignant scene, Sister Jude sits, exhausted, in an all-American diner, the quintessential rest-stop for waifs and strays across cinematic history. It is a transitionary location, a modern-day purgatory. Shachath visits Jude, becoming the literal personification of the hominin 'flirting with death' when she seductively – yet somehow asexually – asks a question which Jude struggles to answer: 'Do you want to come with me?' Jude is tempted, temporarily placing Death in cahoots with the Devil as a manifestation of desire, but she struggles against her need to rest, knowing full well the finality of giving in, and on this occasion, she refuses to seek forgiveness for killing the child, who, in an ironic twist of fate, turns out to be alive. Perhaps the knowledge that Shachath is there should Jude choose to answer her clarion call gives her resilience to keep going. Acquainting oneself with the reality of death is a way of keeping the desire for it away, and perhaps this slowing-down-on-the-highway at the scene of an accident to gawk at someone else's gory misfortune is our way of dabbling with death. A metaphorical toe-in-the-water before running back from the tide, thinking, 'thank goodness this time it is not me'.

## Faith and Modernity

The entire second season of the *American Horror Story* is steeped in religion, which on the surface seems far removed from the reality of modern Western life. But maybe this is a warning about faith. There is a subtext to the convent, to the characters' struggles, both psychological and literal, suggesting that what we are missing is true belief in something higher than ourselves to provide context to our seemingly meaningless lives. And it is here we meet Satan, conveying that, at the very least, there is a hell if not a heaven, and this hell will invite us in if we do not choose good, thereby giving the entire show a depressive warning that if we do not do something to sort our lives out then the only surety is that it will be hell for us here on earth. This is depicted through the character of Sister Mary Eunice McKee (Lily Rabe), who is portrayed as innocent, without sin, but who is still tortured by Satan. She is a tool used to entice and manipulate the Monsignor, who has otherwise committed himself to God, though, like Sister Jude, he arguably makes a conscious decision to align with what could be considered genuine sin in the crimes of Dr Arden, and of acts of the flesh that result in his loss of virginity to the Devil. This is the ultimate metaphor. Not even a man of the cloth can escape.

## Belief and Beyond

Identity, a strong theme of the season, is played out through both morality and religion – with the two being often linked, though certainly not always in positive ways. There is the changing identity of Sister Eunice as Satan beds inside of her soul, warning of what happens when you choose to dance with the Devil, as well as the distorted anonymised identities of the victims of Dr Arden; monsters haunting the woods outside of the asylum. That Dr Arden conducts his experiments in a place of the Lord makes them more sinister, providing a clear message that just because one has faith it does not mean one has the moral high ground. Shachath illustrates that regardless of faith or morality, she equalises all at the point of death. She has no concerns with earthly things, and as she herself says, 'I don't judge. I never judge.' We are all her children, and her acceptance of everyone makes her less judgmental than God himself.

Shachath, therefore, is beyond the reaches of religion, accompanying those who die to an afterlife not spoken about or seen, thus leaving the question of whether there is an afterlife at all unanswered. This ambiguity again posits a relevance for the modern audience who may not have a particular faith but reminds us that, regardless of belief, death will come for us all in the end. Rich or poor, religious or faithless, man or woman, we all belong to Shachath. She has all the time in the world when ours is finite, and her patience is limitless. She is like a nurse; she tends to people and performs her duties. She administers death through the gift of a kiss, a symbol not only of affection but also of the removal of breath, once again linking life and death, sex and innocence (see Figure 28). Her lack of judgement also suggests that her banishing of the Devil from Sister Eunice and sending him back to hell is not because Shachath is inherently good, but it is because she disapproves of meddling with others' moral business. She is neither good nor bad, and it is this neutrality that suggests to the audience that Death is not something to fear but is something to accept. This is a fact. All must die, and the supernatural interference of Satan with Sister Eunice goes against this ethos. This makes Shachath the most powerful of all the supernatural beings depicted in *American Horror Story*. Therefore, the show seems to be saying that the only other thing besides death that we can be certain of is the life we currently live now, and, therefore, we had better make the most of it. Who do we want to be in the here and now, and with what morals, when we know we meet the same fate? We must make every moment count.

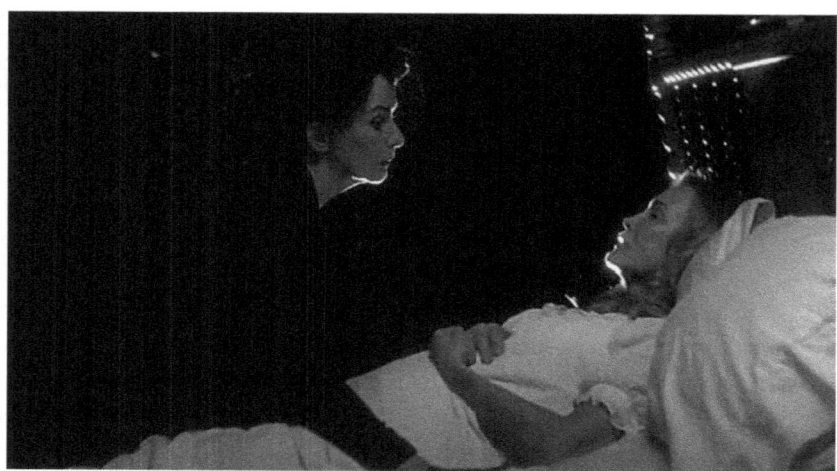

Figure 28. The last embrace of Shachath in *American Horror Story: Asylum*, created by Brad Falchuck and Ryan Murphy (20th Television, 2012–13).

## Conclusion

But after all this, how is Shachath's portrayal relevant to us now, in the technologically driven world we live in? And how can a torture chamber of an asylum have relevance to us today, in a post-pandemic world where death feels closer than ever, yet we are protected behind screens? The depiction of Death in *American Horror Story* speaks to the subconscious animal in all of us, providing a fail-safe, an escape-hatch, reminding us that when life becomes too much one can call on Death and she will always answer. We exist in a time of unrest, with political battlefields drawn and never-ending access to news that pumps fear into our phones. Despite the statistics that we have never been safer (Pinker 2012), we are under an illusion that terror lurks on every street corner (Sharf 2015). We are horrified, but we also can't look away. And why should we? Perhaps it is our curiosity that keeps us riveted to these types of fiction or to the ever-churning juggernaut of true crime as witnessed by its growing popularity (Sayles 2021). Maybe it is terror that we seek by watching shows like *American Horror Story*: to remind us of our shadow, of what we are capable of.

It is this horror, the juxtaposing of the fantastical and of the faith we have abandoned (Voas and Chaves 2016) for the latest celebrity elevated to the level of God in an attempt to fool ourselves that we can live forever, just like Dr Arden, with rudimentary knowledge we have deep inside of us that one day we will die, that makes Shachath, and indeed all of the mythos of *American Horror Story*, hit so close to home. Perhaps the intention of the writers is to show that while fear can be found in faith of many kinds, it is not wise to turn away from the atrocities humans inflict upon their fellow humans. Perhaps, on a fundamental level, we are aware that we run the risk of being lost in the glossy veneer of the online world, and so we seek solace in shows that remind of us how hideous humanity can be, but also, somehow, how beautiful we are because of it.

Robert Mclaughlin

# Mistress Death in the Marvel Universe (Various, 1973–Present)

'Death', represented as one of the Horsemen of Apocalypse, and the pantheons of gods and goddesses of death, such as Nekron or Hela, have throughout comic or comic-centric media appeared on numerous occasions as antagonists for the various heroes of comic book universes. However, the fact that personification of 'Death' itself has appeared in various guises and taken numerous forms – from the trope of the 'manic pixie dream-girl' (Rabin 2007) depiction of Death within Neil Gaiman's *Sandman* to the Silver-Surfer-inspired Jack Kirby-designed Black Racer of the New Gods DC Universe, who is the embodiment of 'death' personified as both male and female characters that interact with other denizens of an established and shared literary comic universe – has become a common occurrence within the pages of recent comic books.

Within the superhero collection created by the American comic book publisher Marvel Comics, the character of Death is presented as a cosmic entity 'born' alongside the universe's other cosmic conceptual abstracts such as Eternity and Infinity. Death as a character within Marvel, sometimes referred to as 'Mistress' or 'Lady' Death, is a fundamental force within the Marvel universe first appearing in Issue #26 of *Captain Marvel* (June 1973). Created and visualised by Mike Friedrich and Jim Starlin apace with these other abstract concepts that are given 'human' form – which also include more bizarre concepts such as 'The Living Tribunal' and master's Chaos/Order – Death alongside these conceptual beings does not technically have an actual physical form but appears within this cosmic ensemble as a human skeleton with 'her' face hidden behind a hood or shroud.

Although Death's appearance within the Marvel Universe varies slightly depending on the artist and storyline, the signs and signifiers – associated with the more-traditional late Middle Ages or memento mori (medieval images of death) which depicts death and its accompaniments of death (such as a shroud and scythe), seen through, for example, the Dance Macabre – are clearly discernible in her initial comic appearances. However, in subsequent storylines, Death is depicted as having a more human-like appearance and even presented as a fully formed flesh-and-blood entity instead of being a skeletal apparition. For example, within the *Infinity Gauntlet* storyline, Death appears to Thanos as a beautiful woman, representing his idealised version of Death. Death has also appeared as the Mexican female personification of death Santa Muerte ('Holy Death' or 'Saint Death') – the ultimate construct of the 'Other' of the Catholic Church again usually depicted as a skeletal figure robed in black, red or white and carrying a scythe.

## Thanos and Death

While best known as the main antagonist within the Infinity Saga of the Marvel Cinematic Universe, Thanos is presented to be a universal threat to existence, a depiction very similar to the character's portrayal within the Marvel Comic Universe. First appearing in *The Invincible Iron Man* (Issue #55, cover dated February 1973), the character was created (again) by Jim Starlin and appeared frequently as an antagonist for the galactic hero Captain Marvel. Throughout his comic appearances, Thanos' main drive and intent was to appease his 'mistress' death, obtaining various cosmic artifacts such as the Cosmic Cube to try and control the universe.

Death's 'romantic' inclinations towards Thanos begin very early in the character's development, appearing to him as an apparition of a young girl while he is being educated on his home planet of Titan. In this guise, Death becomes Thanos' confidant and encourages him to kill for her. This fascination with extinguishing life started with the character killing animals, people and eventually his mother, leading finally to the massacre of entire populations on his quest for galactic genocide.

Within various Thanos-related stories, it is seen that Death abandons the character when she is either bored with him or he is defeated by the heroes of the Marvel Comic Universe. In the fifty years that Thanos has been a major Marvel antagonist, the common thread of the motivation that runs through most of his stories is his attempt to 'woo' Death back with bigger and more horrific gestures, dedications and tributes. In the limited two-part series *The Thanos Quest* (1990) by Jim Starlin and Ron Lim, Death perceives an imbalance in the universe and a gradual shift towards life rather than death; hence, she tasks Thanos to rectify this, which he successfully does so by collecting the Infinity Gems used to redress the imbalance.

By doing this, Thanos attains god-like powers and becomes superior to Death. As a result, Death, fickle as she is, stops speaking with Thanos (a fact relayed via one of Death's minions), and this, in turn, enrages the titan. With this spurning of his love, Thanos' story continues through to the series *The Infinity Gauntlet* (1991). This series' plot forms the basis of the Infinity Saga within the Marvel Cinematic Universe through which the character of Thanos became well known. In this series, Thanos attempts, once again, to prove his love for Death. The plot, as a continuation and culmination of the previous story arc, shows Thanos gathering six Infinity Gems and fixing them into a single gauntlet, which he then uses to kill half of the universe's population, including many of its heroes, to, once again, earn the affection of 'Mistress Death'.

In the finale of the story, Death quietly waits and watches Thanos take on the combined might of Marvel superheroes and defeat them. Once they are vanquished, however, Death, perceiving Thanos to be a threat, joins the other conceptual cosmic aspects of the Marvel Universe in order to try and stop him herself. As with most of Thanos' plans, this one is also eventually thwarted, and he loses the Infinity Gauntlet, because, at his core, Thanos feels he is unworthy of the power and, indeed, Death's love. Scorned by Death and left all alone, Thanos goes on to scheme and plot grander gestures of affection to win Death back.

Through the 1970s until the 1990s, Death's visual coding within the Marvel Comic Universe meant that the personification of death was one of intimidation and foreboding – a character on a cosmic scale who consorts with universal concepts and galactic tyrants and who symbolised both the inevitability of death and the unknown mysteries of the afterlife. It is therefore ironic that her next consort was very much the antithesis of Thanos.

## Deadpool and Death

Over the past two decades, Death seems to have developed a fascination with the mercenary Wade Wilson known as Deadpool. Created by Fabian Nicieza and Rob Liefeld, the character first appeared in *New Mutants* (Issue #98, December 1990, cover dated February 1991) at the height of the 'extreme' phase of Marvel comics of the late 1980s and early 1990s, which saw comic characters become more violent in their framing of 'super-heroics'. A huge fan favourite, Deadpool has gone on to become one of Marvel's most popular characters, but, as Pochapska (2022) describes, the character is a ridiculous champion, a trickster (Lukáč 2019) and comparable to Don Quixote. As such it could be debated that this character is completely unsuited to be Death's companion or love interest.

Across several volumes of Deadpool's comic series, it is shown that Death and Deadpool have a complex relationship. Deadpool as a character breaks the '4th wall' similar to how John Byrne allowed the character She-Hulk to do so in the 1980s. This notion implies that the character is self-aware and understands the comic-related, story-driven narrative that they are part of. This perception allows for the character to engage with or address the 'reader' of the comic book and to add personal opinions to the situation. In the She-Hulk series, her character was portrayed as having light-heated banter with her readership through comments or quips, whereas Deadpool's conversations with his audience are usually portrayed as darker and more reflective. Deadpool is also aware that his love for Death is one-sided, and he is often depicted as engaging in comical and absurd antics to win her affection. He frequently talks to Death as if she were a person and even proposes marriage to her on multiple occasions.

It could be debated that the notion of self-awareness and perception of the meta-context that Deadpool knows he is a comic character could be one of the factors that attract Death to Deadpool (and vice versa). Another possible explanation is his superpower: owing to his superhuman ability to heal himself, Deadpool is technically immortal. It can be argued that Death is in love with Deadpool because, due to his inability to die, she cannot have his soul. With this notion of wanting but never obtaining, Deadpool becomes an object of desire for Death as she knows that she cannot ever possess him. However, while both arguments are valid, there is evidence of a far simpler reason why an omnipotent abstract concept from the beginning of time is attracted to Deadpool: that he makes her laugh.

Initially, Death as an entity is perceived by Deadpool because of the numerous near-death experiences the character finds himself in. An example of this is depicted by the story within the *Deadpool and Death Annual* (1998) by Joe Kelly in which Death helps Deadpool remember his troubled past in the Weapon X facility, the place where he gains his healing ability. In addition, there are numerous examples where Deadpool literally laughs in the face of death, and, surprisingly, Death is amused by him. In one of the most memorable comic panels depicting Deadpool's gallows humour, he is shown explaining to Death that his next attempt at dying is going to be really hard, to which Death responds, 'That's what she said.'

## Thanos and Deadpool: Rivals in Love

In Death's interactions with Thanos, her character has always been portrayed as being cold, aloof and dispassionate, whereas her relationship with Deadpool (who he nicknames as 'sugar-skull') has always been depicted as flirtatious and has thus created a mismatched rivalry between the two characters over Death's affections. During the *Funeral for a Freak* (2002, storyline by Frank Tieri, Buddy Scalera and Jim Calafiore), a jealous Thanos prevents Deadpool from dying and from joining Death forever by cursing him with immortality with a classic comic-book line 'consider yourself cursed ... with life!' However, both Thanos and Deadpool have to put aside their differences during the *Deadpool vs. Thanos* (2015) – a miniseries of comics by Tim Seeley, Elmo Bondoc, Ruth Redmond and Joe Sabino – after discovering that Death was being contained by Eternity in a bid to finally halt the constant loss of life she has caused over the centuries.

Finally confronting Eternity, Death briefly empowers both of her lovers with her own power, with Deadpool realising that this was an elaborate ruse as it was what she wanted all along. While Thanos attempts to destroy Eternity and all life that would ever exist with the power bestowed on him, Deadpool uses the power to defeat Thanos. Deadpool argues through questionable logic that as much as the titan loves Death, Thanos' attempt to stop all life that would ever exist would mean that technically nothing could ever die, and this would inadvertently make Thanos the champion of life rather than Death. This logic in turn causes Mistress Death to turn away from the titan once again and choose Deadpool as her suitor.

## The Winner in the Battle for Love/Death

Deadpool has a unique relationship with Death, with the character depicted as a central part of Deadpool's motivation and character arc. He is willing to take extreme risks and engage in dangerous activities in order to impress her, which elevates the violence depicted in the comics to absurd levels. Although Thanos' nihilistic tendencies and vast gestures of grandeur are on a cosmic scale, the interaction between Death and Deadpool is often comical yet touching, and it is one of the most unique relationships within the Marvel Comic Universe. Unlike Thanos, Deadpool's love for Death is not driven by a desire for power but based on a deep desire for companionship.[1]

The wider image of Death portrayed across the Marvel Universe is that she is rather secretive, both in her appearance and intention. The fact that she

---

1 The relationship between all three of these characters also transcends the pages of the comic book – most notably within the realm of video games. Both Thanos and Death appear in the Capcom fighting game *Marvel Super Heroes* (1995) which is loosely based on *The Infinity Gauntlet* storyline, while Death also featured in High Moon's Deadpool video game (2013).

is not a lover of grand gestures, as well as the inevitable depersonalisation of her function, shows that Death rather prefers the personal over the perfunctory and that she would always choose to engage with someone on her own terms. More than this, and in no small way, because she is a character who is yet to be fully written across the Marvel Universe, she shows that death is never quite what you think it might be.

Maria Giakaniki

# *Suspiria* (Luca Guadagnino, 2018)

Women have been associated with death almost as much as they have been connected to life. From the ancient goddesses of the underworld to the corpse brides of Gothic ballads and from the evil witches of medieval fairy tales to Morticia Addams, a plethora of worldwide female figures and characters from different eras and cultures has been depicted as agents and/or emblems of death.

In twenty-first-century (horror) films and television series, and in the context of contemporary reconsideration of concepts of femininity restricted by socially constructed gender roles, there has been a wide variety of complex representations of female characters as personifications of death and destruction, which range from supernatural evil forces to serial killers, and from victims who seek revenge (often beyond the grave) to mentally unstable characters and powerful matriarchs that defy established morals, sometimes becoming symbols of female empowerment.

A film that seems to embody most of these characteristics into one narrative is the recent remake of *Suspiria* (2018) by Luca Guadagnino. Here in a work centred on women in a woman's world, every part of life is made manifest in the female body: predator/victim, mistress/slave, mother/daughter, life/death. Indeed, at the film's denouement, the narrative purposely inverts the popular trope of woman as life-giver to show the female body at its most powerful and agentic as Death itself.

This chapter will further use the example of *Suspiria* to discuss the motif of women being agents of death instead of life across other recent supernatural texts as a wider (re)examination of concepts of femininity in the post-#MeToo era.

In filming *Suspiria* (1977), Dario Argento was inspired by Thomas de Quincey's invented mythology described in his *Suspiria de Profundis* (1845), a poetic fantasy work based on the author's opium experiences. *Suspiria de*

*Profundis* features three dark female figures: Mater Lachrymarum, Mater Suspiriorum and Mater Tenebrarum, that is Our Lady of Tears, Our Lady of Sighs and Our Lady of Darkness; all three were associated with the ancient roman goddess Levana, were supposed to be of undefined pre-Christian origin and were endowed with dark, sinister qualities (De Quincey 2019: 56–61). Based on this primary literary source, the original 1977 Argento film is a Gothic fairy tale of female monstrosity, with a witches' coven disguised as a prestigious dance academy in Freiburg, Germany, led by an ancient witch named Helena Markos or The Black Queen, who is Mother Suspiriorum. The coven's existence is dependent on its leader's power, who kills anyone considered a threat to its covert exploitative existence; the latter consists of gaining power and wealth by any means possible. Markos is finally put to death by an American student of the dance academy Susie Bannion (played by Dakota Johnson), who is also the heroine in Guadagnino's *Suspiria* (2018).

In the 2018 remake of the film, the story is set in divided Berlin in the autumn of 1977, a time which was politically marked by the RAF (Red Army Faction), a leftist urban guerrilla group that was engaged in armed resistance against the state – which the group considered as a fascist remnant in 1970s Germany – by kidnapping and/or assassinating higher officials. As soon as Susie Bannion (Dakota Johnson) enters the dance academy, she finds it to be a place of danger and death where violent and mysterious incidents take place, reverberating the political fear and turmoil that prevailed in German society at the time. Patricia (Chloë Grace Moretz), a former student of the school, has disappeared after confessing her deepest fears about the academy to her psychiatrist Dr Klemperer (Tilda Swinton), while Olga (Elena Fokina), another student, is horribly disfigured by the supernatural forces employed by the lead choreographer and teacher of the school Madame Blanc (Tilda Swinton) and other matrons during Susie's first rehearsal of the *Volk* dance (German word for people and nation, alluding to remnants of Nazi Germany sentiments). The matrons' aim was to quell any apparent threat that Olga may pose to the hidden agenda of the coven, which is to strengthen Helena Markos (Tilda Swinton), the leader/matriarch of the school–coven. Markos is an old witch with a grotesque appearance, echoing the original film's Mother Markos, who is supposed to be Mother Suspiriorum, a supernatural female entity. Yet, in order to reconsider the hierarchy within the school, the matrons of the cult hold an election, finally choosing Markos over Madame Blanc. In the meanwhile, Susie, the newcomer, becomes the favourite of Madame Blanc, with whom she gradually forms an almost mother-daughter bond, which also reflects a mentorship relationship with some lesbian undercurrents. Sara (Mia Goth), a student at the dance school befriended by Susie, makes some awful discoveries in the secret underway passages of the academy building. Thus she is punished by the matrons of the school who cause a terrible leg fracture while she is also physically manipulated into dancing her part robotically during the performance of *Volk* –whose lead dancer is Susie – which takes place inside the academy (see Figure 29). This powerful dance scene reflects the authoritative character of the school and its female leaders, who wish to exert complete control over their students in an almost mistress-slave relationship while evoking the totalitarian character of the Nazi regime.

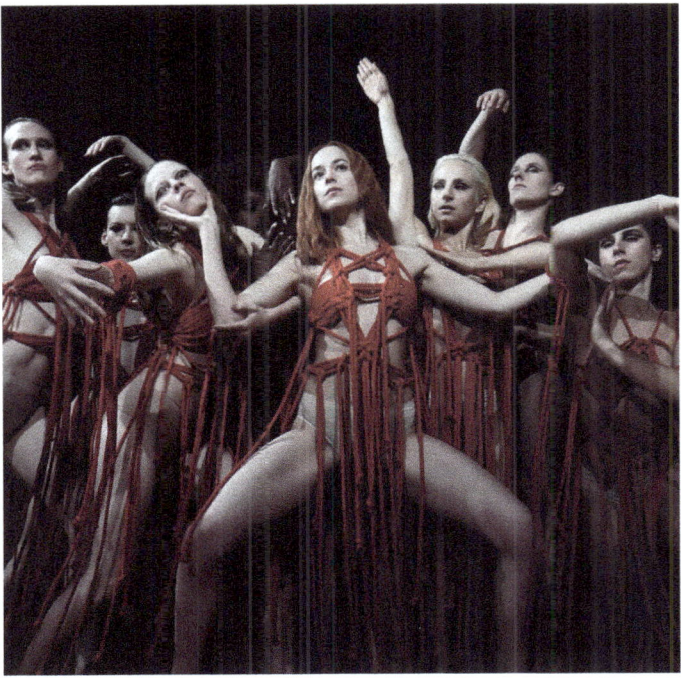

Figure 29. *Volk* dance scene. *Suspiria*, directed by Luca Guadagnino (Amazon Studios, 2018).

Susie is also plagued by strange dreams with flashbacks of her former life in the United States and has haunting visions of her biological mother being close to death; these nightmares/visions are sent to her by Blanc, with whom she is uncannily able to communicate. As the story evolves, Susie gradually becomes more self-assertive and confident among not only her fellow students but also the teachers. In the story's climax towards the closure of the film, a strange ritualistic scene takes place in a hidden part of the school (which the psychiatrist Klemperer is also forced to witness after he was brought there by the witches despite his will), during which Markos is about to inhabit Susie's body, making her the new host for her parasitic existence. Nevertheless, Madame Blanc (see Figure 30) seems to hesitate since she has formed a close bond with Susie, and she pays the price for it as she is almost decapitated by Markos' supporters. Yet Markos, in a totally unexpected twist, is finally defeated by Susie herself, who proves to be the real Mother Suspiriorum; at this point, Susie becomes an agent of death,

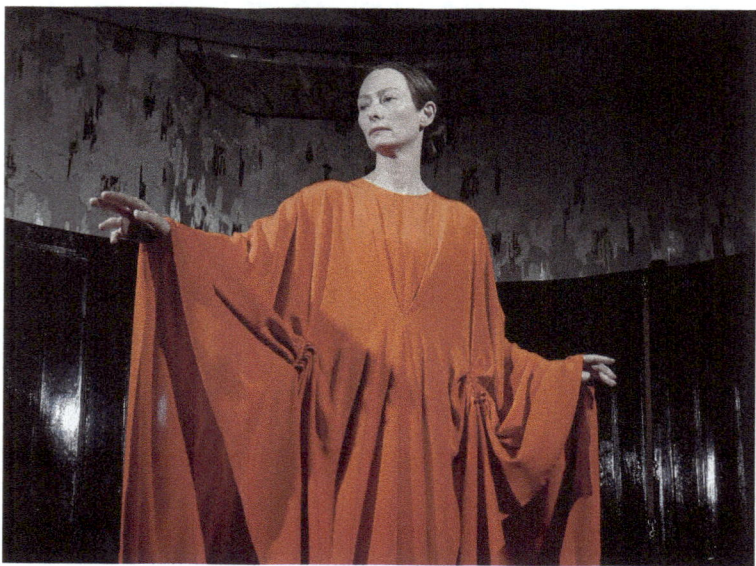

Figure 30. Tilda Swinton as Madame Blanc. *Suspiria*, directed by Luca Guadagnino (Amazon Studios, 2018).

eliminating the supporters of Markos, while offering a merciful demise to Patricia, Sara and Olga, who have endured brutal suffering caused by the arbitrariness of the previous establishment. Thus Susie/Mother Suspiriorum becomes the most dominant figure in the school/cult hierarchy.

*Suspiria* features various supernaturally powerful women, labelled as witches, of different ages and external forms. In horror films and popular culture, the portrayal of witches has shifted through the decades from stereotypical and predominantly one-dimensional depictions associated with evilness, seductiveness or comical elements to more nuanced representations. Historically and culturally, not only patriarchal oppression but also female empowerment are two major concepts that form the basis of female witchcraft (Greene 2021: 2). This is echoed in several recent horror films where the 'witch' is either a victim who seeks retribution or a victimiser who seeks to be self-defined, or sometimes both. Moreover, in films such as *Suspiria* the witch character is loaded with new depth. *Suspiria* revolves around the figure of the witch, whose character is reinvented via the depiction of a conflict of power between and for women, who exist in a somewhat 'post-patriarchal' fantastical realm almost devoid of men's influence; men in *Suspiria* are peripheral or easily defeated.

Markos is an aged witch whose character, verging on caricature, reminds us of the figure of Black Queen in the 1977 *Suspiria*, with its grotesque representation of an evil entity wreathing havoc. On the contrary, Susie Bannion, who gradually evolves into the new witch, is portrayed as mysterious, complex, ambivalent, elusive and almost beyond suspicion or comprehension, while Madame Blanc exhibits a wide palette of traits, ranging from extreme cruelty to protectiveness (see Figure 30). *Suspiria* magnificently blurs the line between good and evil but not only that: it outshines the battle between good and evil, by bringing forth a clash of almost natural forces. The film is not so much about morality as it is about power which can be either good, evil or something in between. Some of the characters exist in a grey zone and the interest is transferred from what is right and wrong to who is the most powerful, efficient and self-assertive. It is a war for power that leads to the extinction of the defeated, with female violence inflicted on female bodies themselves throughout the film. In this respect, in *Suspiria* it is the idea of female (supernatural) force itself that prevails whatever the form it takes – it is a sort of power that is associated exclusively with women, either because women seek it or because it is part of their nature. Also, it is through these supernatural abilities and their power of will that the women in *Suspiria* can bring death and destruction.

Helena Markos, claiming to be Mother Suspiriorum, is a predator seeking the ideal victim to become a host for her spirit. Thus, the soul of the victim must inevitably perish; it is not only physical death but also displacement and demeaning eradication of the self through parasitic exploitation of the old order represented by Markos. In Ari Aster's *Hereditary* (2018), this very idea of the death of the self and one's body being hosted by a demonic entity is presented. This motif is realised by the matriarch of a religious cult who is willing to sacrifice her grandchildren to an otherworldly evil for personal gain; she is an amoral female predator totally reversing any grandmother stereotypes that might still exist in our times. In *Hereditary*, possessing the body of another, and thus enslaving the soul, is an allegory of the shadow cast upon the young by haunting family traumas through the generations.

In Goran Stolevski's *You Won't Be Alone* (2022), an ancient witch and her successor/apprentice have the power to live in other people's bodies after killing them either before abandoning this disguise for another or returning to their own initial form. The novice witch is able to experience human life by using dead humans as hosts by assuming their form, gender and identity. Yet, in this case, through the death of others and her own recurrent 'rebirth' finally comes knowledge and a life she embraces. In *Evolution* (2015) by Lucile Hadžihalilović, an all-female humanoid species preys on young boys, using them as hosts for their babies and then leaving them to perish, in an almost misandrist world, while in the hallucinatory but not overtly supernatural *Midsommar* (2019) by Ari Aster, the theme of human sacrifice is repeated – this time as part of a female-led pagan ritual that results in the empowerment of the heroine. All these representations of female empowerment through human sacrifice subvert preconceptions of femininity by presenting women as powerful agents of death and destruction, as much as males can traditionally be.

In *Suspiria*, there is a strict hierarchy, and it seems that any inferior member of the cult or a student at the school who violates it by questioning or opposing the status quo might find her death through extreme torture. The secret cult may be a collective force, but the lowest members are expected to comply and obey; thus the teacher-pupil relationship takes the mistress-slave form. In *Suspiria*, individual female power must succumb to collective female power, in a fantastic simulation of a female fascist regime. In both *Hereditary* and *Midsommar*, there is the idea of a cult which is constituted by layers of (female) power; the top position of the cult in both cases is occupied by two older matriarchs who lead their subordinates and have the power to cause death if they deem it necessary. In *You Won't Be Alone*, the relationship between the old witch and the female novice is clearly one of absolute power and submission, with the old hag killing everyone her apprentice holds dear. The mistress/slave relationship in *Suspiria* is also paralleled to a mother/daughter relationship; the latter, of course, includes other forms of bonding too. The figure of Markos/Mother Suspiriorum does not conform to what maternity typically means; yet, perhaps, this is the real raw image of motherhood: a mother is a tyrant too, a powerful being who, in a 'queer inversion of maternity' (Kosmina 2023: 198), can both give birth and cause damage to her offspring. The mother/daughter relationship is also depicted through the bond between Madame Blanc and Susie: Blanc is not only authoritative and patronising, but she also develops protective and even erotic feelings towards the young newcomer. Moreover, Susie's real mother's behaviour seems strange and hostile – perhaps a consequence of the suspicion that her daughter is not 'normal' – and depicted as having a conservative religious background. Besides, she resembles a death figure as she is lying on her bed breathing heavily, the scene reminiscent of a similar uncanny portrayal of Helena Markos/Mother Suspiriorum from the 1977 film; the heavy breathing is a sound of imminent death, but in this case, it also suggests menace. In *Hereditary*, the main mother-daughter relationship is deeply problematic, like a trauma that needs to be exorcised, yet it spreads like a disease into the next generation. The grandmother in *Hereditary* is almost a sacrilege to 'woman's nature, as she constitutes a parasite for her offspring, bringing illness and death, in a totally unconventional portrayal of femininity. *You Won't Be Alone* also delineates a mother-daughter relationship that is completely tyrannical, while in Oz Perkins' *Gretel and Hansel* (2020), the mentorship bond between the old crone and the evolving new witch clearly evokes a maternal interest that is both inspiring and dangerous. Moreover, in Kate Dolan's *You Are Not My Mother* (2021) the relationship between mother and daughter is very precarious with the mother being substituted by a beastly entity that is eager to kill her own family, in a metaphorical portrayal of depression, the dark side of motherhood and problematic familial bonds.

In the climactic scene of Guadagnino's *Suspiria*, Susie brings death in more than one way; it is death as retribution and eradication of an enemy (ending the parasitic existence and dictatorial rule of Helena Markos) and death as liberation from suffering. After releasing her true nature from own body, which is the genuine Mother Suspiriorum, Susie then dictates to her own agent of death to kill the followers of Mother Markos, the false Mother Suspiriorum; nevertheless, she herself offers the choice of death to those who have suffered from the witches until now: Sara, Olga and Patricia. Moreover, she later also brings 'death' to the memories of the old psychiatrist who was a potential victim of Markos, since she erases from his mind the facts that are responsible for his feelings of guilt regarding the death of his wife (Jessica Harper) during the Nazi regime. Yet, this is also an ambivalent action on her behalf since it might also insinuate the erasing of history. Nevertheless, at this point, Susie can be seen as an overthrowing force, which in the outside world is somehow analogous to RAF (i.e. the Baader-Meinhof Group). Other allusions such as Patricia being a follower of the radical political activist group and, at the beginning of the film, references to 'Mother Meinhof' draw a parallel between the female head of the extremist group and Mother Suspiriorum, perhaps anticipating the emergence of the original version of the latter, that is Susie Bannion.

Susie seems to be the most enigmatic, ambiguous and nuanced version of the witch/matriarch and also the most powerful one (see Figure 31). Being the final girl, she embraces the 'evil' side but on her own terms: by opening a new path through death and catastrophe since destruction can also bring rebirth (Kosmina 2023: 126).

Luca Guadagnino's *Suspiria* portrays the power balance within an autonomous sisterhood, indicating that women can be as dominant, transgressive and self-sufficient as men; yet, the fact that all this is happening in a particular space is a microscopic reflection of the power battles and interactions in the broader social sphere where men are still in charge, especially in the field of politics. In this respect, it seems that, according to modern horror films distinguished by feminist concerns and endowed with symbolism, it is mostly through the supernatural element that women can overcome the limitations of their sex;

*Suspiria* (Luca Guadagnino, 2018)

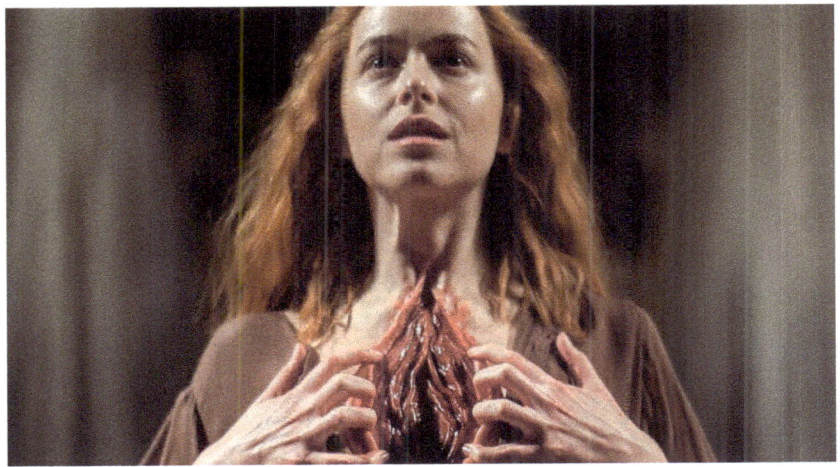

Figure 31. Dakota Johnson as Susie Bannion/Mother Suspiriorum. *Suspiria*, directed by Luca Guadagnino (Amazon Studios, 2018).

unlike men who maintain power more easily in real life, women's voices are still not placed at the core of society but rather at its peripheries.

Octavia Cade

# Deathface Ginny (Kelly Sue DeConnick, 2014–20)

## Multiple Mortalities in *Pretty Deadly*

The comic series *Pretty Deadly*, written by Kelly Sue DeConnick and with art by Emma Ríos, currently consists of fifteen issues published from 2014 to 2020. It is a magical realist narrative strongly focused on multiple personifications of death, with a number of ostensibly subordinate reapers overseen by the figure of Death. Regarding the many images of Death that have been created over history and by different cultures, Guthke asks 'if imaginative personification of the unknown is one of the characteristic features of our species, why does it operate in such contradictory ways?' (1999: 19). There are a number of possible responses to this, but in *Pretty Deadly* that response is one of method. The reapers of the comic exist in multiples because of the specialised manner of the deaths – such as thirst, war or obsession – for which they are responsible.

On the death penalty, Canuel notes that critics 'decline to explain how any law whatsoever could avoid the taint of dehumanized ritual, or how any law could ever be made to account for the infinite variety of human subjects' (2007: 170). While the analogy between executioners of the death penalty and the reapers is not exact, *Pretty Deadly* uses multiple reapers to confront the individual with a figure who is in some way reflective of their own choices. In this, *Pretty Deadly* overlays the idea of personalised justice on reapers such as Deathface Ginny, the reaper of vengeance; Rosenbaum comments that 'when performed to perfection, vengeance and justice can and should serve the same societal purpose and fulfil the same human need' (2013: 190).

More frequently in speculative fiction, the moral status of the dying, or of the recently deceased, is linked to their experiences of the afterlife. Characters who have behaved morally experience a different afterlife to those who have not; an argument for personal responsibility, or the justice of the world, which occurs post-death. In *Pretty Deadly*, it is the representation of death – not solely the subsequent experience of the afterlife – that primarily critiques justice within the text. Issue #6 to Issue #10 of the series, comprising the graphic novel *The Bear*, are set largely in the trenches of France during the First World War. Soldiers are killed in a number of terrible ways, including a gas attack, but their deaths are less a judgement of the individual than of society as a whole. The reapers of war and fear hold sway, but a conversation between Ginny and Big Alice, the reaper of cruelty, indicates that here, too, responsibility is a critical factor. Of the soldiers, Alice asks 'When they dig their trenches, do you think they know that they're digging their own graves?' 'I do', Ginny answers (DeConnick et al. 2016: #8), and it is a horribly accurate observation; one of the disadvantages of trenches, in chemical warfare, is that the chlorine gas sinks to the lowest point, and those sheltering within the trenches have the least protection from it.

That the reaper of cruelty can recognise the harshness of this reality – a brutality both inflicted on the soldiers and inflicted by them, even on themselves – is painful to read. The individual soldiers may have little choice, given the consequences to themselves and their country of not fighting, but they do have some choice, as do their communities and their nations. That choice is underlined by the presence of the reaper of war, who presumably cannot facilitate the dying of those who exist outside of his own particular remit. This is, arguably, a form of justice, albeit an exceedingly hard one derived from choices that are both poor and limited.

The choices that result in these reapers are clearly linked, on a number of levels, to individual history. Ginny's mother, referred to within the text simply as Beauty, is confined in a tower by her jealous husband, Mason. Beauty's plea to her husband that she would 'die from despair if you put me in there!' (DeConnick et al. 2014: #1) is ignored, and her agency is disrespected. Miserable and alone, she prays for death. What arrives is Death himself, and this is presented as unusual. It quickly becomes clear that Death is in love with Beauty, but the latter's desire to die does not abate. Death facilitates that desire – although 'he wept as she passed' (#1) – giving Beauty the choice, and the agency, that her marriage denied her.

Beauty's choice takes place in exceedingly unusual circumstances, in that she has a relationship with Death that, admittedly, may just be one-sided. The inserted panels that show her initial suicide attempt within the tower have her ripping at her wrists with her own teeth. That desire does not abate over time. Beauty has little control over her own life and is capable only of choosing an end to it – but she does choose, and her choice not only appears to be respected and actively facilitated by Death, but it also produces a second agent of mortality.

Before she dies, Beauty gives birth to a daughter, who is subsequently raised by Death to be 'a reaper of vengeance, a hunter of men who have sinned' (DeConnick et al. 2014: #1). The most interesting element of these introductory panels is the question of Ginny's biological father. Cooper (2020: 54) argues that Ginny's paternity is established in the third issue, but the possibility of ambiguity remains – 'You are not the girl's father', Death proclaims to Mason, in defence of his own role as Ginny's parent (DeConnick et al. 2014: #3) – yet fatherhood can be adoptive as well as biological.

It is difficult to imagine that a Beauty who has fallen in love with Death, and who has given birth to his child, would still be so set on suicide. The alternative is that her husband confined her to the tower while pregnant and that she could not face raising the child or risking another romance with yet another individual who had power over her. That Death, who loved the mother, might choose to take in the child for that mother's sake, instead of returning her to the abusive biological parent, seems plausible. The skeletal elements of the adult Ginny's face could be attributed to her role as a reaper, rather than a biological parent; it is notable that, as an infant and later a child (and therefore before she became the active reaper of vengeance), these elements do not exist. That Ginny is raised to reap men who are like her mother's husband, and that she can be called by those who are victims as her mother was a victim – 'If you done been wronged, say her name, sing this song, sound the bell's knell that calls her from hell … Ginny rides for you on the wind' (DeConnick et al. 2014: #1) – may indeed be a slightly more vengeful vindication of the second paternal possibility but is not sufficient to be certain. What is certain is that the reaper of vengeance has been raised as a conscious repudiation of abusive relationships.

Barton argues that institutionalised revenge – and the inclusion of a reaper of vengeance within Death's wider purview is surely institutionalisation – is morally permissible, in that it validates 'victim resentment and anger' and acknowledges the 'moral legitimacy of victims' needs for retributive justice' (1999: 85). That Ginny's role is heavily influenced by her mother's victimisation is certain, but she is a reaper of vengeance and her role does not include prevention. The initial presentation of agency, as applied to Beauty's mortality, is quickly subverted, in a manner which speaks to the lingering influence of trauma within the narrative. Death may facilitate Beauty's passing, but once dead she belongs to him entirely, and the prison of her previous relationship is repeated in the lands of the dead. Aware that Death's time to die is also approaching, Beauty asks that they go on 'into the black' together (DeConnick et al. 2014: #4). This is a clear compromise on her part, and one that she appears to be unwilling to offer, as her daily requests to be able to go alone are continually rejected. 'I ask you to let me go', she says, as 'I have asked of you every day since you took me from his prison and brought me to yours' (#4).

Death, while initially presenting as respectful of Beauty's choice, has taken on the role of her former abuser. He has also, in the meantime, raised Beauty's daughter to be the reaper of vengeance. It is no surprise, then, that the relationship between Death and Ginny is fractured. This conflict between aspects of death has, at this point in the text, been prefigured in the fight between Ginny and Big Alice. Cruelty and vengeance might be thought, by some readers, to be naturally aligned, and, in some cases, they certainly would be. The text indicates that this alignment is, at least to some extent, expected: 'They were meant to be a pair, Ginny and Alice. Cruelty and Vengeance. But Ginny preferred to ride alone. And Alice ... Alice was never one to forgive a slight. The irony was lost on no one' (DeConnick et al. 2020: #4). Sometimes vengeance is cruel, but alternately, sometimes cruelty is visited upon those who don't deserve it. When this occurs, and a suffering child sings the song that calls Ginny to his family's aid, the reapers engage in combat.

That the reapers can enter into violent conflict on behalf of their charges underlines the importance of dialogue, agency, and the potential for chosen justice within the work. As the narrative continues, however, it becomes clear that the envisioning of death in *Pretty Deadly* is concerned not only with agency and justice but also with transformation. If an individual may invite a death, or a reaper, of peculiar and gruesome aspect, may they not earn another sort of death as well? *Pretty Deadly* appears to argue not only that they might but also that their choices can even cause them to transform into the very deaths that they have invited. This determined engagement with death, and the ability to engage differently with death, is illustrated in two separate storylines within the series.

The first concerns Beauty's abusive husband Mason, who returns to the tower in which he imprisoned his wife only to find her dead. His remorse is enormous, but remorse is not enough. He travels to the lands of Death in order to trade his life for Beauty's, and although Death does not allow this, he does offer him the hope of seeing her again if Mason will hunt down and kill an infant girl called Sissy. Mason locates the child but chooses instead to raise her himself. It is possible to argue that, having been confronted with Ginny as a young girl being raised by Death, he is trying to replace the potential daughter he has lost with another child. Though this argument has merit, it is overshadowed by the fact that Sissy is supposed to be Death's replacement.

Mason's love for the child is admittedly spurred on by remorse, but raising her kindly and doing his best to protect her is active atonement on his part. His abusive treatment of Beauty can never be remedied, but his determination to ensure that the next Death realises the value of love and compassion is both choice and transformation. It also, although this is never explicitly stated within the text, ensures that Sissy will become a Death who will never imprison someone as both Ginny's fathers did to Beauty. As a result, while Ginny may hold substantial resentment for Mason's treatment of her mother, his death does not come at her hands. In Issue #10 of *Pretty Deadly*, Mason's life and death have resulted in him becoming a reaper himself – the reaper of grace – and he is shown bringing a gentle death to a woman who has earned one.

The second storyline concerns a young woman, Clara, who after her death has been trapped by the reaper of obsession. When Ginny confronts this reaper, she and Clara are used as bait, in order to lure Sissy into the reaper of obsession's grasp. This further underlines the potential for conflict between reapers, and between the reapers and Death – the reapers may exist as functionaries of Death, and have specific roles to act out in relation to the dead and dying, but they exist as independent actors with their own motivations and ability to choose. As Sissy points out, however, that agency has limits, and one of those limits is the agency of others: Clara is able to free herself from the reaper of obsession and move forward in her own death through the act of forgiveness. 'If you can forgive, there ain't a rope in any realm what can bind you', Sissy advises her (DeConnick et al. 2020: #5). What follows is admittedly a general, rather than a specific, act. It is difficult for Clara to forgive the reaper of obsession, so she forgives easier personalities – including the uncle who never made enough time for her and the film director who exploited her work. She also forgives herself, and this allows Clara the freedom to escape the reaper that came for her, in much the same way as Mason's own choices allowed him to embrace an end which is different from that of vengeance. Ginny, who as the reaper of vengeance is intrinsically unable to forgive, remains entangled with the reaper of obsession at the current conclusion of the series. Arguably, this indicates that, as functionaries or aspects of death, the reapers are potentially incapable of change. Ginny, however, is a liminal creature, one who exists on the borderlines of the natural and supernatural worlds, and this may prefigure a yet-to-be tapped transformative capacity on her part.

In *Pretty Deadly*, then, visions of Death are both individual and transformative. Death has a number of functionaries, divided by vocation, and these reapers are responsible for facilitating the deaths of humans within their remit. Those humans, however, are capable of altering their experiences of, and interaction with, their assigned reaper through both active identification and invitation – as with the child who calls Ginny for aid – and through their own moral choices. Through the primary character of Deathface Ginny, this ability to choose is reflected in the reaper as well as those who are reaped, and the visions of death become, ultimately, visions of the self as well.

Bethan Michael-Fox and Renske Visser

# *Mrs Death Misses Death* (Salena Godden, 2021)

## Readdressing Erasure and the Personification of Death

In poet Salena Godden's debut novel, *Mrs Death Misses Death* (see Figure 32), death is personified as a series of Black women – older, younger, overworked and without work, famous and powerful, compared to Billie Holiday, Grace Jones and Nina Simone, and anonymous. As Godden writes:

> There is no human more invisible, more readily talked over, ignored, betrayed, and easy to walk past than a woman; a poor old black woman, a homeless black beggar-woman with knotty natty hair, broken back, walking ever so slow, slow, slow, pushing a shopping trolley full of plastic bottles. (2021: 2)

Godden's poetic, rhythmic literary portrayal challenges dominant representations of death as a skeletal figure, sometimes hooded and with milky white bones, which implies that death is white and probably male. It also counters the representation of death as a fully fleshed-out white man, as played by Fredric March in *Death Takes a Holiday* (1934) or by Brad Pitt in *Meet Joe Black* (1998). What Godden's challenge reveals is the extent to which the personification of death as white and male is normalised, and to which depictions of death are political.

Achille Mbembe (2003) has defined necropolitics as the social and political power that decides how some may live and how some must die in a broad genealogy of global inequality, terror, militarisation, racism and fascism. Godden's envisioning of death can be understood as engaged in representational necropolitics which both advances and reflects a broader push to diversify and decolonise discussions about death within and outside

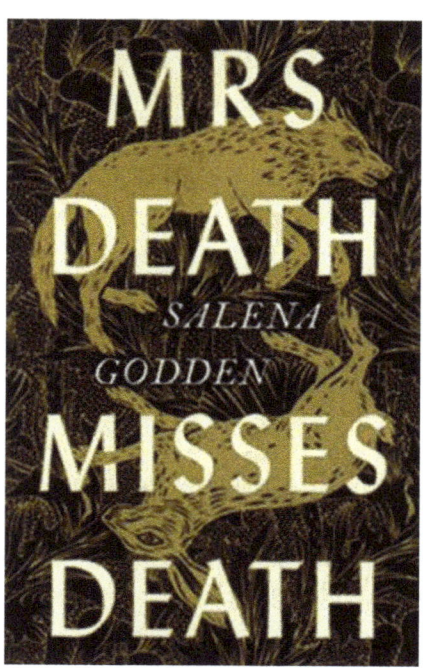

Figure 32. The cover of the hardback edition of *Mrs Death Misses Death*. Photo courtesy of Salena Godden.

of the burgeoning academic field of Death Studies. Theories within Death Studies, such as experiences of grief, bereavement and personal accounts of dying, have predominantly been based on the experiences of white middle-class people. While death and dying is a universal phenomenon, experiences will vary widely across the globe. As Maurice Jackson has emphasised, 'All people die, but not all people die alike' (1977: 82). This is why, for example, the Collective for Radical Death Studies' 'mission is to interrogate the field of Death Studies to decolonize and de-center whiteness while calling to radicalize death practices, all in theory and in practice from a variety of angles' (CRDS 2023). As noted by Renske Visser, 'in many ways Godden's work falls within the remit of Radical Death Studies. Her novel is a social critique of whose lives are acknowledged in death, which lives, and deaths are marginalized, unmarked, or seemingly unremarkable' (Visser 2021). Death

Studies, like other academic disciplines, is one in which increasing calls to decolonise need to be acknowledged. As Khyati Tripathi (2021) has noted, there is a 'great need' for greater diversity within the field. Whilst, as Visser writes, 'envisioning death as a black woman is the type of intersectionality that the academic discipline of Death Studies craves' (Visser 2022). Godden's novel is not explicitly academic and though it has been popular with the academic audience, it has far greater reach. The novel has been met with critical acclaim, winning both the Indie Book Award for Fiction and the People's Book Prize in 2022. With its broad popular appeal, *Mrs Death Misses Death* speaks and responds to broader calls to decolonise culture in myriad contexts as well as to give voice and presence to voices that have been ignored or erased (see Appiah 2020 for the case for capitalising the B in Black). The personification of Mrs Death as a Black woman can in this sense be understood as part of a broader political project to readdress cultural erasures.

One of the cultural erasures that *Mrs Death Misses Death* readdresses is that of women, and Godden enacts this through language. It is widely recognised that language itself is political, shaping how people see and experience the world. Death is a good example of this. As Grazyna Drzazga and Magda Stroinska (2012) note, the grammatical gender of death may in fact have far-reaching effects at the level of discourse and conceptualisation. It can also offer a challenge to those who translate texts from a language with a different gender allocation. In some languages, for example, Portuguese and Polish, death is female, and in German death is male. Other languages, like English, do not assign gender to nouns, though Death personified is predominantly portrayed as male, and called 'he', demonstrating patriarchal ideologies that underpin the tendency to default to masculine personal pronouns. In *Mrs Death Misses Death*, the title of the book utilises the gendered 'Mrs' to signify a woman. Yet 'Mrs' is a title denoting a woman who is married in the English language, and this opens up the possibility that Mrs Death is not Death, but Death's wife. It is throughout the novel that Godden utilises the personification of death as a literary device for exploring the social construction of gender, of death, in addition to the broader issues of inequality, explicitly positioning Mrs Death not as the wife but as Death herself. Godden begins by questioning the dominant designation of death as male, writing in the first person from the perspective of death:

> The greatest trick man played was making you believe I was a man. They erased me and made you all believe that Death was male in spirit – the Grim Reaper in a black hood with a scythe. Remarkable that nobody questioned it really, don't you think? For surely only she who bears it, she who gave you life, can be she who has the power to take it. The one is she. (2021: 2)

Godden emphasises the life-giving biological capacity of (some, not all) women, ties this to female power (the power to give life and to take it away) and reiterates the gendered pronoun in stating 'the one is she' (2021: 2). As the novel develops, she also draws attention to the social and cultural marginalisation of women, and arguably of death (for debates about whether death is 'denied', see Tradii and Martin (2019) and Martin and Tradii (2019)). As Godden explains:

> Mrs Death is the woman we hardly see, the woman we do not care to see. She is the person we ignore, she is the pause in the silence, she is the invisible woman. She is the refugee at the border. She is the cleaner. She is the cab driver. She is the backing singer we never bother to learn the name of. She is nobody and she is everybody. She is the homeless person begging for change at the train station. Mrs Death is the spirit of the ignored and the saint of the betrayed. She is the first woman. Mrs Death is the first mother of all mothers. She is calling to us all now. He is weeping. She is cradling her crumbling world. She is holding this toxic and wounded planet to her cold breast. She is sitting next to you on the bus. She is amongst us. I got it wrong. Mrs Death is not the wife of Death. No. And she is not the mother of Death. No. She is Death, and she gets the final say. (2021: 36–7)

Godden makes references not only to women as a broad category but also to socioeconomic inequality within the context of engrained global capitalism and to the intersectionality of gender discrimination, emphasising women who are marginalised, discriminated against and ignored not only for their gender but also for their status as refugees, low paid workers and those in the background of the sociocultural landscape. She goes on to produce an image of a nurturing, loving Mrs Death cradling a toxic planet gendered linguistically as 'he', suggesting the role of patriarchal ideologies in ecological destruction and social inequality – signalling the notion of 'toxic masculinity' (see Giannini 2022 for a discussion of this term). The extract above closes with the confirmation that Mrs Death is not the wife of death, or the mother of death, but Death herself. By giving the 'final say' to Mrs Death, Godden can be seen to readdress the disregard and exclusion of women historically and in the present, both socially and culturally. Godden is explicit about this in the below extract, which explores the positioning of women as having only a reproductive function – a life-giving function – and not what is constructed as the masculine function and power to take life away:

> We are programmed to believe that the female is here for birth, she is mother, she is here to nurture a soul inside her body and to feed the infant at her breast. That the woman may house new life and soul, and feed and care for a soul, but she may not be the power that takes a soul. I am here. Death is a woman. Surely by erasing me we have erased this power. By never portraying a woman as the representative of Death, the boss of Death, the figure of Death itself, one could debate that an important and fundamental disempowerment takes place. Perhaps this is what erasure looks like. (2021: 162–3)

Godden explicitly challenges the dominant personification of Death as a man in this extract, and she suggests that the erasure of women and of the possibility of women as sufficiently powerful to be Death itself is disempowering. In doing so, her personification of Death as a woman comes to function as a form of re-empowerment, a call to women to identify themselves with power, and to bring about change.

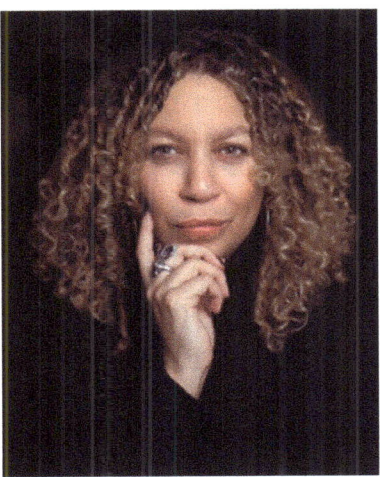

Figure 33. Photograph of Salena Godden. Provided by the Author.

Godden (see Figure 33) has reflected in an interview with *The Death Studies Podcast* (2022) on her motivation for writing the book and on her interest in death, as well as the connections she makes in the novel between the personification of Death as a woman and broader themes of social justice. Godden explains that she has 'always been drawn to the way death is portrayed in art and in poetry and in song and theatre' (Godden 2022). She also shares that she has always had 'quite a relationship with death […] from being quite empathic as a young child' and in relation to her father dying when she was aged nine (written about in her memoir *Springfield Road*, 2014). Godden suggests that it is 'healthy to be friends with death', and the novel itself has been popular with the global Death Positive movement. It is because the book was written over a long period of time (around a decade) – not for a publisher or a deadline but, instead, because she was drawn to the ideas – that it came to include explicit and implicit references to 'different stories in the news', 'real time injustice and crimes' as well as experiences of 'personal loss.' A bulk of the writing took place in 2015 and 2016 when the stories of Grenfell Tower, Prince and David Bowie's death, were 'whirling and swirling around in her subconscious and her dreams' (Godden 2022). Godden imagined 'conversations with death and what she'd say to us' in response to these events. Emphasising the social justice themes central to *Mrs Death Misses Death*, Godden articulates that in the novel 'death is in protest', 'angry' and telling readers that 'if we carry on like this everything will be gone' (Godden 2022). The vision of Death here is one that is willing to 'fight for us' and 'to find more balance, and justice, and voice' as she walks in the guise of 'people that we walk past in society, or people that we don't value, invisible people, unheard people. Someone homeless in a doorway or an old lady on the bus that we're ignoring' (Godden 2021). In this sense, the personification of death in the novel can be understood to readdress broader erasures – of difficult losses, of social injustices and of evidence of global climate crisis.

Godden has explained that there are many reasons she took the decision to make death specifically a Black woman in the novel, with the most obvious being that she herself is a Black woman. Another, she has explained in her interview with *The Death Studies Podcast* (2022), is to do with the context in which the character of Mrs Death came to her. She heard it first as a voice in her head as she walked through Whitechapel at Christmas, saying the words

'I know a lot of dead people now' (Godden 2022) – in hindsight, she wonders if this voice emerged from one of her ancestors, perhaps her maternal great-great-grandmother in Jamaica. There may be 'some of her in there' (Godden 2022), in the character of Mrs Death, who is a strong Black medicine/healer woman like her ancestor was. Godden explains that there are both political and personal reasons for the fact that Godden is a Black woman. She suggests that, on reflection, she is herself 'in the middle somewhere of it, in that I think Wolf is the confused suicidal teenager I once was and then Mrs Death the wise old woman I hope to become – I am neither of those things now, so in some ways it's a conversation' (2022). The character of Wolf, a non-binary young person who is visited by Mrs Death after a near-death experience in a fire, also functions to explore dominant gender constructions and their potentially suffocating nature. Again, the readdressing of erasure is evident in the novel, which not only personifies death as women and specifically Black women who have historically, culturally, socially and at present suffered erasure but also explores the erasure of different gender identities.

Godden has explained that she wanted the book to be concise, and not a 'massive, great big heavy book', because she understood that 'some of the messages and meanings and thoughts and dreams and visions were pretty heavy anyway' (2022). Godden did not envisage the book being so successful and was 'prepared for it to bomb', especially given the fact that it was being published during a pandemic when people might want 'happy happy clappy Salena, jokey joke around Salena' (2022), rather than a mediation on grief and loss – Godden is often described as one of Britain's best-loved poets, and many of her poems are humorous and/or joyful. Yet the success of the novel has been evident, and the book rights to *Mrs Death Misses Death* have been purchased by Idris Elba's production company, Green Door Pictures. This suggests that a visual representation of Mrs Death is imminent, and will no doubt bring fresh audiences to the novel and its themes. The novel and its success are evidence of a clear appetite for personifications of death that challenge normative and dominant ones. Godden, who describes her work as 'full of hope and seeking hope' (Godden 2022), offers in *Mrs Death Misses Death* the hope of more dynamic, politically engaged, socially just and powerful personifications of death.

Part V

# Global Pandemics: Contagion, Mental Health and Dementia

# Image Intervention VI: The Source

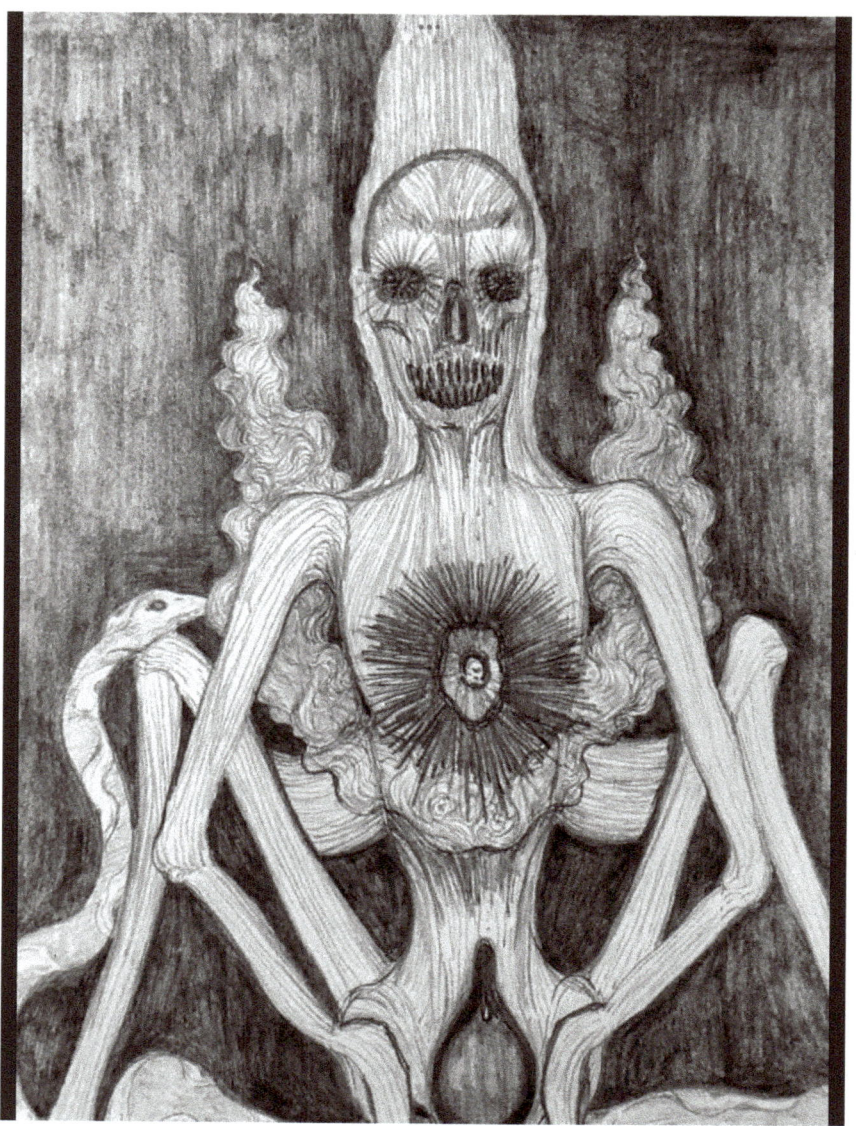

Artwork by Gemma Files
(Reproduced with the permission of the artist)

Cath Davies

# Coco (Lee Unkrich, 2017)

## 'Not bad for a dead guy': Conceptualising the Corpse

How the deceased occupy the spaces and experiences of the living despite their ontological absence is at the heart of Disney/Pixar *Coco* (Unkrich 2017). This animated feature film is a reminder that tensions between bodily presence and absence in discourses on death are frequently assessed in popular culture. Media texts are valuable platforms signposting conceptualisations of death, mourning and memorialisation (Hallam and Hockey 2001, Aaron 2013, 2014, Penfold-Mounce 2018). These are mediums that formulate and interrogate presumptions about mortality and, in the process, highlight thematic and visual techniques that shape representations of the deceased. This chapter will evaluate the film's narrative devices that foreground posthumous identity, with specific attention to the composition of the cadaver. Meanings inherent in bodily forms are investigated to evaluate an array of design features that materialise the dead.

*Coco* interrogates symbiotic relationships between the living and deceased, reimagining visual culture's significance in preserving and restoring a tangible presence for the dead (Bronfen 1992, Walter et al. 1995, Mulvey 2006, Aaron 2014, Troyer 2020). The film's primary narrative focus is on remembrance rituals that substantiate posthumous presence. However, it is also a significant text in its conceptualising of the corpse as a material entity existing beyond the territories of the living. The film probes how the body in death assumes 'two different shapes' (Benkel and Meitzler 2019: 235), synthesising the corpse's biological form and sociocultural construction. This chapter deconstructs the cadaver as a character in *Coco* by identifying how the dynamics of bodily preservation and decay are illuminated in the landscapes of the film.

## 'So their spirits can cross over': Designing the Deceased in the Spaces of the Living

*Coco* is a study on how the living cope with the loss of loved ones. How the deceased retain an identity within the domain of the living is the central premise of the film. Set in Mexico, the film follows our pre-teen protagonist Miguel's adventures into the afterlife to restore an equilibrium between his deceased and living relatives. Preparations for Mexico's traditional remembrance ceremony Day of the Dead is the pivotal plot motivator. This carnivalesque celebration, where skeletal surrogates are embellished and blend seamlessly with the living, provides a catalyst for the film's dissection of posthumous regeneration.

In this context, the film specifically highlights mourning and remembrance strategies. Photographs, audio recordings and family tales express familiar memorialising discourses that ensure the deceased are interwoven into the spaces and routines of the living. Love and respect for the dead are exemplified in artefacts that secure a recognisable presence within domestic spaces. We are reminded that these are meaningful objects that 'guide our ancestor's home' (Unkrich 2017). They become agents that stimulate memories and storytelling and keep the deceased very much alive in family history. This is especially notable when Miguel informs us of the family trauma relating to his great-grandmother Coco and her estranged father Hector. Hector's shameful abandonment of his family when Coco was a child has resulted in his presence being vehemently erased within memorialising traditions. He is not remembered fondly by subsequent generations and is almost not remembered at all. It is only Coco who has retained a photograph of him, and this is hidden to quell any family shame.

*Coco* thus documents the function of material objects in inscribing a tangible presence for the dead (Hallam and Hockey 2001, Meyer and Woodthorpe 2008, Gibson 2011). The deceased are, in effect, reimagined through artefacts that perform as counterpoints to the demise of the mortal body (Belting 2011). Disintegration and bodily decomposition are subsequently disavowed with effigies that regenerate and embalm the deceased – a process of 'technological taxidermy' (Davies 2010). Material culture re-animates, generating a cohesive identity, 'a stable image/sign of that body' (Bronfen 1992: 46). In *Coco*, these mementoes are expressions of love and affection, and they provide a posthumous framing of a life well lived. This is especially pertinent when Miguel's Day of the Dead adventure catapults him accidentally into the afterlife. Here he encounters the disgraced great-great grandfather who has a very different story to tell about his disappearance from Coco's life. As the film progresses, Miguel unearths the historic injustice that explains Hector's hasty retreat from the family unit when Coco was an infant. The storyline is thus actively preoccupied with Miguel's quest to restore Hector's posthumous identity. This is expressed visually in the final scenes when his surrogate presence is reinstated and his photograph adorns the wall alongside other relatives.

Convergences between death, embodiment and image cultures are, however, not only interwoven in the remembrance rituals of the storyline. *Coco* develops its narrative preoccupations with shaping the deceased by also foregrounding the corporeality of the cadaver itself. Drawing on the notion that the corpse encapsulates 'a particular set of bodily characteristics' (Hallam et al. 1999: 62), this film interrogates the conceptual tropes that materialise the deceased, which are evident when we encounter them as characters in their afterlife.

## 'I miss my nose': The Cadaver as an Animated Figure

*Coco* responds to the traditions of material objects as posthumous avatars by highlighting the value of remembrance to the cadaver's physical existence elsewhere. Rather than focusing only on how the living interact with the dead, we see an alternative perspective in this film as the concept of materialising posthumous identity is further scrutinised. When Miguel travels into the afterlife, we become privy to how the deceased interact in their domain, and it is evident that their life is shaped by memories in the land of the living. The cadavers' conversations pivot on the thoughts of their loved ones still grieving for them, and they are completely reliant on a memorialising process. Furthermore, material entities assume a remarkable significance to the dead as photographic images of them alive are necessary passports for transit to physically participate in the Day of the Dead celebrations. Being remembered by their relatives is their currency to ensure legal refuge for the day. These practices are even more significant because the preservation of their surrogate forms in memories and objects is actually keeping them alive in the afterlife. Photographs and aural recordings embalming their living incarnations literally constitute preserving their corporeal substance elsewhere.

The film's afterlife scenes foreground the cadaver as a tangible entity, predicated on its surrogate presence in the land of the living. This substantiates how a posthumous form is constructed. Each cadaver is personalised, and their characters are designed in their emotional responses to their previous living incarnations. Characters are composed through the interplay between materials. The dead are designed as a skeletal frame reliant on sartorial embellishments to construct identity. Clothing and props are devices that inscribe individuality to indistinguishable skeletal bones in this film. Adornment practices thus replicate the dressed body of the living and act as a connective tissue to their past identities embalmed in photographs of them when alive. Clothing contributes to the skeletal body's composition of personhood by mirroring memorial traditions in the land of the living. Remembrance rituals, from gravestones' inscriptions, personal possessions and monuments for example, signpost a preoccupation with preserving subjectivity and disavowing the facelessness of the corpse (Aries 1974, Bronfen and Goodwin 1993, Davis 2004, Benkel and Meitzler 2019). Remnants of the deceased's living incarnations are not only foregrounded in sartorial practices in this film. Skeletal bones are also dressed in the corporeal matter of hair and eyes, features that directly embed the character with emotion and individuality. *Coco*'s cadavers have clearly maintained some material essence of the living body despite their dissipated flesh. Such devices position the corpse as maintaining a direct correlation with their once living form. This is achieved by integrating additional materials within the skeletal frame to emulate a life-like physiognomy.

Nevertheless, despite comforting indicators of the self within sartorial practices, *Coco* does not completely avert its gaze from highlighting the reality of the corpse's penchant for decomposition. We are still reminded of bodily dissolution when Hector's eyes fall out in front of Miguel, providing a terrifying confrontation with a form that has lost its individual character and soul.

Here, Miguel confronts the realisation of the dead body as unruly and fragmented as Hector scrambles to relocate his eyeballs apologetically in order to continue the conversation. As an agent of 'dysfunction and disorder' (Howarth 2007: 186), the cadaver's gradual decomposition diminishes facial characteristics that once inscribed recognisability. Collapsing flesh naturally destabilises the individuality residing in the face (Howson 2004, Shilling 1993). In a comic moment, the film thus acknowledges the dead body's material deterioration, corporeal decay and threat to physiognomy.

In its recognition of material unruliness, the film also transgresses the borders of a benign representation of the corpse by suturing moments of existential dread into the narrative trajectory. It appears that the deceased share the living's dread of the passing of time. The mortal body's disintegrating capabilities (and subsequent anxiety) are equally embedded in cadavers' character dispositions. The passing of time is also crucially inscribed on their bodies in the afterlife. This landscape directly mirrors the somatic vulnerabilities experienced by the living characters as the cadavers' remaining matter is precariously hovering between the territories of the afterlife and the domain of complete obliteration. It is evident that the afterlife is not the final destination for the dead after all. They are permitted to exist as a tangible entity only when they are alive in the memories and artefacts belonging to the living. As these surrogate avatars diminish, so do the corpse configurations dematerialise, and this is known as 'the final death' (Unkrich 2017).

This is the fate of Cheech, whose skeletal form and matter evaporate into dust when the last of his loved ones dies. This understanding motivates Miguel's quest to restore Hector's presence in the memorialising rituals of the family. Hector is threatened with extinction in the afterlife as Coco nears her death. She's the only figure keeping him alive as a tangible skeletal body because the rest of the family have erased him. The corpse as material matter thus correlates directly with preservation practices in their corresponding surrogate human form. Despite designing the dead as already having experienced the decomposition of flesh, the cadavers suffer further anxieties about the dissolution of their limited bodily frame. They yearn to embalm their bodies, to exist as matter however incomplete this may be.

Tensions in maintaining a fixed bodily shape in the face of deteriorating flesh are also reflected in Miguel's personal race against time. His mortality is threatened as he lingers too long in the afterlife. The afterlife is a terrain that erodes healthy living flesh, and Miguel witnesses his own gradual decomposition which signifies that life is draining away from him. This is composed as an interplay between a solid somatic silhouette allowing him to continue interacting with the dead, but his clothes are concealing the dissolving flesh beneath the fabric. Unlike the makeup he uses to camouflage the healthy textures of his youthful body earlier in the film, the reality of the dead body is characterised by translucent surfaces, exposing the bones beneath as he's transitioning into a full-fledged liminal form.

The medium of animation successfully accentuates the body as physical matter thereby presenting different variations of corporeality: alive and dead. Reflections on the aesthetic and material credentials of the dead body are therefore explicitly addressed. The body of the deceased is aesthetically liminal, further highlighting the presence/absence paradox of death. Somatic unruliness is integral to the design of the body at different stages of life and death in the film. Subsequently, *Coco* provides an effective mediation on corporeal configurations in documenting the deceased.

### 'I woke up dead': Conceptualising Death's Paradox

*Coco* contributes significantly to the discourses on designing the dead in popular culture, interrogating tensions that 'recover the disappearing body' (Hallam and Hockey 1999: 23) in its multiple configurations of posthumous bodies. The 'recovery' process permeates the narrative in an account of remembrance practices that pivot on restoring the absent body of the deceased with material signifiers. Thus, the disappearing body is reframed and subsequently embalmed in audio recordings and photographs as the deceased assumes a posthumous presence in the domain of the living. The film accentuates the integral role that material culture plays in synthesising emotional responses to death. It exemplifies the symbiotic relationship between loss and restoring a surrogate bodily presence in memorialising practices.

Moreover, this presence/absence paradox in discourses of death and dying is explored by observing the reconstruction of the bodily form from the perspective of the deceased. The dead exist as a physical matter only when composed in surrogate forms by the living and rely on such practices to exist as cadavers. The film significantly extends observations on recovering and regenerating a tangible presence for the absent body of the dead. It sutures the disappearing body itself into the narrative, foregrounding an array of compositions of decomposition. The cadavers provide alternative posthumous bodies to those embalmed in the artefacts of the living, thus destabilising tropes of somatic integrity that infuse these material objects. The disappearing body of the dead is effectively shaped in its many stages of disintegration.

*Coco* has imaginatively interwoven the social body of the deceased with its organic counterpart. Whilst the occupants of the material world and the afterlife would initially imply a territorial binary, the film is significantly preoccupied with eroding such distinctively drawn boundaries. The cadavers are sentient beings – reflective entities with an awareness of their own existential predicament. They express emotional bonds to their living relatives and experience loss with a similar yearning to be reunited. The dead are designed with memories that shape their personalities, and their living experiences are at the forefront of their identity. These skeletal bodies possess a consciousness, which motivates them to keep living in the afterlife, to exist as matter and to be present whilst evaluating their past lives. By humanising the cadaver, they are designed as mirroring the living, aligned through tropes of recognisable subjectivity. Consequently, there is an embalming procedure preserving personhood and individual personality inscribed within a cadaverous body whose physical materiality continues to diminish.

*Coco* evaluates thematic preoccupations and design features that conceptualise the corpse in visual culture. Posthumous identity is predicated on discourses of preservation sutured with configurations of dematerialisation. A textual autopsy reveals that the dead are composed of tropes connoting material restoration and decomposition concurrently. The film thus exemplifies an interplay between discourses of tangibility and dissolution in the dynamics of the corpse. In doing so, it makes a valuable contribution to popular culture's capacity for animating and reconfiguring death in the twenty-first century.

Simon Bacon

# *The Thing* (Matthijs van Heijningen Jr, 2011)

This chapter will consider the depiction of the Covid-19 microbe in popular news media during the height of the pandemic to propose that its ubiquity and non-human representation saw it resonate more closely with popular horror narratives than medical ones. Subsequently, by examining the unique representation of alien and deadly microbes in selected horror films, it will be suggested that the depiction of the coronavirus resonated with other images within the popular imaginary to give the microbe even more deadly connotations seeing it not just as an image of contagion but of Death itself.

## Introduction

Whilst all viruses are spread by microbes, it is with the recent Covid-19 pandemic that an image of the microbe has come to represent the disease itself. As the virus began to spread across the world with varying responses from the nations involved, the one image that seemed to unite all of them was the now familiar orb covered in barbs – these are actually protein spikes, whose crown-like, or corona-like, appearance has given the disease its name of 'coronavirus'. In lieu of images of the source of the outbreak – such as an animal or definite location – the inhuman microbe seemed to take on a malevolent life of its own appearing on all news updates hovering on our screens like an alien life-form come to earth to wreak havoc upon humanity.

Although the existence of microorganisms has been known since about the sixth century BC, they were observed under the microscope by Antonie van Leeuwenhoek only in the 1670s. More well-known is Louis Pasteur's work when he discovered the connection between microbes and food spoilage in the 1850s, and importantly for this study, it was in the 1880s that Robert Koch found that microorganisms caused tuberculosis, cholera, diphtheria and anthrax. While knowledge of the existence of microbes became more common, images of them or how they worked were not, and certainly not beyond the medical community. It is of particular interest then as to how they have made their way into the narratives of popular entertainment media such as cinema.

Of interest here is the film *Nosferatu* (Murnau 1922), which is not a movie you would necessarily link to the idea of disease, even though they make much of the vampire being a plague carrier. In fact, the scene in question does not involve contagion but rather the vampiric qualities of nature – as shall be seen, microbes are often framed in very vampire-like ways. In the film, we see a professor surrounded by students as he tells them about predators in nature: the first is a Venus Fly Trap, while the second is a polyp attacking a water flea (see Figure 34). The latter is very interesting as the image shown is in extreme

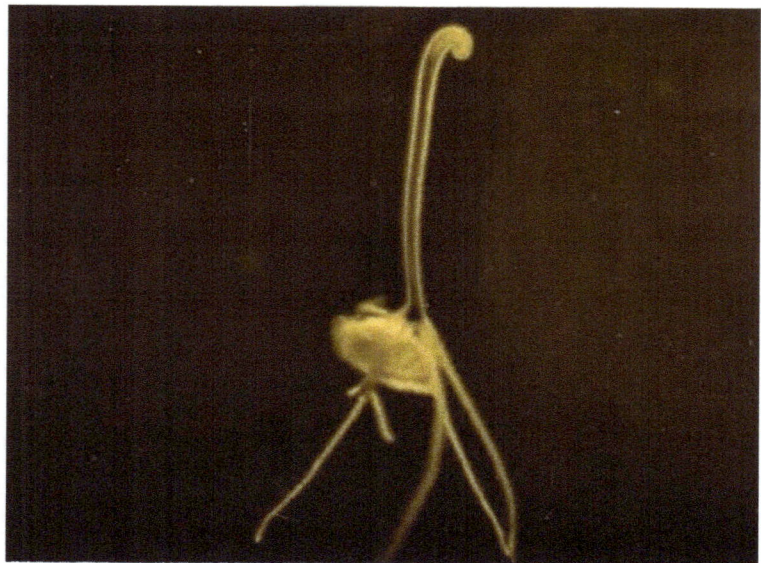

Figure 34. Microscopic vampires. *Nosferatu*, directed by F. W. Murnau (Prana Film, 1922).

close-up and almost at a microscopic level, and though not a microbe, it works in a very similar manner to more recent images to be discussed in this chapter.

The image of the polyp we see seems more like an outline next to the tiny water flea. The 'legs' of the polyp wrap itself around the creature readying it for consumption. The professor describes a vampiric world of 'phantoms' that consume lives to survive, as demonstrated by the amoeba-like polyp enveloping its prey. This idea seems to have a strong influence on the next movie of note *House of Dracula* (Kenton 1945), especially in its depictions of vampire blood. *House of Dracula* is a curious film that tries to medicalise both the vampire and the Wolf Man – the werewolfism seemingly caused by pressure building within the brain and Count Dracula's condition originating from some kind of blood disease. To study this, the scientist in the film, Dr Edelman, while trying to treat the count, collects a blood sample and examines it under a microscope (see Figure 35). We are shown what the doctor observes: round human blood cells being attacked by things that look not dissimilar to the polyp from *Nosferatu*; the image we see in the film is obviously a hand-painted one and hence shows no movement.

Of note here is the idea of trying to cure vampirism via blood by creating some kind of antibodies that have the ability to cure those afflicted. Although here it is the vampiric microbes that might spread the disease, it is Count Dracula who remains the central attraction as a figure representing Death.[1]

*The Andromeda Strain* (Wise 1971), our next important example from the 1970s, shifts its focus away from supernatural sources to the extra-terrestrial by portraying potentially catastrophic microbes originating from outer space. In the film, a returning space probe that crashes into the earth near a remote town in a desert carries an otherworldly microbe that turns its victim's blood into dust. The film spends a great deal of effort in its attempts to visualise the alien invader on screen rather than just showing its effects on the human body, which is the recourse of many films on diseases and pandemics. More so, in contrast to other films of the period like *Fantastic Voyage* (1966), it eschews

---

1   It should be noted that although Richard Matheson's novel *I Am Legend* (1954) does feature blood and the medicalisation of the vampire, the 2007 filmic adaptation of this book, *I Am Legend* (2007) as well as films such as *The Last Man on Earth* (1964) and *The Omega Man* (1971) never show microscopic representations of blood.

236                                      Simon Bacon

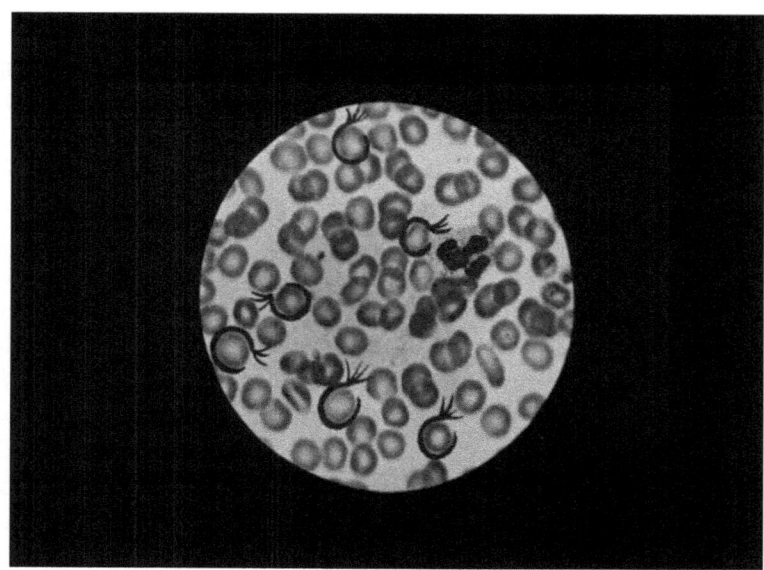

Figure 35. Alien microbes vampirising human blood cells. *House of Dracula*, directed by Erle C. Kenton (Universal Pictures, 1945).

'realistic' representations of the inside of the human body for those that are more dependent on technological interpretation emphasising the conceptual symbolism of the disease. In *The Andromeda Strain*, scientists soon arrive at the crash site, equipped to collect samples, which they transport to a secure underground laboratory specifically designed to handle potential biological warfare scenarios – this was Cold War America after all. Unlike other films, this one offers us two versions of what the microbe looks like, and both are very different from what has previously been portrayed. The first one is more akin to a computer code – and is very much related to the early days of computers – in which the microbe is represented by a series of numbers (0, 1, 2, 3, 4). Whilst this bears no comparison to a real cell, it does contain something akin to the idea of DNA and cellular coding (see Figure 36).[2]

2    Although the existence of DNA was proven in 1869 by Freidrich Miescher, modern microbiology developed only later, and the DNA's double-helix structure was not confirmed until 1957.

Figure 36. Veracity given to the representation of deadly microbes through cutting-edge technological representation. *The Andromeda Strain*, directed by Robert Wise (Universal Pictures, 1971).

The second image is completely different and is more of a layered animation of blue-green crystalline shapes that bear little relation to anything organic, but does show the shifting, mutating, alien nature of the contagion. The film ends with the microbe mutating into a form that is not harmful to humans.[3]

The next film *The Thing* (Carpenter 1982) combines science fiction with horror, synthesizing various earlier concepts into a narrative tailored to the audience's preconceptions of how the microbe should appear and behave. The 'disease' in *The Thing* exhibits monstrous mutations but enters its victims via the blood stream. Its presence can be detected by testing the blood of the affected person.[4] At one point the doctor at the Antarctic outpost where the

---

3   This is an interesting feature that rarely makes its way into later examples and certainly not in relation to the recent Covid-19 pandemic, which is curious given how important mutations have become in its ongoing narrative.

4   In this sense, it mirrors films of the 1980s and beyond, such as *The Hunger* (1983), which deal with real diseases such as AIDS but depict only the effects of contracting it rather than representing the disease via blood cells. The recent *120 BPM* (2017) portrays this

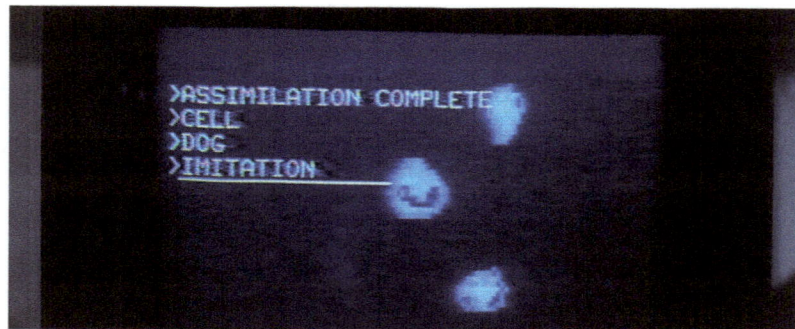

Figure 37. Alien microbes and blood disease as an arcade game. *The Thing*, directed by John Carpenter (Universal Pictures, 1982).

outbreak has occurred conducts some tests on a blood sample he has procured and displays the results. As with *The Andromeda Strain*, the computer screen is the preferred viewing device. The image mirrors the visual quality of 1980s graphics, which presents the vampirism enacted in a manner reminiscent of an arcade game (see Figure 37), particularly the game Asteroids which was released in 1979.

In many ways, it looks less realistic than its much earlier representation in *House of Dracula*; however, to the popular audience of the 1980s, this would have appeared more believable due to the use of modern means of representation; this idea is further consolidated in the film when the computer is used to calculate infection rates thereby lending it a form of mathematic veracity. The film also symbolises the notion of curing disease as a fight against an alien invader, a theme that permeates not only the depiction of blood cells but also the entire narrative.

However, by the 2000s such representations were not sophisticated enough for the audience, at least in terms of the kinds of visuals they were used to not just via film but also through computer games and other kinds of image manipulation. This takes us to the next film called *The Thing* (Hiejningen Jr, 2011), which is not a remake but rather a prequel to the earlier film. This

---

in a slightly different manner through a 'realistic' depiction of blood cells as seen in *The Thing* (2011).

2011 film is much more 'realistic' in its representation of microbes and, perhaps equally important, in its portrayal of the outbreak narrative. It has not been mentioned much so far, but many of the films described above follow something of an established outbreak narrative, which has become central to how things like pandemics are packaged, explained and understood. To explain this better, it is worth quickly looking at the film *Contagion* (2011) by Steven Soderbergh. *Contagion* follows a very expected pathway, indeed pretty much the same outbreak narrative that can be found in Priscilla Wald's book *Contagious* (2008). Here then, once an outbreak is identified, it is followed by specific stages and/or tropes: the discovery of the point of origin, the search for 'patient zero' who carries the disease out into the world, contact tracing and implementation of quarantine, the capture and study of the disease itself, and the production of vaccines and their subsequent distribution. Something similar can be seen in *World War Z* (Forster 2013) though more so in the book by Max Brook (2006) from which the film is adapted.[5] *Contagion* neatly wraps up its narrative as a discrete and contained event by revealing the true 'patient zero' of the entire outbreak at the end of the story – it was an infected bat that dropped some half-eaten food into a pig pen, and the pig that ate it subsequently passing it on to humans. However, we never actually 'see' the microbe that is the disease but only the effects it has on the world around it. *The Thing* follows a very similar outbreak narrative except for two differences: first, we 'see' the contagion, and, second, it is a story that never ends.

*The Thing* sees the members of an Antarctic research station encroach into alien territory and bring something back to their base camp. This 'patient zero' quickly begins to infect the members of the group which prompts the female anthropologist to investigate the cause and find a way to defeat the deadly disease. She does this by taking samples from one of the infected patients and examining them under the microscope. As in the earlier films, we are shown healthy cells and alien microbes, although this time not on a computer screen, but directly through the lens of the microscope (see Figure 38). Here we not only see the easily recognisable circular human blood cells, very

---

5   *Contagion* also rather presciently includes an extra part of the narrative around misinformation, which is eventually dispelled in the film but is far more resistant in real life as seen during the Covid-19 pandemic.

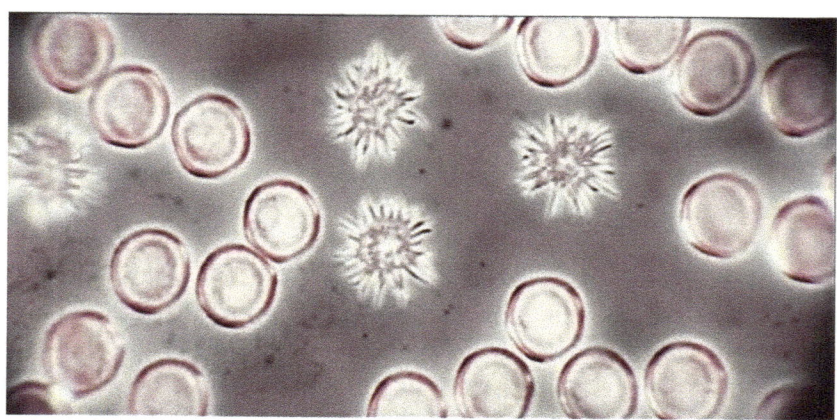

Figure 38. Polyp, corona-like alien cells that mutate to become indistinguishable from our own. *The Thing*, directed by Matthijs van Hejningen Jr (Universal Pictures, 2011).

much harking back to *House of Dracula*, but alongside them, we are able to spot the spiky globes that constitute the alien cells, which in appearance are oddly not much different from the polyps in *Nosferatu*, though much closer to what the recent coronavirus looks like – a coincidental yet interesting detail.

We then observe these alien cells attach themselves to the human cells, 'consume' them and then replicate them so that the human cells are not destroyed but become alien themselves. The doctor then realises that the contagion does not always present itself in those it has infected and is extremely mutational; this narrative is borne out through the rest of the film. She further deduces that the contagion cannot 'infect' non-biological matter and that all parts of it are alive, and hence even contaminated blood will react to preserve its life. Armed with this knowledge, she enforces a regime of quarantine and testing but to no avail. Although the film ends with the researchers tracing the contagion back to its source, a spaceship buried under the snow, the narrative does not offer a neat conclusion as *Contagion* did, and the disease is shown mutating faster than any cure can be found. Indeed, the mutations of the disease are so extreme that Death has no face or shape but becomes diffused into the environment itself.

Real-life events, of course, are very different from fictional narratives, but as noted by Wald (2008: 2), films and popular media often provide frameworks that help us make sense of the world around us, and consequently, the formula of the outbreak narrative has been continually applied to the ongoing pandemic. Covid-19's place of origin was quickly determined as China and probably in the environs of Wuhan but details beyond that are contested with original cases potentially being as early as September 2019. This is coupled with the ongoing uncertainty as to whether it had natural origins, was it an infected animal or did it spread from a specimen that escaped from a scientific laboratory (there is one in the environs of Wuhan). The fuzziness of the start of the outbreak narrative seems to plague its ongoing unravelling; the contagion can be seen by its effects, yet they can vary greatly with many being infected but not showing any symptoms; testing, tracing and quarantine are easier in theory than practice with only quarantine having any real effect. Although studying the disease and creating vaccines have occurred at a phenomenally fast rate, we are continually running into coherent issues over distribution – some require incredibly low temperatures to be maintained during transportation thereby making it difficult in all but the most-developed countries. In addition, the disease keeps mutating which calls into question the efficacy of the vaccines created as well as the number of doses that might be required. Last, the unexpected level of resistance from the general population to vaccines due to misinformation results in the inability to meet the levels of immunity required within the population to effectively 'kill' the disease, and consequently, the disease continues to circulate and mutate. Oddly, the one stable thing through the pandemic has been the image of the microbe itself: the orb wearing its corona of spikes (see Figure 39).

Whilst all else changed and wavered – the efficacy of masks, or face shields, the minimum safety distance that needs to be maintained between people, length of lockdowns, maximum number of people allowed in enclosed spaces – the hovering, emotionless microbe was consistent. In its blankness and ubiquity, it was not so much an image of the disease but a symbol of its effects, including the daily count of the infected and dead, and the number of available hospital beds and respirators; of lost loved ones and family members; of make-shift hospitals and mortuaries. In this sense, it stopped being a microbe and morphed into a signifier – not just of death, but of Death itself. With a corona-enclosed face, like Death, it has meant something slightly different to the almost 4 million people it has ushered from this world to the

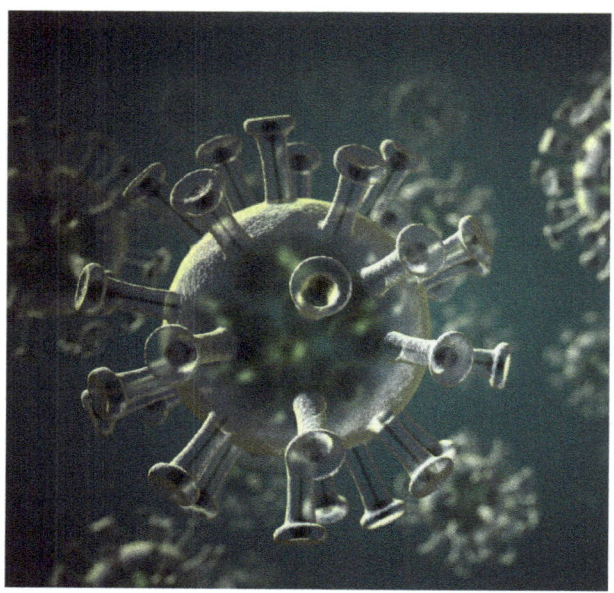

Figure 39. Corona virus Covid-19. Whilst details might change slightly, the symbol remains the same faceless, emotionless Death. Image in the public domain.

next. Indeed, it is this air of consistency around the microbe that identifies many of the issues around the ongoing response to Covid-19. In many ways, it speaks to the consistency that was required but missing from the outbreak narrative; the reliable microbe reflected the need for a consistent narrative from start to end, thus showing a disease that was identifiable and, therefore, eradicable. However, life is far fuzzier than that, and so the microbe has come to represent something far more abstract than the ever-mutating disease – indeed the only constant is the figure of Death. This is evidenced by the fact that as vaccination has started to have meaningful effects on the spread and mortality rate of the contagion, and, even in the face of vaccine resistance, the image of the microbe has largely disappeared from news stations and other information media outlets whose focus has turned towards sites specifically about the pandemic. It would seem that Death is no longer the central image of the outbreak and that the disease, as in *The Thing* and *The Andromeda Strain*, has mutated beyond it. We can but hope that it stays this way.

Debaditya Mukhopadhyay

# *Ludo* (Anurag Basu, 2020)

Death as the Game-Player in Post-Covid India

The personification of death (*Mrityu* in Sanskrit) in Indian popular films has centred chiefly around the mythical entity Yama. However, Death and Yama are not exactly the same throughout the entire corpus of Hindu culture. In some iconographic representations of Yama, Mrityu appears as one of the assistants of Yama (Ondračka 2022: 1802), and there is also a tale in the epic *Mahabharata*'s 'Shanti Parva' in which Yama and Mrityu appear as separate beings engaged in a debate (Ganguli 1883–96, section CXCIX). Besides, *Mrityu* is also referred to as a female entity in *Kalki Purana* (Chaturvedi 2008: 10, Das 2006: 6). Instead of taking these historic iterations into account, popular Indian films have predominantly personified death through the male deity Yama. Interestingly, even this male avatar of Yama has also gone through significant alterations in popular Indian films. Anurag Basu's film *Ludo* (2020) will be taken up as a case study in this chapter to analyse one such manifestation, which remarkably bears traces of the Indian popular imagination's responses to both life and death during the pandemic of 2020. Keeping in mind the chapter's focus on Yama, the discussion will begin with an outline of Yama as a mythical entity.

## Yama in Indian Myths

Etymologically the word Yama means 'twin', and Yama owes his name to the fact that he was born with a twin sister Yami (Chandra 2001: 371). Since both his parents were divine beings (the sun god in Hindu mythology known as Martandya and his wife Saranyu), both Yama and Yami should ideally be divine entities. Yet, Yama is known as 'the first of the mortals that died' (Handa 1983: 53). Indeed, Indo-Iranian creation myths feature an account of Yama's death at the hands of Manu, the first man (Ondračka 2022: 1799). Alternatively, in *Brahma Purana*, Yama's death is attributed to Shiva's rage (chapter 35). Though Yama's death makes him arguably the only major character in Hindu mythology to be bereft of immortality (Ondračka 2022: 1799), his death does not only show his weakness. Rather, his arrival at the world of the dead, despite being an entity of divine origin, endowed him with the throne of the underworld and the duty to guide dead souls (1800). This throne and duty have turned him into the god of death in Hindu mythology and correspondingly created a much sterner image of Yama.

At Yama's court in the underworld, he is assisted by another god named Chitragupta who maintains a database regarding the activities of each human being which is consulted while judging a dead soul (Chandra 2001: 372). Being a fearsome judge, especially to the sinners, Yama is said to appear with a rope noose and mace, riding on a large black buffalo (371–2, see Figure 40).

Yama, however, is not simply a punisher. Instead, he is popularly known as *Dharmaraj* or the King of *Dharma* (meaning the king of justice) for his impartiality to the dead souls (Ondračka 2022: 1800, Chandra 2001: 371–2). In addition, a popular story from the *Mahabharata* shows Yama's kindness as well. In this story about prince Satyaban and his wife Savitri, Yama returns Satyaban's life from the underworld after witnessing the genuineness of Savitri's love for her husband (Chandra 2001: 373). Though popular Bollywood movies have utilised these aspects of Yama's appearances in varying degrees, they have also added some extra details which have mostly made him into a more comic figure.

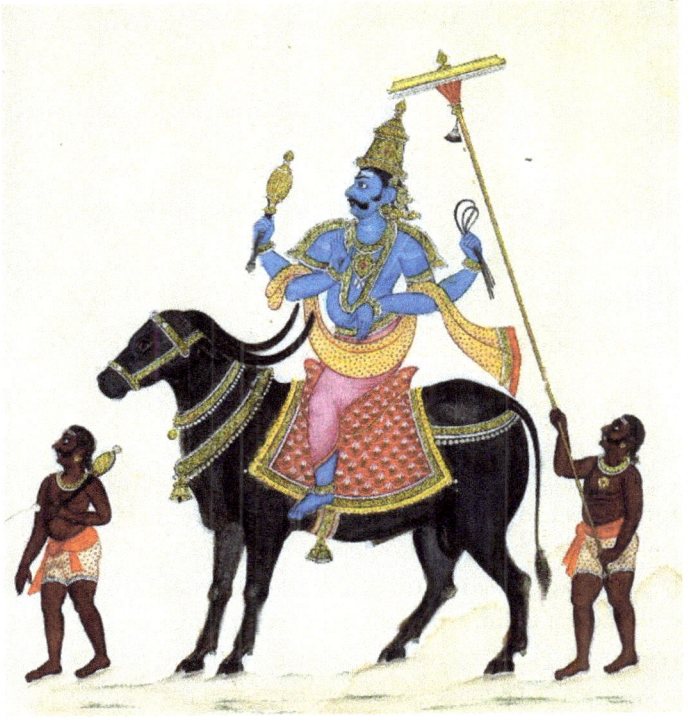

Figure 40. Yama riding a black buffalo. Image in the public domain.

## Yama in Bollywood: A Comic God of Death

Though Yama has appeared in a significant number of regional films, keeping in mind the present chapter's focus on *Ludo*, this section will limit itself to discussions on only Bollywood movies that feature him. Other than *Ludo*, two major Bollywood films have shown Yama playing important roles: *Taqdeerwala* (1995, see Figure 41) and *Vaah! Life Ho Toh Aisi!* (2005). In both films, Yama comes to the earth to live amongst mortals to solve a problem of some sort, and during his stay, as he becomes a part of their daily lives, his comic side is revealed. In *Taqdeerwala*, both Yama and his assistant

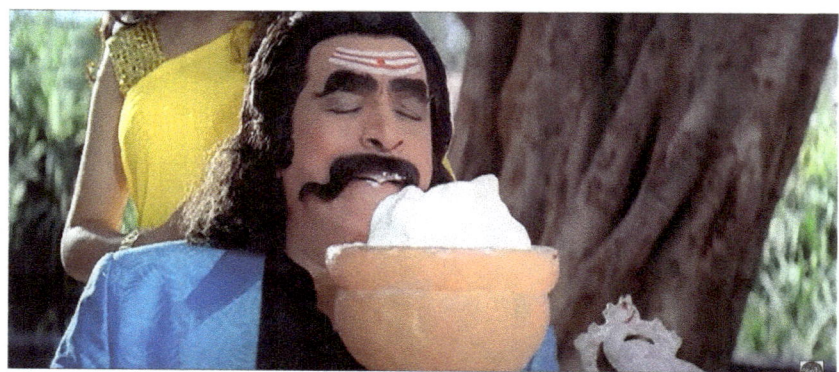

Figure 41. *Taqdeerwala*, directed by K. Murali Mohana Rao (Suresh Productions, 1995).

Chitragupta chase the hero Suraj who, because of a mistake made by Yama, gets hold of a divine book of prophecies. Both during the chase and in the scenes where Yama experiences the pleasures of the mortal world, he is shown to behave like a man-child, especially his craving for ice cream. Though Yama and Chitragupta appear in their traditional clothing in most of the scenes and Yama carries a huge mace (*Gada* in Sanskrit), their antics make them a constant source of fun.

The ending of the film strongly alludes to the Satyaban-Savitri story mentioned above as it shows Yama making an exception to his rules by returning the soul of Suraj's mother.

Likewise, in *Vaah! Life Ho Toh Aisi!* (see Figure 42), Yama is portrayed as a very colourful character. He is seen collecting dead souls while driving a flying car and wearing fashionable clothing. Yama meets the hero Aditya and his orphan nephew Parth after they both get killed in a road accident. Though Yama initially cites his rule of never making an exception regarding the collection of dead souls, when he hears the story of Aditya's extremely sad life, he becomes emotional and helps the man by giving him the power to go back to the mortal world, once again, ignoring the rules. While accompanying Aditya to the mortal world, Yama goes to a night club, drinks heavily and dances to the song 'Teri Yaad' (Your Memories) – a typically peppy Bollywood dance number.

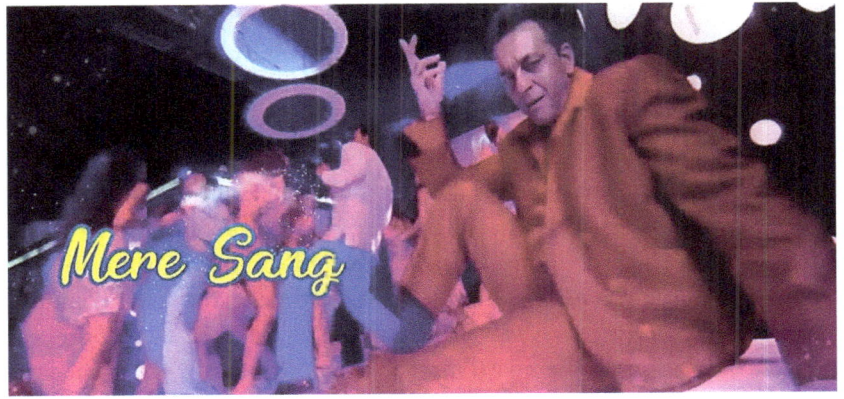

Figure 42. *Vaah! Life Ho Toh Aisi!*, directed by Mahesh Manjrekar (Aavishkaar Films, 2005).

The plots of both films reveal the respective directors' intentions to show Yama as a comic character. In *Taqdeerwala*, the famous comedian Kader Khan is cast as Yama, and in *Vaah! Life Ho Toh Aisi!*, it is Sanjay Dutt who plays the part of Yama – his role in the movie is reminiscent of his earlier comic portrayals in the immensely popular *Munna Bhai* series of films. However, *Ludo* introduces an alternative representation of Yama by distancing the character from the comic image established by these two previous films and by associating the character with a game that is described as one similar to life itself. The following sections will analyse this subversion by focusing on the portrayal of Yama and the film's use of the game of Ludo as symbolising life and death.

## Yama in *Ludo*

In *Ludo*, Yama is not played by any comic actor but by the film's director Anurag Basu and is shown as a much more serious character from the start. Along with his sidekick Chitragupta (Rahul Bagga), the two appear very much like any other citizen of India going about their daily activities, and although they appear in person only in two sequences, they are an integral part of the film as they provide commentary on several characters throughout the narrative. In the two sequences that they appear – the opening scene and climax – they are shown to be near places and events where a large number of casualties are going to occur. Despite being divine in nature, the duo never interferes in these events. Instead, they treat these as routine occurrences and simply visit the places afterwards to count the number of dead bodies. However, before doing that they play Ludo, a traditional board game of Indian origin (Bell 1960: 12). Ludo involves four sets of pawns/counters (four in each set), with each player rolling dice to get their own counters to the final destination on the board marked as 'Home' first. During the game, Yama reveals his philosophical nature during his conversation with his opponent, Chitragupta.

During the first round of Ludo, prior to the unfolding of the opening sequence, Yama tells Chitragupta: 'Life is Ludo, Ludo is life.' He goes on to explain the metaphor by pointing at the board game that is visible on the digital device carried by Chitragupta. Pointing at the pawns of four different colours on the board, Yama explains that human beings are exactly like these pawns, and the trajectory of their respective lives is determined by the rolling of dice by 'Him'. This opening line suggests Yama is more a philosopher of, rather than a judge of, humanity, which is contrary to how his nature is depicted in mythical accounts. Instead of having any control over the fate of humans, he simply visits the mortal world with his assistant regularly to count the number of casualties. Yama's lack of involvement regarding the judging of a man's doings is further revealed when Chitragupta asks him to explain *Karma*, referring specifically to the case of a murderer, Sattu (played by Pankaj Tripathi), who is shown as being prosperous.[1]

To this query, Yama nonchalantly replies with a question asking Chitragupta to explain whether all the people who died from Covid-19 were sinners. Noting the puzzled expression on Chitragupta's face upon hearing this, Yama uses another allusion to explain the impossibility of unravelling the

---

1  Karma is a Sanskrit word meaning 'action'. In Indian metaphysics, this word signifies a universal law by which every individual's life is shaped by her/his doings in the present and past lives.

mystery of life. Subsequently, when Chitragupta raises the question again prior to the film's climax, during their second game of Ludo, Yama asks Chitragupta to explain the intriguing ending of the *Mahabharata* where the apparently vicious Kauravas were shown to enjoy the pleasures of heaven, while the heroes of the epic had to suffer. Yama's strategy to answer questions with counter-questions baffles Chitragupta, who clearly functions as a surrogate of the audience in these scenes. After this, Yama adds with a smile that even one entire life is not enough to understand the puzzles of Karma – and sin and virtue. It is here that the film's portrayal of Yama has moved dramatically away from the mythical portrayals of the deity, and, more so, from the previous comedy films.

Instead of being a judge of humanity or a punisher of the wicked, the Yama of *Ludo* is an amused spectator of humanity. He does not believe in maintaining any order or discipline for human life because, for him, their lives are as unpredictable and chaotic as the board game. This chaos is explicitly shown in *Ludo* through the lives of the film's characters, particularly in those scenes that show their close encounters with death – and in some cases, the scenes where they meet death – and which resemble the randomness of the game of Ludo.

## Close Encounters of the Deadly Kind

Four sets of couples (representing the four sets of pawns of different colours of the Ludo game) meet each other by chance in *Ludo*. While each set has their own unique story arc, their respective narratives are further shaped by their encounters with each other and the criminal Sattu, who functions metaphorically as the dice that affects the movement of all pawns of the game. During the majority of the inter-couple encounters, they face deadly situations, and yet none of these moments is shown to highlight the inherent violence or gore. Rather, these scenes are shown in a comic and playful manner, highlighting their accidental nature. In the film, there are three such sequences and though each leads to singular or multiple deaths, the audience is encouraged to note the absurdity, rather than the horror, of these situations.

The first sequence takes place at the den of Sattu where the blue pawn Rahul (played by Rohit Suresh Saraf), the red pawn Bittu (played by Abhishek Bachchan) and the yellow pawn Akash (played by Aditya Roy Kapoor) gather together, as they are connected in different ways to Sattu. At the den, Akash accidentally turns the gas oven on and the blast caused by the subsequent fire kills many of Sattu's henchmen. Instead of exploring the fierceness of the blast, the cinematography and narration draw attention to the chaotic manner in which the incident happens. The blast also brings Akash close to Sheeja, the other blue pawn (played by Pearle Maaney) and the background score to this chance meeting brought about by the explosion foreshadows the pair's love.

In the second sequence, which takes place at a hotel, the green pawns Alu and Pinky (Rajkumar Rao and Fatima Sana Shaikh) are shown caught in a crossfire with some corrupt policemen. The crossfire causes bullets from the shooting to ricochet into the next room where Akash and his love interest Shruti (Sanya Malhotra) are trying to resolve their romantic crisis. Although multiple policemen are killed during the gunfight, in the chaos that ensues, the actions of the characters – biting each other or losing wigs – bring the comedic, and random, aspects of the scene to the fore. Just like the first sequence, playful background music accompanies these scenes.

The final sequence is the most chaotic and brings all the pawns together (except the little red pawn Mini), and each of them faces death during another crossfire started accidentally by Sheeja who shoots first after being startled by Bittu's car being broken into. During the shooting, Bittu and a majority of the henchmen get killed and each of the characters in the scene escapes death by the narrowest of margins. The absurdity of this chaotic scene is reinforced by a love song crooning in the background, featuring the refrain of *Lo Aise Hua Pyaar* 'And that's how love happened'.

In an interview with Anupama Chopra, the actors observed that the director had deliberately kept all of them in the dark about the other characters, with the aim of capturing their confused expressions at the chaotic turn of events more naturally (Chopra 2020). The music composer for the film, Pritam, also offered insights into the film's unusual choice of background score to the same interviewer, stating that Basu's brief required him to compose soothingly sweet romantic songs in order to set the background score in contrast to the violent scenes. According to Pritam, Basu adopted an approach that is different

*Ludo* (Anurag Basu, 2020)

from directors like Quentin Tarantino, who uses songs to compliment the violence of the scenes (Chopra 2020). These sequences and the accompanying soft background score, together, encourage viewers to experience the deadly scenes while remaining calm. This calmness resonated significantly Indian society's response to the pandemic and contributed significantly to the film's popularity, as shall be discussed next.

## Echoing a Pandemic-Ridden Society

Maintaining a complete lockdown in India during Covid-19 turned out to be more challenging than expected due to the unforeseen impact it had on the finances of the majority of Indians. Research on the impact of lockdown reveals a decrease in income of almost 63.4 per cent of Indians between the age group of thirty-five and fifty years (Kochhar et al. 2020). As a result, the majority of people had to resume going outside to work despite the health risks involved. Another survey reveals that no less than 60 per cent of its respondents went outside for their work during lockdown (Ghosh et al. 2021). It is possible to imagine how the larger section of Indian society gradually started viewing the threat of Covid-19 as a part of their daily lives.

The central government of India imposed lockdowns in four phases between 25 March 2020 and 31 May 2020, and by the time of phased reopening which commenced in June 2020, India was witnessing more than 2 billion cases of Covid a day and more than 7,000 daily deaths (The Wire 2023). Accepting death as a part of everyday life thus became an important aspect of India's cultural response to the pandemic. *Ludo*, which had its release postponed due to the pandemic, resonates with this response and the portrayal of Yama strongly manifests this acceptance.

Though Basu's film was given its title before the pandemic (Quint Entertainment 2019), the decision to release the film on a streaming platform instead of a theatrical release gave the director the scope to incorporate references to the pandemic itself. The direct mention of Covid-19-related deaths in the Yama-Chitragupta scene and the portrayal of ludo using the 'Ludo King' game that had become immensely popular during the lockdown (Lakshmanan 2020), for example, reveal how the character of Yama and his liking for Ludo were shaped specifically in relation to the Indian popular imagination during the pandemic. In an interview with Sankhayan Ghosh, Basu describes the Yama-Chitragupta scenes to be a homage to *Waiting for Godot* and admits having similarities to the film *The Seventh Seal* (The Film Companion 2020). Taking into consideration Basu's allusions and the film's purposeful resonance to the geist of India under Covid lockdown, *Ludo*'s Yama becomes a distinctive portrayal of Death and one that sees the new normal of a pandemic-stricken society as being exactly the same as the old normal.

Heidi Kosonen

# *13 Reasons Why* (Brian Yorkey, 2017–20)

## Romanticised and Medicalised Suicide

In spring 2017, the presses stopped at the release of the first season of the Netflix series *13 Reason Why* (2017–20, henceforth *13 Reasons*), created by Brian Yorkey and based on Jay Asher's novel (2007) of the same name, which narrates the reasons for a young girl's suicide through guilt-tripping thirteen cassette tapes delivered to her peers and her could-have-been-sweetheart. In question is a young adult's high school drama, posthumously studying the ups and downs in the life of seventeen-year-old Hannah Baker (Katherine Langford) and her peers, both through her narration in the tapes and from the perspective of her schoolmate Clay (Dylan Minnette), who secretly loved her. As revealed by the tapes, Hannah's suicide is caused by a cumulation of social factors related to rape culture and gossip at her high school and is tied to her social ostracisation and loneliness. Her suicidal spin is depicted according to the pattern of developing depression and told through the parallel narrative (see Figure 43) of Clay's self-destructive mourning. Beyond the volatile topic of self-willed death, the next three seasons focus on Clay and Hannah's other peers outliving her.

The tensions and volatile discussions surrounding the series, and meriting suicide the hyperbolic title of 'last taboo' (Tatz 2017) in the media, make *13 Reasons* an interesting case study to contemplate self-willed death's cultural position. In its first week of streaming, the series became the most tweeted Netflix show of 2017 (Bruner 2017). Soon after, several agents from mental health experts to parents and suicide survivors criticised the series for, among other factors, its romanticisation of suicide (Skehan 2017), the triggering nature

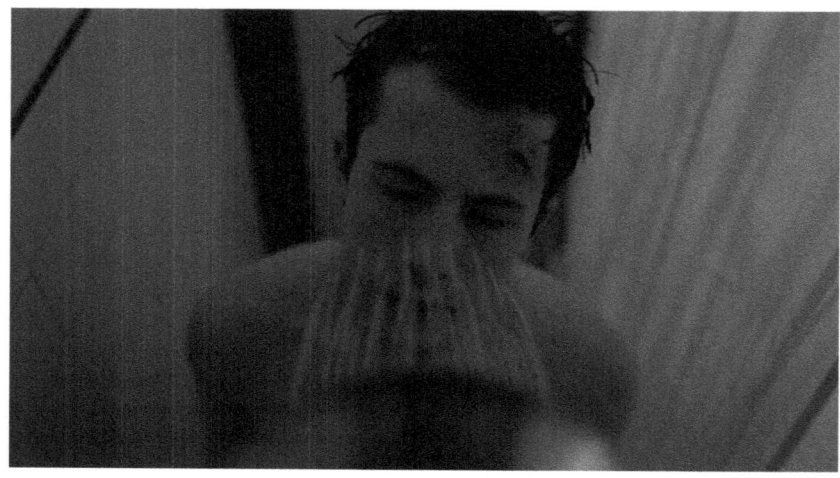

Figure 43. Suicide is often depicted through parallel narratives. In the first season (2017) of *13 Reasons Why*, Clay (Dylan Minnette) travels through a similar trajectory of self-harm to Hannah (Katherine Langford), who committed suicide, and yet he survives. *13 Reasons Why*, created by Brian Yorkey (Netflix, 2017).

of the graphic rape and suicide scenes (Gilbert 2017) and the downplaying of the role of mental health and recovery (Jacobson 2017). As a result, the series was argued to encourage 'suicide contagion' among the audiences, and actions were taken: warning letters were sent to parents, trigger warnings with mental health service hotline numbers were added to the opening texts and Netflix's viewing age limits were raised; in some places, even discussions of the series were curbed by schools. In 2019, after two years of streaming, the final episode of the first season was edited to censor the visual representation of Hannah's suicide.

In many ways, the narrative of Hannah's self-willed death does not stand out from among other audiovisual representations of suicide, but it rather crystallises many of the conventions through which the taboo-natured death is depicted in Anglophone entertainment. At the same time, the treatment of suicide *13 Reasons* is made unique by the show's reception and subsequent censorship, pointing to particularly sensitive elements and their volatile combinations in suicide's audiovisual depiction. Both in its conventional and scandalous elements, *13 Reasons* points to self-willed death's status as a taboo, pivoted between hypervisibility and fear-based regulation. This essay will discuss the show's first season to reflect on suicide's position in the twenty-first-century Western culture and imagination, especially in film and television. It will focus on the dynamics between suicide's romanticisation and medicalisation, and their relation to the suicide taboo, which were at the core of the series' media reception.

## Suicide, a Contagious and Romanticised Death?

According to the movie database IMDB, Anglophone cinema produces over 200 titles featuring suicide annually, and between fifty and eighty-five titles for television. Unlike *13 Reasons*, where a representation of a teenage girl's self-inflicted death caused fears of suicide imitation, most of these titles are released without controversies. One could even argue that most of them are not seen as including representations of suicide. Why such a number of on-screen suicides might fly off the radar is that rarely do these films or television series study self-willed death thematically (Kosonen 2020a, Aaron 2014, Saddington 2010). Instead, most of the represented suicides are, in varied ways, instrumental, serving some narrative or affective function as a fleeting image of the shocking and symbolically invested death (Kosonen 2020a). Only sometimes, like in *13 Reasons*, does suicide interest the creators as a topic of its own.

At the same time with this proliferation, suicide is feared as a contagious death, transmitted through media discussions and representations (Phillips 1974) and through both vertical and horizontal influences: from parents to children (Cerel et al. 2018) or within peer groups (Randall et al. 2015). In particular, in considering the fact that young adults constitute a major part of the series audience, the fear of suicide's contagion among the young has been strong (see Gould et al. 2003, Marshall 2006): the decision to edit out Hannah's suicide scene was based on a paper reporting an increase in the suicide rates among American boys aged ten to seventeen after the release of the show's first season (Bridge et al. 2019), a finding that was later contested by another study (Romer 2020).

At its core, suicide contagion is about the fears surrounding suicide as a death that is historically seen as inexplicable, sinful and bad. It first surfaced as Werther Effect after Goethe's eighteenth-century romantic novel *The Sorrows of Young Werther* (1774), which was connected to a large number of copycat suicides. As with Goethe's novel, the accusations of suicide's contagion are especially related to representations that romanticise or glamorise self-willed death. In film and television, this romanticisation takes varied and often gendered forms. For instance, ideas of glorification and martyrdom repeat in the depictions of the suicides of male artists (Stack and Bowman 2009), invoking the mythology of the suffering creator (Wittkower and Wittkower 1969). Narratively distanced from suicide proper, male self-endangerment also roots several action genres with heroic, reckless or even death-desiring male protagonists portrayed through varied 'mortality-testing, death-defying, and martyr-invoking moments' (Aaron 2014: 19) which flirt with self-destruction and connect it to masculine heroism. Rarely do these characters die, though, and rarely are they female – two narrative contours defied by *13 Reasons*. One could argue that the reason this series stands out, at least partly, is because it is a high-profile drama that features a female protagonist who commits suicide, and that this death in some way deviates from the way suicides are often depicted.

Relating to the romanticisation of male suicides, the conventional representation of female characters' suicidality can be described through film scholar Michele Aaron's concept of 'necromanticism' – the manner in which cinema's mortal and erotic economies are intertwined in the image of the dead woman. As Aaron argues, the dead or to-be-dead woman is 'figured as beguilingly and prophetically ethereal' as she 'embod[ies] a romance with death [...] as beloved spectacle, muse, and, or rather as, inevitable projection of male desire and despair' (2014: 52). Necromanticism simultaneously romanticises death and eroticises woman within the regime of suicide. In this, suicide cinema repeats the gendered division, discovered by Laura Mulvey (1989) as those who look and those who are looked at, and implicates economies of desire in the spectacle of the taboo death (Kosonen 2015). This regime, too, is prevalent in *13 Reasons*, especially in the scenes where a mourning Clay pictures

*13 Reasons Why* (Brian Yorkey, 2017–20)

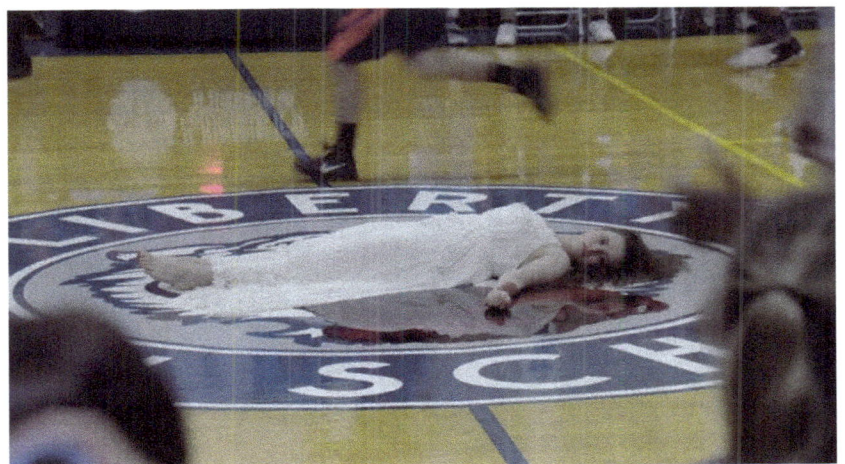

Figure 44. Spectral Hannah lying on the basketball court in a pool of blood in Clay's imagination. *13 Reasons Why*, created by Brian Yorkey (Netflix, 2017).

Hannah lying on the basketball court in a pool of blood in a white nightshirt (see Figure 44) – an image reminiscent of Ophelia, the art historical embodiment of the suicidal woman. The difference between women's suicides' 'necromanticisation' and men's romanticisation is that the former does not often glorify suicide itself, like the regime of the artist suicide connecting to male genius. Its romanticisation rather works through sexual titillation in the image of the dead woman (Kosonen 2018).

Another manner in which necromanticism is prevalent in *13 Reasons* is through the story arc of romance and the theme of young, unfulfilled love (see Figure 45), similarly introduced through Clay's perspective as the spectral images of Hannah. Altogether, necromanticism in *13 Reasons* works through the centring of the male protagonist's mourning of his high school crush, a journey complicated by guilt, longing and disenfranchised grief (Doka 1999). In parallel narratives (see Figure 45) like these, which are common to suicide cinema, a side character's suicide is often revealed in flashbacks that are veiled by elements of nostalgia. Their decisions to die are also defied by the protagonists, who travel through similar trajectories to the 'suicide victims' – and yet survive (Kosonen 2020a). Survival also

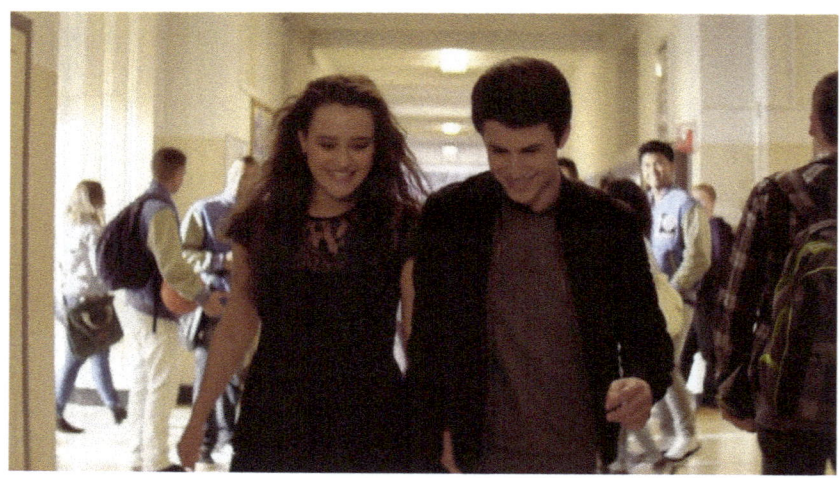

Figure 45. Hannah represents Clay's unfulfilled desires – here depicted in a montage representing what could have been – but a happy ending is guaranteed through Clay discovering a new love. *13 Reasons Why*, created by Brian Yorkey (Netflix, 2017).

takes place in *13 Reasons*, whose male protagonist Clay struggles to get over Hannah's suicide and eventually finds a new love in a happy ending to the first season. To counter the messages related to Hannah's guilt-tripping tapes and the glossing of her death through necromanticism, Hannah's fatality is – next to Clay's survival – conjoined with a storyline focused on Hannah's parents, involved with a legal case against her school in their tremendous grief, and defied by Clay's actions with his new sweetheart, another girl with a history of self-harm.

## Suicide's Medicalisation: Biopower and the Regulation of Self-Willed Death

The fears of suicide's romanticisation and subsequent contagion were, in the case of *13 Reasons*, closely related to the topic of suicide's medicalisation. As mentioned, one of the criticisms directed at the show was its downplaying of the role of mental health and recovery. In the words of the authority on film classifications around the media coverage of *13 Reasons*, suicide should never be presented 'as something resulting from reasoned thinking' (Office of Film & Literature Classification 2017) but should instead be depicted as a question of mental health, represented with a suitable array of medical solutions, and this was also demanded of *13 Reasons* in other statements as well (Bostan 2017, Jacobson 2017).

It is interesting to note these criticisms, presented mainly by mental health professionals, because the storyline of depression is not missing in the series. Although not diagnosed and labelled as depression, Hannah's slide from a state of forward-gazing resistance into murky hopelessness reflects the recognisable conventions of how depression is represented in both lay discussions and media, leaving her possible depression to thus be subject to interpretation. Moreover, Hannah does seek help from the school counsellor; however, she gets no help and also faces victim-blaming for her sexual assault. Furthermore, both depression and medical solutions are present in Clay's storyline as a diagnosis from his past and a bottle of pills (duloxetine, a medication used to treat major depressive disorder) given to him by his parents. The parallel narrative, mentioned above, instead ensures that not only death but also recovery is central to the narrative, although it salvages only the male protagonist, and not the female.

In looking at how self-willed death is presented elsewhere in audiovisual culture, its medicalisation is evident: suicides are often made sense with diagnoses, which are pertinent to medical knowledge production, or through vernacular depictions of madness. The medicalisation of suicide is made manifest through dialogue, settings and emblems (e.g. bottles for pills) in varied ways reminiscent of medical institutions, depression or other mental illnesses (Kosonen 2018, 2020a, b). Audiovisual entertainment frequently studies suicide in institutionalised settings, like the drama film *Girl, Interrupted* (Mangold 1999), which is set in a psychiatric institution. The film follows the protagonist's recovery from a borderline disorder by juxtaposing it with the suicide of another girl with bulimia and obsessive-compulsive disorder.

Suicide's habitual connection to mental illness is almost one of the axioms connected to self-willed death in late-twentieth and twenty-first-century Western knowledge production, and it pervades not only film and television but also other media as well. Philosopher Margaret Pabst Battin, for instance, comments:

> For much of the twentieth and on into the twenty-first century, thinking about suicide in the West has been normatively monolithic: suicide has come to be seen by the public and particularly by health professionals as primarily a matter of mental illness, perhaps compounded by biochemical factors and social stressors, the sad result of depression or other often treatable disease – a tragedy to be prevented [...] the only substantive discussions about suicide in current Western culture have concerned whether access to psychotherapy or improved suicide-prevention programs, or more effective antidepressant medications should form the principal lines of defense. (2005: 164)

Battin is not the only one to recognise the way philosophical and theological discussions of suicide (Minois 1999) have been largely displaced by the discussion of suicide as a public health issue and a societal risk. Ian Marsh (2010) notes how the wealth of different kinds of discourses that present suicide as a 'tragic act of a mentally unwell individual' (27), work as a manifestation of knowledge production of suicides under Western biopower. Biopower refers to the use of normative techniques and practices that aim at the subjugation of human bodies to state control. To biopower – which seeks 'to foster life or to disallow it to the point of death' (Foucault 1990: 138–9) through normative discourses in the medical world and other institutions of knowledge – suicide has been argued to appear as a dangerous form of resistance (141). Instead of appearing simply as a danger to self, suicide represents dangers to the 'social body' (Douglas 1970), and this is reflected in the ways that the Western imagination makes sense of voluntary death (Kosonen 2020b).

Suicide's medicalisation under Western biopower can be seen as an exemplary case of voluntary death's control under the taboo as well. The connection to taboo manifests particularly clearly in the reception of *13 Reasons*, where the arguments related to a work of fiction's insufficient medicalisation led to fears of its contagion as well as the series' censorship and the curbing of discussions of suicide in certain North American schools. According to Mary Douglas' line of scrutiny of the taboo (Douglas 1996, 2002, Douglas and Wildavsky 1983), this societal 'danger structure' (Radcliffe-Brown 1979, Steiner 1999) is empowered by ideas of dirt and contagion in instances where classificatory borders and collectively agreed values are threatened or breached (Douglas 2002, Kosonen 2020a). In *13 Reasons*, which in many ways is a conventional example of cinematic and televisual suicide fiction in the late twentieth and twenty-first century, this symptomatic fear of contagion surfaced in relation to its representation of suicide as a reasoned, albeit depressed, action (See. Kosonen 2020a, b).

To be alarmed by the idea of suicide's representations generating their imitation is understandable; however, the phenomenon of suicide contagion continues to be contested among and denied by the scholars studying it (Cheng et al. 2014, Evans et al. 2021, Ferguson 2019, Hittner 2005). From a humanities perspective, this contagion too easily takes the form of the hypodermic needle theory, where audiences are seen as non-autonomous victims of media's messages, removed of their psychological, social or other reasons for contemplating suicide. This contagion's regulation via suicide's representation through stigmatising and marginalising ways, rather than empathetic depictions, is also questionable. Contrary to the alarming reports about suicide's contagion, recent studies have also shown that *13 Reasons* has brought about a decrease in thoughts related to harming or killing oneself (Arendt et al. 2019, Zimerman et al. 2018) as well as an increase in empathy among its viewers and has also augmented respondents' willingness to discuss mental health issues with others (Northwestern 2018).

## Concluding Remarks

This essay has considered suicide's uneasy status in the Western imaginary and culture through the Netflix series *13 Reasons Why* that both repeats and defies some of the existing conventions used for depicting self-willed death. As the series' reception was marked by controversy as well as the medical authorities' criticism of suicide's romanticisation and its insufficient connection to depression, it has been meaningful to discuss suicide's gendered and medicalised representation and its persistent taboo in Western culture as a death seen as dangerously contagious and subjected to regulation. This chapter has discussed the representative regimes that more often feature suicide on screen as 'necromanticised' images of the suiciding women and sometimes glorify it through male genius and recklessness or connect suicide to mental illness, rather than thematically study suicide, its motivations and reasons. In *13 Reasons*, both necromanticism and medicalisation persist and yet its connection to female agency is seen as problematic. The fact that the series presents controversial elements and has opened a discussion about suicide and its on-screen representation has made *13 Reasons* a worthy case study.

Rae Hargrave

# *Land of the Lustrous* (Takahiko Kyōgoku, 2017–17)

## Death of the Self

How do you define death? Is it the moment your cells die – the physical collapse of the body? Or could the loss of memory and identity mark its own death, the death of the personality or soul that occupies the physical body even if the body lives on? And if we accept that loss of memories and identities can become a death of its own, at what point do we cross the line from *me but missing some memories* to *something else*? Interrogating these questions through media can help us process the complicated feelings that come with dealing with the loss of memory and self in real life, such as with dementia. We often think of death in our media as physical death – frequently violent, often tragic – but some stories deal with the more abstract form of death of the self. The Japanese manga and anime *Hōseki no Kuni*, translated as 'House of Jewels' or 'Land of the Lustrous', forces readers and viewers to confront their own definitions of identity and self as the main character, Phosphophyllite, loses formative memories that define their personality and personal beliefs, resulting in a drastic personality shift over the course of the story that echoes real-life parallels in memory-based diseases such as dementia.

*Land of the Lustrous*, based on Haruko Ichikawa's manga of the same name, was adapted into an anime in 2017. The story centres on the Lustrous, humanoid life-forms made of gemstones, who are engaged in war with the Lunarians, who use the Lustrous' bodies for jewellery. As non-organic life-forms, the Lustrous hold their memories in the crystalline structure of their bodies instead of in their brains – they do not age and have no gender, and so this chapter will use neutral pronouns for the Lustrous. In battle, they can be shattered; when they shatter, they can be repaired but any memories held in a missing piece will not be recovered. The protagonist Phosphophyllite, known as Phos, is the youngest and softest of the Lustrous with a hardness of only 3.5. This makes them unsuitable for battle – clearly illustrated in the first episode as Phos shatters when Master Kongo, their leader, yells at two other Lustrous. Phos sustains extensive damage throughout the series, including losing their legs and replacing them with agatised snail shell, losing their arms and replacing them with gold and platinum alloy, and losing their head and having it replaced with another Lustrous' head. This results in a significant loss of memory over time – more significant than any other Lustrous present in the show has experienced, making Phos' change stand out amongst the other older and largely unchanging Lustrous.

In the third episode of the anime, Phos is broken down and absorbed by a giant snail; after their body dissolves, they become part of the snail shell and lose 'consciousness'. Ultimately, Phos must be chipped out of the shell and reassembled. As they are reassembled, there is an artistic scene of Phos' body fluidly reforming and then their moment of regained consciousness once enough pieces are put back together. This depiction emphasises the idea that there must be enough of the original body present to form consciousness and that consciousness has a threshold for the Lustrous. After a subsequent fight with the Lunarians leads to the loss of Phos' legs, Phos replaces the missing pieces with pieces of the agatised snail shell, which increases Phos' speed, but causes the first noticeable loss of memory; they are unable to remember the fight with the Lunarians that resulted in the loss of their legs, including key information about the origins of their world and their species that was learnt during that fight. The Lustrous are generally unconcerned by Phos' shattering; shattering does not typically kill a Lustrous but just damages them, and so it is shocking but not worth grieving. They do not have a concept of death in the traditional sense as mortal wounds for a human would simply result in repairs for a Lustrous – unless the piece of their body is lost or taken. They may not conceptualise the loss of their shards as death, but they do recognise that a Lustrous without their head is lost to them. For non-organic, crystalline beings like the Lustrous, death is not necessarily predicated on major bodily harm; therefore, what is death to the Lustrous if not loss of self?

*Land of the Lustrous* (Takahiko Kyōgoku, 2017–17)

The question of whether or not death of the self has occurred is a more complex one than whether or not physical death has occurred. In *Plutarch's Lives*, Plutarch asks: if the ship on which Theseus sailed has been so heavily repaired and nearly every part replaced, is it still the same ship – and, if not, at what point did it stop being the same ship? The Ship of Theseus thought experiment challenges us to question at what point Phos stops being theirself. Chomsky acknowledges that 'our concepts just don't give an answer' to the Ship of Theseus question because it is not an issue of physicality but rather one stemming from the very nature of the human mind (2010: 382). Given this, he notes that we should trust the authenticity of our experience: if we understand the object to be the Ship of Theseus, then it is the Ship of Theseus, even if our cognitive systems are not designed to deal with this concept (UCD 2013). Phos is Phos as long as they continue to view their body as their own – that is, as long as there is a time/space continuity between the parts of themselves, then it is Phos. Phos continues to perceive themselves as 'Phos', but their memory loss complicates this question: if Phos loses enough memories, but is told they are 'Phos' and accepts that fact, can they still be trusted to recognise themselves? Further, is memory the precondition for a sense of self or is Phos' identity immutable regardless of their memories? One could argue that whatever Phos becomes through the changes in their personality is simply the new 'Phos' – that the changes are natural and should be accepted as part of who they are in the same way we accept personality changes after a major experience or event. However, when we colloquially discuss loved ones with dementia, we often speak in phrases such as 'this isn't them', 'they aren't acting like themselves' and so on. This indicates that we *do* see a functional difference between personality changes that come from growth and experience over time versus personality changes that come from memory loss.

Essentially, *Land of the Lustrous* is challenging viewers to engage with a concept many humans find deeply uncomfortable: the possibility that your 'self', your 'identity', could potentially die before your body – a concept familiar to anyone who has experienced or witnessed the ravages of memory-based diseases such as dementia. When we analyse the portrayal of death in media, we traditionally focus on physical death. However, Phos' character arc opens up the space to interrogate an Ego Death: the loss of their sense of identity. If your ego is the idea of who you are and your sense of individuality, then Phos' lost memories impact their understanding of theirself – they can no longer remember formative moments that had previously been focal points of their growth and goals. Your ego is a combination of memories, experiences, desires and goals. All of these are eroded each time Phos loses a part of their body. When Phos is consumed by the snail, they physically melt away and lose their conscious sense of self. This scene is the perfect representation of Phos' loss of ego at that moment. Eventually, they physically reform and regain consciousness: they regain a sense of self alongside their physical self, underscoring the continual theme of the Lustrous' identities being closely tied to the well-being of their physical bodies. This parallels the way progressive memory loss can erode a dementia patient's recognition of themself and those around them. Many cases of dementia get more severe with time, meaning that there are stages of change within the person and their memories in the same way that Phos experienced stages of change with each subsequent loss of their original body. Unfortunately, with dementia, there is no hope of reintroducing memories the way Phos and the other Lustrous can potentially regain their lost limbs; in reality, these losses are more permanent and heart-breaking.

Death in pop culture is often violent and almost always physical, regardless of how sanitised the violence is rendered. While plenty of great literature has interrogated the concept of the Ego Death, it is a less common theme to find addressed in more accessible popular media. Hayley Campbell argues that we are 'surrounded by death' in her novel *All the Living and the Dead*. She states,

> It is in our news, our novels, our video games – it is in our superhero comics, where it can be reversed on a monthly whim … it is in our nursery rhymes, our museums, our movies about beautiful murdered women. But the footage is edited, the decapitated head of the journalist is pixelated, the words of the old songs are sanitised for modern youth. Death is everywhere, but it's veiled, or it's fiction. (2022: 5)

It is present but never directly addressed because death makes most people uncomfortable, despite it being the ultimate end for all of us. Some people may even become numb to the visual representations of death in media yet still never confront what death means to them personally – nor confront non-physical types of death. *Land of the Lustrous* goes beyond just demanding that we confront the reality of physical death; it challenges us to think of a more nebulous, non-traditional death through the death of the self. The loss of what makes someone 'themselves' is a deep-seated fear for many people, especially if they have watched a loved one succumb to a disease like Alzheimer's. There are 10 million new cases of dementia each year, with 55 million people living with dementia worldwide (World Health Organization 2022). Both physical death and loss of identity are central tragedies of the human condition.

Interrogating questions of memory, self-identity and what makes us who we are is necessary to better understand human nature and our core fears. It is uncomfortable to be confronted with the dramatic, clear-cut loss of memory and identity in *Land of the Lustrous*. Each viewer or reader may come to a different conclusion about when Phos crosses the line from *Phos but missing some memories* to *is this even Phos anymore*, but the question is always there. It is even starker in the manga, where Phos' current arc sees them enacting a level of betrayal against Master Kongo and the other Lustrous that the original Phos never would have dreamed of. The best media, however, challenges us to confront what makes us uncomfortable. I am left thinking of a line by Don DeLillo in his novel *White Noise*: 'How can you be sure it is death you fear? Death is so vague. No one knows what it is, what it feels like or looks like. Maybe you just have a personal problem that surfaces in the form of a great universal subject' (1984: 187). Death can take many forms, and while we are often fearfully preoccupied with physical death, it's important to confront the possibility of the death of the self as well. In her Afterword, Campbell realises that everyone she interviewed dealt with death by determining their own personal limits on what they could handle, and she directly encourages readers to determine their own limits rather than allowing 'arbitrary, institutionalized assumptions' to guide our perceptions of death (2022: 231). She argues that 'as long as you have carefully considered [your limits] rather than allowed them to be dedicated by cultural norms, they are right' (231). She experienced things that continued to haunt her long after her research was complete, yet she knew that the work she had done – professionally and personally – was important. Death is the end for everyone, and most of us will not know what form it will take until it is already upon us. Making peace with death, of one form or another, helps us move through our lives with peace and purpose instead of fear. We cannot know what we fear until we confront it, and when we find media poignant enough in its portrayal to make us uncomfortable, we do ourselves a disservice if we turn away from that discomfort.

Catherine Pugh

# *Unus Annus* (Mark Fischbach and Ethan Nestor, 2019–20)

Memento Mori: The Thanatological World of *Unus Annus*

In November 2019, streamers Mark Fischbach ('Markiplier') and Ethan Nestor ('CrankGamePlays'[1]) launched *Unus Annus* ('one year') – a YouTube channel that would exist for only one year before being permanently deleted. Posting one video a day – every day – for a year, Fischbach and Nestor created a series of videos that explored death and the unstoppable march of time, made more significant as the vast majority of the series coincided with the Covid-19 pandemic. The channel was originally set up with the intention of creatively freeing Fischbach and Nestor, allowing them to make whatever kind of videos they wanted because of the temporary nature of the channel. However, *Unus Annus* quickly captured the imagination of fans; the community began generating art, stories and memes as lore and characters organically formed. Through the channel, Fischbach and Nestor created alter egos: Unus (Nestor) and Annus (Fischbach) who increasingly interrupted the entertainment in order to remind the audience of the inevitable demise of the channel, and therefore, Unus and Annus.. As the series progressed, Unus and Annus were interpreted as manifestation(s) of death: a balanced and fatalistic pair leading the audience towards an end that many fans begged them to change.

Many episodes featured Fischbach and Nestor attempting a wide variety of new experiences, from trying unusual foods and products to activities

---

1 Nestor has since changed his social media handle to 'Ethan Nestor'.

and challenges – including dance, mime, fire-eating, axe-throwing, cryotherapy, aerial hoop and silks, film combat and, in one infamous episode, pepper spray. Other episodes involved DIY recreations of various death rituals – Viking funeral, mummification and so on – as well as discussions on difficult subjects, including their own fears and traumatic experiences. The series also heavily featured Amy Nelson, a visual and interactive media maker and Fischbach's partner. Although she rarely appeared on screen, Nelson was integral to the formation of the show, taking on numerous creative and production roles, with her voice often heard behind the camera. A significant part of *Unus Annus* took place during quarantine in the United States, while in August several episodes were filmed on location at 'Camp Unus Annus', a 1980s-style summer camp that gave dubious advice on surviving in the wilderness (1.281–9). Due to the topic of the series, it frequently utilised horror tropes and themes, with several episodes explicitly set in the genre. However, other episodes featured different styles of film-making, such as 'Hunting HeeHoo' (1.288): a pseudo-documentary during the 'Camp Unus Annus' era. The series itself was not without risk and numerous physical activities resulted in injury, while more introspective episodes explored painful or complex subjects, including traumatic events in Fischbach's and Nestor's lives. *Unus Annus* culminated in a twelve-hour livestream on 13 November 2020; at midnight on 14 November 2020 PST, the channel and all of its content and social media were permanently deleted by Fischbach, Nestor and Nelson. The stream was watched live by over 1.5 million viewers and, alongside analysis and reminiscences of the series, featured an improvised ritual where Fischbach, Nestor and Nelson took turns lying in a bespoke coffin as the others eulogised about them.

The format and content of *Unus Annus* invoke Ruth Penfold-Mounce's framework of thanatological imagination: 'a space to explore the social potential of death' that allows popular culture and those who consume it to form a '"morbid space" to explore their "morbid sensibilities"' (2020: 52, see also Penfold-Mounce 2018). Penfold-Mounce argues that this morbid space allows for engagement with the undead, as well as the posthumous careers of celebrities, thereby 'highlight[ing] how interests of sociology into mortality have spread beyond the confines of the discipline and contribute to the transformation of expectations and understandings of sociology' (2020: 54). Thanatological imagination can be direct or indirect, explicit or left to the spectator's imagination, but it frequently appears in consumer culture – everything from media to fashion and even children's products.

## Death Iconography

Devaleena Kundu speaks of the twentieth century's 'obsessive fascination with death', as 'visual imageries of death continue to infiltrate our domestic spaces' (2020: 103). As both Kundu (2019) and James Walvin (1982) explain, for Victorians, death was inextricably tied to life, influencing *Unus Annus*' culture of memento mori ('remember death' or 'remember you must die'). The culture of death in the nineteenth and early twentieth centuries incorporates what Deborah Lutz calls a 'resurgence in relic culture' arguing that it speaks 'of a desire to see death as not permanent, in that material remains might be proof that the loved one still exists somewhere, somehow' (2011: 128) rather than keeping the relic as a 'memento mori' (130). Whereas memento mori is a reminder of the inevitability of death, relics 'work as traces of a life and body completed and disappeared, in this sense something like last words, but they also serve as frames or fragments of the moment of loss' (128). The merchandise created for *Unus Annus* – clothing, posters, figurines and so on – inadvertently became a type of memento mori and relic culture: tangible reminders not only of a show and time that met its unavoidable demise and can never be revisited or recreated but also of the fact that everything must end.

*Unus Annus* employs death iconography familiar to Western audiences, particularly in their framing narrative, to create a recognisable and striking aesthetic: a black-and-white contrasting colour palette; the clock that loudly ticks down the remaining seconds of the channel's life; and the Gregorian chant ('Unus. Annus. Unus. Annus!') that opened each episode, in effect becoming a funeral lament. As the series continued, other iconography and memento

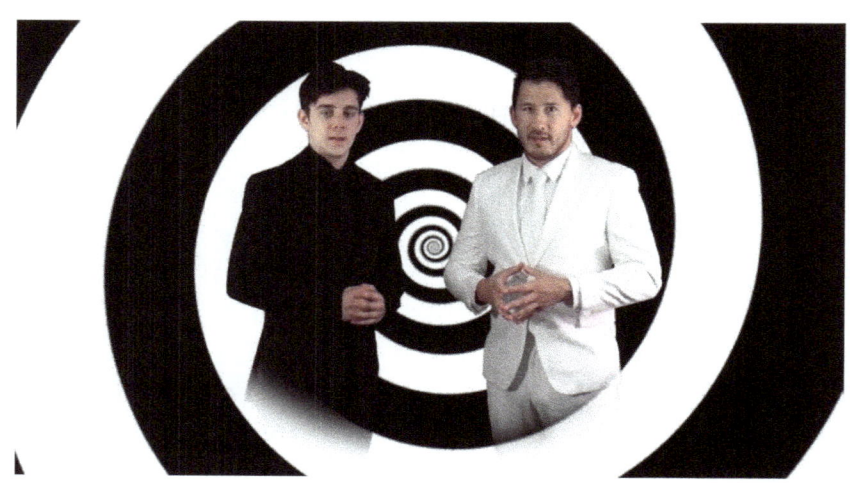

Figure 46. Unus (Ethan Nestor) and Annus (Mark Fischbach) introduce the series *Unus Annus*, created by Mark Fischbach and Ethan Nestor (2019–20).

mori were adopted, either by fans or by the creators themselves, such as skulls, clocks, hourglasses, flowers and, the *Unus Annus* casket.[2] The suits worn by Unus and Annus, the spiral background used in framing scenes where they address the audience and the call-and-response maxim of 'Memento mori. Unus annus' became important signifiers within the series (see Figure 46). The importance of these recognisable rituals – and how eagerly the fan community adopted them – serves as a reminder of 'our still-deep-seated need for rituals, ceremonies, and celebrations whenever death strikes' (Jacobsen 2020: 29).

Although the central action of individual videos could take any form the creators desired, the series featured an overarching framing narrative where alter egos Unus (Nestor) and Annus (Fischbach) could directly address the audience. The two characters, separate from Nestor and Fischbach themselves, actively reminded the viewer of the fate of the channel, coming to represent death despite the series itself being about their own inevitable demise (see Figure 47). Unus and Annus acted as one, yet they represented different

---

2   The casket is technically a coffin (six sides, taped towards the end) but is primarily referred to as a casket throughout the series.

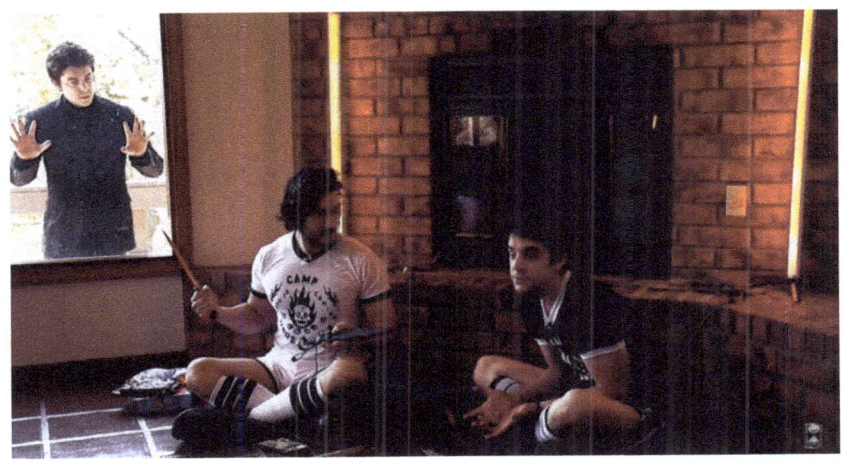

Figure 47. Unus watches as Fischbach prepares to kill Nestor in the episode 'How to Start a Fire ... (Except Don't)'. *Unus Annus*, created by Mark Fischbach and Ethan Nestor (2019–20).

personality archetypes, based on complementary self-identified attributes of Nestor and Fischbach, respectively:

UNUS: Our kind heart, our compassion, our driven nature [...] you can tell when people are feeling down and you try your best to bring them back up with you. You're creative and your heart – you wear it right on your sleeve.
('Only Unus-es May Watch This Video', 1.195A)

ANNUS: Annus-es speak from the heart. They speak their truth. They let people know how they feel. And they don't let anyone walk over them. Ever [...] The defining traits of an Annus: Boldness. Brashness. Confidence.
('Only Annus-es May Watch This Video', 1.195B)

The boundaries between the framing narrative of Unus and Annus and the real world of Nestor and Fischbach became increasingly blurred as the series neared its end. Nestor and Fischbach frequently 'died' in the series only to be resurrected offscreen, suggesting a symbiotic relationship between them and their besuited doppelgängers. In the video 'How to Start a Fire (Except Don't ...)' (1.286), Fischbach appears to contemplate killing Nestor, at which point

Unus steps into frame, watching from a window (see Figure 47). Exactly two weeks before the series ended, Nestor and Fischbach officially 'transformed' into Unus and Annus during the episode 'The Truth of Unus Annus' (1.351) The episode itself is a dramatic short, as Nestor and Fischbach are taunted by the realisation that their time has almost come to an end. Slick editing, horror film techniques and a score made up of discordant strings and other sounds suggest voyeurism and doppelgängers as the pair separately explore an abandoned, dark and decrepit building, guided only by taunting voices on a walkie-talkie. Reflections, shadows and even Nestor and Fischbach themselves begin to merge, seamlessly blending into one another from shot to shot. The pair are reunited at the *Unus Annus* casket, which they reluctantly open (see Figure 48). When the lid of the casket is replaced a few seconds later, Nestor and Fischbach have been substituted with Unus and Annus, completing the transformation, emphasising that there is no going back. The remaining videos in the series focus on introspection and reminiscences with Nestor/Unus and Fischbach/Annus continuing to wear the iconic suits until the end: an amalgamation of death and life, reality, and mythology.

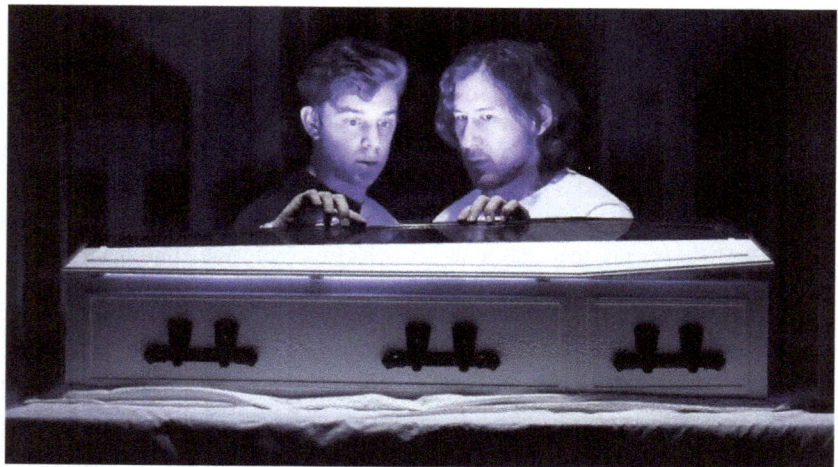

Figure 48. Nestor and Fischbach open the casket before their final transition into Unus and Annus in the episode 'The Truth of Unus Annus'. *Unus Annus*, created by Mark Fischbach and Ethan Nestor (2019–20).

Like other examples of thanatological imagination in popular culture, *Unus Annus* generates a morbid space that 'embraces death with the intent to entertain, divert, and amuse the consumer' (Penfold-Mounce 2020: 54). Like the Victorian memento mori, this morbid space is distanced enough from the physical realities of death to allow 'a safe imaginative environment in which consumers can consume mortality without direct consequence or full sensory exposure' (Penfold-Mounce 2020: 55; see also Penfold-Mounce 2018). An example of this occurs during the episode 'Mark and Ethan Go Casket Shopping' (1.58) in which Fischbach and Nestor discuss different kinds of coffins and caskets with a funeral director, speaking frankly about various issues including the fear people have of the practicalities of death. Fischbach explains:

> Fischbach: One important thing that we try to get through to people is that [preparing for death] isn't something to be afraid of […] it's something that's a reminder that we have to live as best we can while we have the time we can. And even if you have to think about the 'morbidity' of casket shopping or something like that, it is important to remember that we all go through the same end, every single one of us, we just don't know when. But given the time we have, we have to enjoy it while we can.

The duo eventually settles on a bespoke casket: a toe-pincher style half-black, half-white coffin with satin lining. This casket ultimately becomes an important symbol for the channel. Although it does not appear on screen again until 'The Truth about Unus Annus', it plays a significant role in the last few episodes, particularly during the finale 'Goodbye' (1.364) as well as in the afterlife of the channel.

The morbid space of *Unus Annus* destabilises the gravity and solemnity of potentially weighty issues through both its structure and its use of humour. From the beginning, *Unus Annus* is simultaneously presented as an introspective channel and an opportunity for its presenters to take part in light-hearted experiences or challenges. The fundamental question of 'What would you do if you only had one year?' allows for the chance to indulge in activities or desires as well as provides a space to reflect on difficult personal or existential questions that may not have an answer. Challenge-based or light-hearted videos are frequently juxtaposed with more serious topics or discussions ('A Serious Conversation under the Stars' (1.257); 'Was 2020 a Bad Year for Unus Annus?' (1.290)). Furthermore, many videos that begin in a more light-hearted way either naturally become contemplative ('What Was the Most

Painful Thing We've Ever Endured?' (1.38); 'Emotional Pain vs Physical Pain … Which Is Worse?' (1.45); 'How NOT to be the Perfect Boyfriend' (1.150)). While humour in *Unus Annus* is a fundamental part of the channel, it is also used to undermine moments where tension is high or in instances where the issues discussed are in danger of becoming too philosophical or morbid.

## The Impact of Covid-19

The function, effect and meaning of the thanatological space nurtured by *Unus Annus* changed during 2020 as the Covid-19 pandemic spread across the world. On a practical level, Fischbach and Nestor were unable to continue the kinds of activities or experiences they had throughout the series so far, particularly during lockdown. However, in a year where death, grieving and isolation became prominent and immediate concerns of everyday life, *Unus Annus* offered both comedic distraction and a space where death was discussed in a palatable way; paradoxically allowing space for release and confrontation from world events. Nestor notes that the year was 'so crazy and so ruthless in a bunch of different ways and I think that 2020 was the perfect year for *Unus Annus* because it really showed that. And it made it more special because we did it in a year that threw everything at us' ('Memento …'). As well as offering content during a time when entertainment was particularly important, many viewers found comfort in the stability of the series; the knowledge that there would be a video every day invited consistency in uncertain times as well as access to a community complete with in-jokes, fan art and merchandise during a period where, as Fischbach notes, the 'world was incredibly alone' ('Mori …'). The ending of *Unus Annus*, therefore, was not simply the end of an entertainment series; it was the ending of a sense of safety and community in a time of worldwide trauma, and this evoked intensified feelings of grief in the audience as would be expected at the end of a beloved series (see Figure 49).

The sense of loss was further exacerbated by the deletion of the *Unus Annus* channel, social media and so on; unlike other beloved products such as television series, the videos could not be revisited or remade – the death

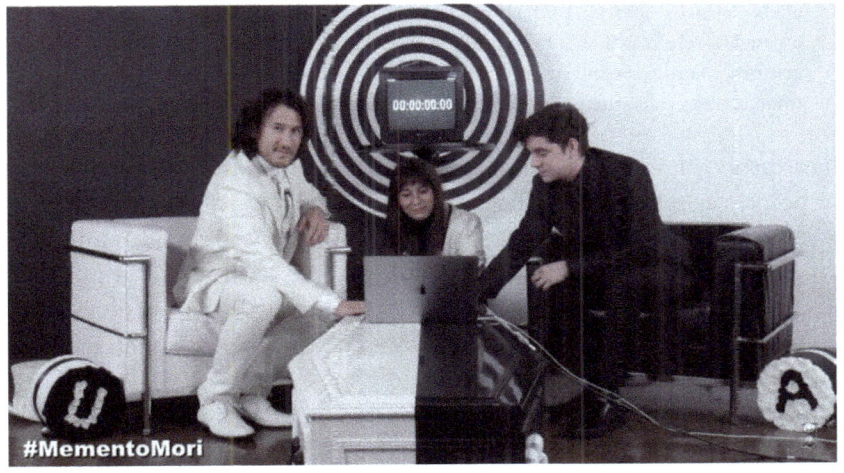

Figure 49. The final shot of Unus Annus before the channel is deleted, featuring Fischbach, Nelson and Nestor in episode 'Goodbye'. *Unus Annus*, created by Mark Fischbach and Ethan Nestor (2019–20).

of *Unus Annus* was swift and permanent. Fischbach and Nestor repeatedly warned viewers against attempting to archive or re-upload episodes; their 'last wish' and 'parting gift' was for viewers to 'Stay true to the purpose of our final year or we shall lay down wrath upon those that attempt to escape the end' (*Unus Annus* channel description). For a time, mentions of *Unus Annus* and its content were 'redacted' or censored in other works by the creators, reinforcing the permanence of its demise. Fischbach later notes that while many viewers attempted to cling on to the series or to the hope that it would be resurrected somehow, others 'lean[ed] into humour and [...] inside jokes' possibly to 'compensate for the pain of it being gone' ('Mori ...').

## Afterlife

*Unus Annus* and its legacy conducts and operates within a thanatological space; a 'morbidly inclined' space that enable[s] an exploration of the boundaries surrounding mortality and how these can be crossed or reinforced [...] exemplif[ing] how corpses and death are far from taboo but are instead ordinary and normalized whilst also becoming popularized, eroticized, and even at times celebrated alongside societal ambivalence. (Penfold-Mounce 2020: 54)

The creators acknowledge this, with Fischbach explaining thus: 'The loss was the point, the emotions of that was the point of it. The feelings, the conflicted emotions. The reluctance to let go of it. I wanted to make something that was so important that people would hate to let it go' ('Postmortem'). Nestor agrees, noting, 'I think there was something so beautiful about the willingness to let it go and that's something that made it so much more special [...] it was special because it had to die.'

While the creators expressed satisfaction, contentment and a rejuvenation of creativity following the end of the series ('Unus Annus – Post Mortem' (Fischbach); 'The End of Unus Annus' (Nestor)), there was an outpouring of grief amongst fans. At the time of writing, the last videos by Fischbach and Nestor which explicitly discuss the series were released on the respective anniversaries of its passing. The first anniversary videos in 2021 show the duo as they separately approach the casket in the woods to lay a rose and offer their thoughts (black for Nestor, white for Fischbach, naturally, see Figure 50). The second set of anniversary videos, released in November 2022, feature reminiscences between Nestor and Fischbach about the impact of the series. However, the pair are seated back-to-back with a sheet in between them and therefore cannot see each other. In each segment, only half of the conversation can be heard, with the volume on the 'other side' lowered to a mumble. For either of the two videos to make sense, they must be played simultaneously; while Nestor and Fischbach have moved on to other projects, Unus and Annus do not make sense without each other even after their demise.

*Unus Annus* invites viewers into the complex and emotive reality of death. It creates a 'morbid space' where 'sensibilities about death can be explored without concern of being censured or criticized for being overly macabre' (Penfold-Mounce 2020: 55). Much like the black-and-white colour themes used in the show, *Unus Annus* provides supposedly conflicting techniques to create a thanatological or morbid space that is safe enough to experience and express this complicated subject. Death is presented as a constant reality yet mythologised through the characters of Unus and Annus. Sombre, introspective or difficult

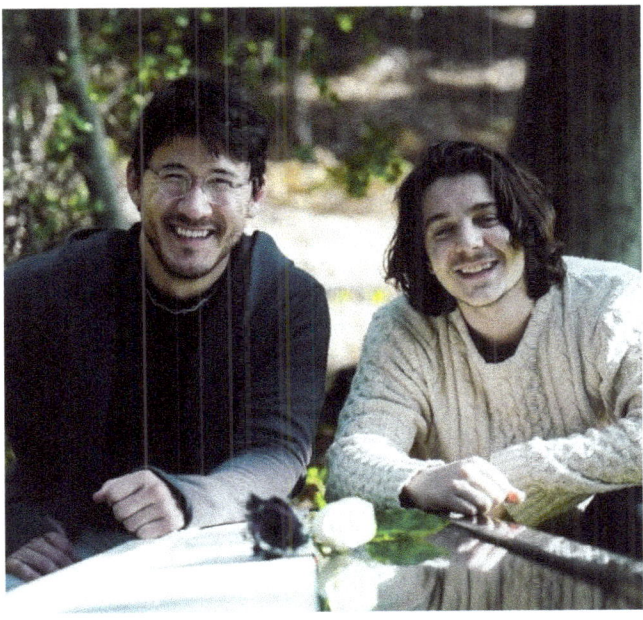

Figure 50. Promotional shot of Unus (Ethan Nestor) and Annus (Mark Fischbach) celebrating one year after the ending of *Unus Annus*.

subjects are explored alongside humour, clowning and adventure. The anniversary videos allow creators and viewers alike to reflect on memories of *Unus Annus* and its legacy, and potentially to grieve what it gave them or the time in their lives it represented (see Figure 51). Nestor and Fischbach observe that although *Unus Annus* has an established legend and lore on YouTube as well as other social media, there will 'be less and less people every year [who remember it]. But for those that it had meaning it *really*, really had meaning. It's beautiful that people are willing to share' (Fischbach, 'Mori ...', emphasis added). However, despite the temporality, potential and joy of making the show (Fischbach, 'Mori ...'), the pair acknowledge that there are more endings to come, although, in typical *Unus Annus* style, this sombre note is quickly undermined:

Fischbach: You know what's an even sadder thought though? Is if we were to do this every year – which, who knows, maybe we will – if we were, there'll come a year someday where one of these chairs will be empty. And then, both. [Pause] Probably because one of us will be cancelled, let's just be honest!

The story of *Unus Annus* is not quite finished; this undead Scheherazade arguably has more stories to tell. Despite the death of the channel, it is still talked about in YouTube videos, social media, references and in-jokes amongst fans. The final image of the *Unus Annus* story so far is, appropriately enough, Fischbach, Nestor and Nelson companionably talking around a fire – a reminder that, even with the permanence of death, stories must continue, and life must go on.

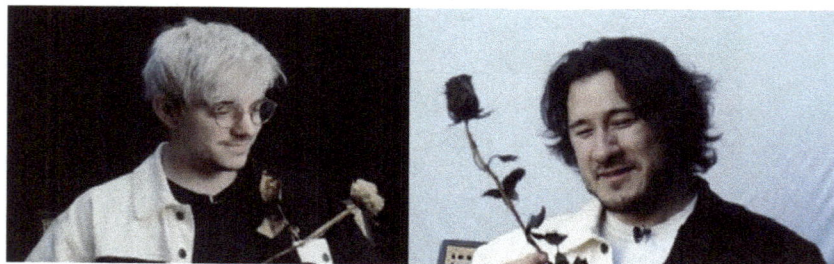

Figure 51. Nestor and Fischbach receive the roses they left for each other the year before 'Memento …'/'Mori' (Second anniversary of *Unus Annus*).

Lisa Morton

# Afterword: The Tomorrow of Death – Dia de los Muertos

As a Halloween expert, one of the things I'm routinely asked to opine on during interviews is the holiday's future. Twenty years ago – before we had terms like 'cultural appropriation' – I routinely answered that I foresaw Halloween and its Mexican cousin [Day of the Dead] merging more and more. At the time (circa 2005), Dia de los Muertos was still largely a regional observation in the United States, and few Americans knew of it or understood it.

Now, twenty years later, I've seen that prediction coming true. Large chains like See's Candies now carry Dia de los Muertos treats; on the shelves of their shops, little skull-shaped candy containers are nestled in next to jack-o'-lantern truffles. Movies like Pixar/Disney's *Coco* (Molina 2017) have introduced audiences around the world to the central themes and iconography of Mexico's Day of the Dead.

Why did I make that prediction all those years ago, and why have big American companies decided to appropriate this holiday and profit from it?

Dia de los Muertos offers a rendering of death that is both sombre and playful. On the one hand, it has made a queen of artist José Guadalupe Posada's early-twentieth-century etching 'La Calavera Catrina'; this classic image of a grinning skull wearing an elegant hat bedecked with plumes and flowers tells the viewer immediately that death is equitable, that it holds dominion over both the poor and the rich (see Figure 52).

On the other hand, Dia de los Muertos – unlike the Celtic-based Halloween – kept many of the traditions of the Catholic All Saints' Day (1 November) and All Souls' Day (2 November), with honouring loved ones who have passed taking the central positions. Mexican families celebrate Dia de los Muertos by making ofrendas – elaborate altar-like collections of photographs,

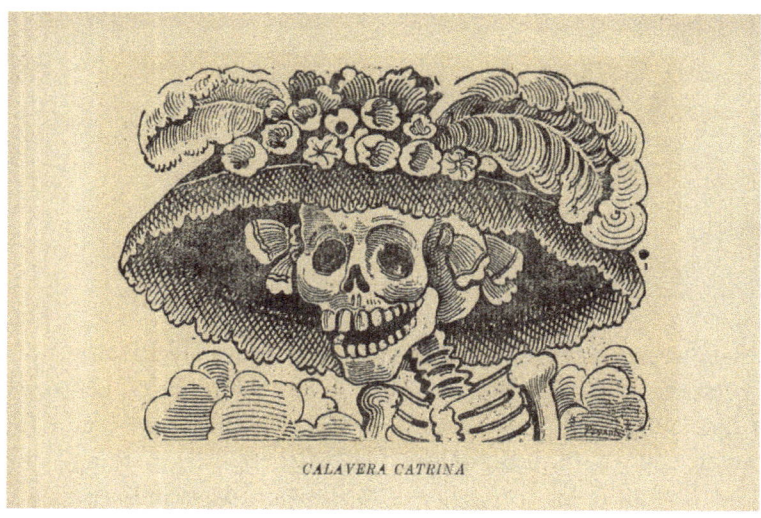

Figure 52. *Calavera de la Catrina* (Skull of the Female Dandy), from the portfolio 36 Grabados: José Guadalupe Posada, published by Arsacio Vanegas, Mexico City, c. 1910, zinc etching. Image in the public domain.

food, drink, trinkets and orange marigolds – in remembrance of their late family members (and to provide the visiting spirits with sustenance), and they venture out to the graveyards to clean and decorate graves and tombs (this latter practice also takes place in much of Europe and even a few parts of the United States, principally Louisiana). In Dia de los Muertos, then, death is something to be mocked and accepted but not feared.

Americans, of course, are well known for their fear of death. Books like Jessica Mitford's *The American Way of Death* (1963) and Elizabeth Kubler-Ross' *On Death and Dying* (1969) brought the American discomfort with death and dying out into the open.

Things are changing, however; recent surveys show that over half of Americans no longer report greatly fearing death (see *Statista Surveys* 2019). The world has changed for recent generations and so has the way death is regarded. When funerals cost more than what many people earn in several months and shows like *Six Feet Under* (2001–5) entertain by limning the realities of the funeral business, death becomes a far more practical matter. Add to that the ways that younger people are forced to confront death in America on a daily basis – whether from mass shootings or ecological disasters – and death can only be more accepted … and finally mocked.

Which brings us back to why Dia de los Muertos is gaining popularity throughout North America. The question of cultural appropriation must surely arise, what with massive American corporations lifting the playful sugar skull and calaveras designs wholesale in the name of the dollar. However, the argument could be made that they are also marketing these products to North America's significant numbers of Latinx consumers as well as others.

Perhaps this is less about cultural appropriation and more about timing. Americans, as we see in both surveys and depictions of death in popular culture, are moving on; for many, acceptance of death has replaced fear. It is surely no coincidence that one of the hottest Halloween items in years was Home Depot's twelve-foot-tall skeleton with 'LifeEyes™ LCD Eyes' which appear to move and blink. First issued in 2021, these skeletons sold out immediately (a feat repeated in 2022) and became highly sought after, drawing three times the original retail price in second-hand markets. This huge recreation of the ultimate image of Death was first sold just over a year into the pandemic; Halloween 2021 was still largely lacking in traditional Halloween rituals like trick or treat, but homeowners could install a cyclopean and playful image of Death in their front yard (and many chose to simply leave the skeleton up throughout the year, given the difficulties of disassembly and storage). Death had now become a kind of status symbol, a prize gained only by the luckiest shoppers; it was a product that could be seen from hundreds of yards away. Death now towers over many American suburbs.

The twelve-foot-skeleton is a close cousin of Dia de los Muertos' whimsical skeletons, with their grinning skulls painted in bright colours and floral designs. It is surely more than mere coincidence that this product was introduced – and proved to be immensely popular – at the same time that the Mexican Dia de los Muertos has been embraced by American consumerism.

This book has presented essays that have explored death's various representations, mainly in horror movies, television and comics/manga. These media depend upon prodding our fears – of technology, of nature, of change, of our own bodies, of disease, of what lies beyond death. Is death itself still the central object of fear in these films? Or have we moved beyond that to be afraid of what comes before death (physical pain, confusion, loss of sanity/identity/memory, isolation)? Several of the chapters contained herein refer to death in the *Harry Potter* series, suggesting that death is transforming into a concept that adults are less likely to consider taboo for children.

As we move forward into our increasingly dangerous future, one split wide open by almost daily environmental, medical and ideological disasters, death – or big-D Death – will surely become more accepted, expected and even mocked. North American culture may not embrace the *other* side of Dia de los Muertos – the one that honours the dead and feeds their visiting spirits – but it is already taking in and spitting out the whimsical image of the bony spectre who grins back at us.

Death, in other words, is here to stay … and we are fine with that.

# Image Intervention VII: The Guardian

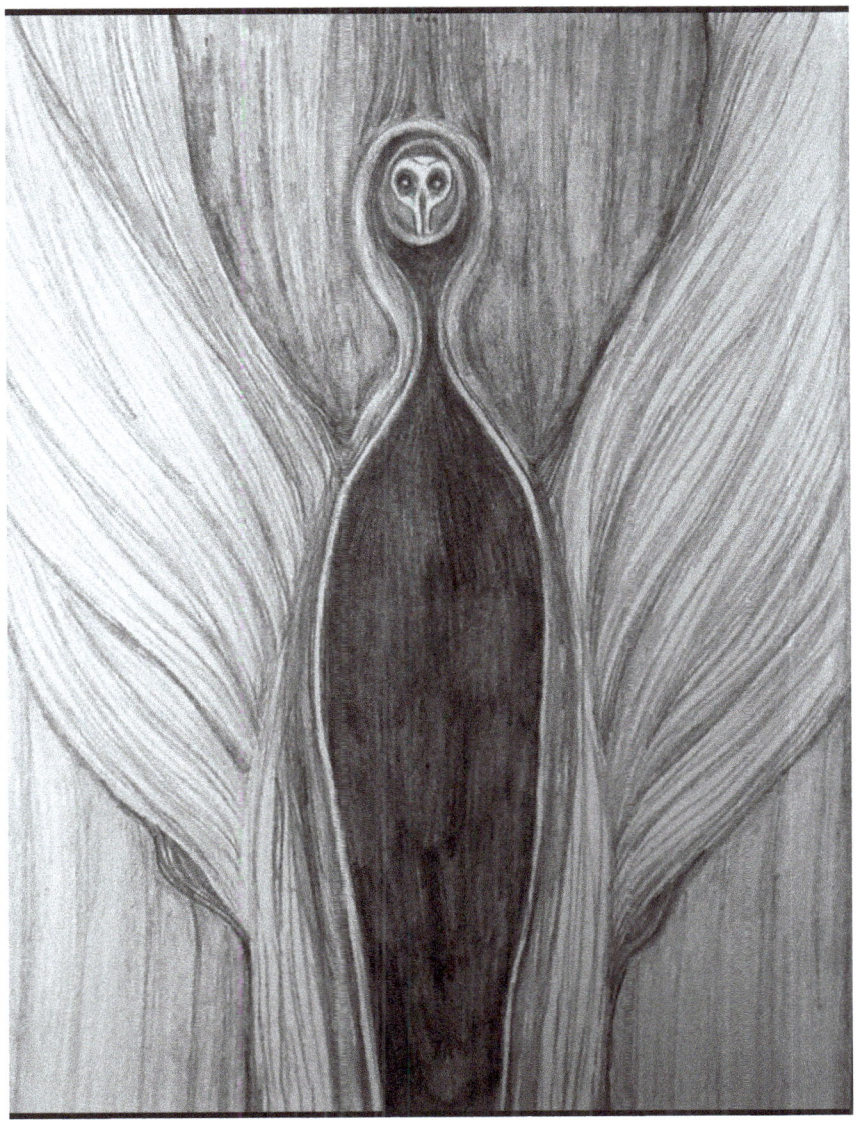

Artwork by Gemma Files
(Reproduced with the permission of the artist)

# Bibliography

*2012*, dir. Roland Emmerich (Hollywood: Columbia Pictures, 2009).

*28 Days Later*, dir. Danny Boyle (London: Fox Searchlight Pictures, 2002).

Aaron, Michele, *Death and Moving Image: Ideology, Iconography and I* (Edinburgh: Edinburgh University Press, 2014).

Aaron, Michele, ed., *Envisaging Death: Visual Culture and Dying* (Newcastle: Cambridge Scholars Publishing, 2013).

Abbott, Stacey, *Undead Apocalypse: Vampires and Zombies in the 21st Century* (Edinburgh: Edinburgh University Press, 2016).

Achebe, Chinua, *There Was a Country: A Personal History of Biafra* (New York: Penguin, 2012).

*After.Life*, dir. Agnieszka Wojtowicz-Vosloo (Beverly Hills: Anchor Bay Entertainment, 2009).

Alimi S. A. (2012). 'A Study of the Use of Proverbs as a Literary Device in Achebe's things fall apart and Arrow of God'. *International Journal of Academic Research in Business and Social Sciences*, 2 (3), 121.

*Amazing Grace*, dir. Michael Apted (Yoronti: Momentum Pictures, 2007).

American Civil Liberties Union (ACLU), 'LGBTQ Rights', 2023a. <https://www.aclu.org/legislative-attacks-on-lgbtq-rights>. Accessed 21 February 2023.

American Civil Liberties Union (ACLU), 'Mapping Attacks on LGBTQ Rights in U.S. State Legislature', 2023b. <https://www.aclu.org/legislative-attacks-on-lgbtq-rights>. Accessed 21 February 2023.

*American Horror Story: Asylum*, created by Ryan Murphy and Brad Fulchuk (Los Angeles: 20th Television, 2012).

*Amistad*, dir. Steven Spielberg (Hollywood: Dreamworks Pictures, 1997).

*Andromeda Strain, The*, dir. Robert Wise (Universal City: Universal Pictures, 1971).

Antonio, Edward, 'Religion and the Environment', in Elias Kifon Bonmba and Jacob OLuona, eds, *The Wiley-Blackwell Companion to African Religions* (Oxford: Wiley Blackwell, 2012), 140–52.

Anugwom, Edlyne, 'Memory as Social Burden Collective Remembrance of the Biafran War and Imaginations of Socio-Political Marginalization in Contemporary Nigeria', in A. Dirk Moses and Lasse Heerten, eds, *Postcolonial Conflict and the Question of Genocide: The Nigeria-Biafra War 1967–1970* (New York: Routledge, 2018), 387–411.

Appiah, Kwame Anthony, 'The Case for Capitalizing the B in Black', *The Atlantic*, 18 June 2020. <https://www.theatlantic.com/ideas/archive/2020/06/time-to-capitalize-blackand-white/613159/>. Accessed 1 October 2022.

Arata, Stephen D., 'The Occidental Tourist: "Dracula" and the Anxiety of Reverse Colonization', *Victorian Studies*, 33/4 (Summer 1990), 621–45.

Arendt, Florian, Sebastian Scherr, Josh Pasek, Patrick E. Jamieson and Daniel Romer, 'Investigating Harmful and Helpful Effects of Watching Season 2 of *13 Reasons Why*: Results of a Two-Wave U.S. Panel Survey', *Social Science & Medicine*, 232 (2019), 489–98.

Arendt, Hannah, *The Origins of Totalitarianism* (1951; London: Penguin, 2017).

Aries, Philippe, *Western Attitudes towards Death* (London: Marion Boyars, 1974).

Armstrong, Megan A., ' "A Nation Reborn": Right to Law and Right to Life in the Purge Franchise', *Journal of Intervention and Statebuilding*, 13/3 (2019), 377–92.

Aschheim, Steven, 'How Did Josef Mengele Become the Evil Doctor of Auschwitz', *New York Times*, 29 January 2020. <https://www.nytimes.com/2020/01/28/books/review/mengele-david-g-marwell.html>. Accessed 10 January 2022.

*Autopsy of Jane Doe, The*, dir. André Øvredal (London: Lionsgate & IFC Pictures, 2016).

Bar-On, Tamir, 'Richard B. Spencer and the Alt Right', in Mark Sedgwick, ed., *Key Thinkers of the Radical Right: Behind the New Threat to Liberal Democracy* (New York: Oxford Academic, 2019).

Barton, Charles K. B., *Getting Even: Revenge as a Form of Justice* (Chicago: Open Court, 1999).

Bataille, Georges, 'The Mask', trans. J. Biles, *LVNG: An Independent Journal of Poetry, Fiction, & Art*, 10 (2002), 63–7.

Battin, Margaret Pabst, *Ending Life: Ethics and the Way We Die* (Oxford: Oxford University Press, 2005).

*Bay, The*, dir. Barry Levinson (Beverley Hills: Baltimore Pictures, 2012).

*Beach House, The*, dir. Jeffrey A. Brown (Cleveland: Low Spark Films, 2019).

*Beasts of the Southern Wild*, dir. Benh Zeitlin (New York: Cinereach, 2012).

Behr, Kate, ' "Same-as-Difference": Narrative Transformations and Intersecting Cultures in Harry Potter', *Journal of Narrative Theory*, 35/1 (2005), 112–32.

Bell, Corey, 'From Victim to Kira: *Death Note* and the Misplaced Agencies of Cosmic Justice', in Sarah Pasfield-Neofitou and Cathy Sell, eds, *Manga Vision: Cultural and Communicative Perspective* (Clayton: Monash University Publishing, 2016), 70–86.

Bell, R. C., *Board and Table Games from Many Civilizations*, Vol. I (London: Oxford University Press, 1960).

*Belle*, dir. Amma Asante (London: BFI, 2013).

Belting, Hans, *An Anthropology of Images: Picture. Medium. Body* (Princeton: Princeton University Press, 2011).

Benkel, Thorsten, and Matthias Meitzler, 'Materiality and the Body: Explorations at the End of Life', *Mortality*, 24/2 (2019), 231–46.
Bennett, Alice, 'Unquiet Spirits: Death Writing in Contemporary Fiction', *Textual Practice*, 23/3 (2009), 463–79.
Benshoff, Harry M., *Monsters in the Closet: Homosexuality in the Horror Film* (Manchester: Manchester University Press, 1997).
Bentley, Christopher, 'The Monster in the Bedroom: Sexual Symbolism in Bram Stoker's *Dracula*', in Margaret L. Carter, ed., *Dracula: The Vampire and the Critics* (Ann Arbor: UMI Research Press, 1988), 25–34.
Berger, J. M., *Extremism* (Cambridge: MIT Press, 2018).
Bhatt, G. P., ed, *The Brahma Purana* (New Delhi: Motilal Banarasidas Publishing House, 1955).
*Blackfish*, dir. Gabriela Cowperthwaite (Atlanta: CNN Films, 2013).
Blake, Linnie, The Wounds of Nations: Horror Cinema, Historical Trauma and National Identity [2008] (Manchester: Manchester University Press, 2013).
Boon, Kevin, 'Part Introduction', in D. Christie and J. Lauro, ed., *Better Off Dead: The Evolution of the Zombie as Posthuman* (New York: Fordham University Press, 2011).
Bostan, Sarah-Nicole, '13 Reasons Why We Need to Talk about Clinical Depression', *Psychology Today*, 21 May 2017. <https://www.psychologytoday.com/us/blog/greater-the-sum-its-parts/201705/13-reasons-why>. Accessed 19 September 2022.
Botting, Fred, 'Zombie London: Unexceptionalities of the New World Order', in Sarah Juliet Lauro, ed., *Zombie Theory: A Reader* (London: University of Minnesota Press, 2017).
Branson, Susan, 'Phrenology and the Science of Race in Antebellum America', *Early American Studies*, 15/1 (2017), 164–93.
Breen, Lauren, Daisuke Kawashima, Karima Joy, Susan Cadell, David Roth, Amy Chow and Mary Ellen Macdonald, 'Grief Literacy: A Call to Action for Compassionate Communities', *Death Studies*. 46/2 (2022), 425–33.
Bridge, Jeffrey A., Joel B. Greenhouse, Donna Ruch, Jack Stevens, John Ackerman, Arielle H. Sheftall, Lisa M. Horowitz, Kelly J. Kelleher and John V. Campo, 'Association between the Release of Netflix's *13 Reasons Why* and Suicide Rates in the United States: An Interrupted Time Series Analysis', *Journal of the American Academy of Child & Adolescent Psychiatry* (28 April 2019), 236–43.
Bronfen, Elizabeth, *Over Her Dead Body: Death, Femininity and the Aesthetic* (Manchester: Manchester University Press, 1992).
Brown, Jeffrey A., *The Modern Superhero in Film and Television Popular Genre and American Culture* (New York: Routledge, 2016).
Brown, Mark, 'Tomb Raider's Grisly Death Animations Are Outdated', *Polygon*, 23 October 2018. <https://www.polygon.com/2018/10/11/17961496/tomb-raider-death-animations>. Accessed 3 September 2022.

Bruner, Raisa, 'This Is the Most Tweeted-About Show of 2017 So Far', *The Time*, 21 April 2017. <https://time.com/4751256/13-reasons-why-twitter-conversation/>. Accessed 4 August 2022.

Bub, Vera, '"The Last Enemy That Shall Be Destroyed Is Death", Christian Elements in Harry Potter?', in Marion Gymnich et al., eds, *'Harry – Yer a Wizard': Exploring J.K. Rowling's Harry Potter Universe* (Baden-Baden: Tectum, 2017), 107–17.

Bucher, Cornelius J., *Three Models on a Rocking-Horse: A Comparative Study in Narratology* (Tübingen: Gunter Narr Verlag Tübingen, 1990).

Bulgakov, Mikhail, *The Master and Margarita*, trans. by Katherine Tiernan O'Connor (New York: Overlook Books, 2021), 107.

Bundrick, Christopher, '"Covered in Blood and Dirt": Industrial, Capital and Cultural Crisis in Red Rock and *Dracula*', *Southern Literary Journal*, 47/1 (Fall 2014), 21–34.

Byers, Steven, *Introduction to Forensic Anthropology* (Oxford: Routledge, 2016).

Caciola, Nancy Mandeville, *Afterlives: The Return of the Dead in the Middle Ages* (Ithaca: Cornell University Press, 2016).

Caetano, Kalie, 'The Nuances of Mastering Death: Murder, Capital Punishment, and Assisted Suicide in Harry Potter', in Cecilia Konchar Farr, ed., *A Wizard of Their Age: Critical Essays from the Harry Potter Generation* (Albany: State University of New York Press, 2015), 113–27.

Caffrey, Stephanie, 'Exploring the Roles of Women on Supernatural', Hidden Remote, 22 September 2017. <https://hiddenremote.com/2017/09/22/exploring-roles-women-supernatural/>. Accessed 10 August 2023.

Callus, Ian, '(Auto)Thanatography or (Auto)Thanatology: Mark C. Taylor, Simon Critchely, and the Writing of the Dead', *Forum of Modern Language Studies*, 41/4 (2005), 427–38.

Campbell, Hayley, *All the Living and the Dead* (New York: St. Martin's Press, 2022).

Camus, Albert, *The Plague* (London: Hamish Hamilton, 1947).

Canuel, Mark, *The Shadow of Death: Literature, Romanticism, and the Subject of Punishment* (Princeton: Princeton University Press, 2007).

Carlisle, Rodney, *One Day in History: September 11, 2001* (United Kingdom: Harper Collins Publishers, 2007).

Carter, Elisabeth, 'Right-Wing Extremism/Radicalism: Reconstructing the Concept', *Journal of Political Ideologies*, 23 (2018), 157–82.

*Cast Away*, dir. Robert Zemeckis (Novato: Image Movers, 2000).

Castillo, David R., David Schmid, David A. Reilly and John Edgar Browning, *Zombie Talk: Culture, History, Politics* (London: Palgrave Macmillan, 2016).

Centers for Disease Control and Prevention, 'Racial and Ethnic Disparities Continue in Pregnancy-Related Deaths', 6 September 2019. <https://www.cdc.gov/media/releases/2019/p0905-racial-ethnic-disparities-pregnancy-deaths.html>. Accessed 14 December 2022.

Cerel, Julie, John R. Jordan and Paul R. Duberstein, 'The Impact of Suicide on the Family', *Crisis*, 29/1 (2008), 38–44.
Chaim, Bentorah, 'HEBREW WORD STUDY – PASS-THROUGH', Chaim Bentorah.com, February 19, 2020. <https://www.chaimbentorah.com/2020/02/hebrew-word-study-pass-through/>. Accessed 28 October 2024.
Chandra, Suresh, *Encyclopedia of Hindu Gods and Goddesses* (New Delhi: Sarup & Sons, 2001).
Chaturvedi, B. K., trans., *Kalki Purana* (New Delhi: Diamond Pocket Books, 2008).
Cheng Qijin, Hong Li, Vincent Silenzio and Eric D. Caine, 'Suicide Contagion: A Systematic Review of Definitions and Research Utility', *PLoS ONE*, 9/9 (2014), 1–9.
Chikamatsu, Monzaemon, 'The Love Suicides of Amijima', trans. Donald Keene, in Karen Brazell, ed., *Traditional Japanese Theatre: An Anthology of Plays* (New York: Columbia University Press, 1998), 333–63.
Chomsky, Noam, *Chomsky Notebook* (New York: Columbia University Press, 2010).
Chomsky, Noam, YouTube, 9 April 2013. <https://www.youtube.com/watch?v=iR_NmkkMmO8>. Accessed 21 August 2023.
Chopra, Anupama, 'Anurag Basu and Pritam Interview', YouTube, 7 November 2020. <https://youtu.be/k8hRxIUc9LI>. Accessed 14 June 2023.
Chopra, Anupama, 'Team Ludo in Conversation with Anupama Chopra', YouTube, 11 November 2020. <https://youtu.be/4NX6h2yEEcM>. Accessed 14 June 2023.
Chuku, Gloria, 'Woman and the Nigeria-Biafra War', in A. Dirk Moses and Lasse Herten, eds, *Postcolonial Conflict and the Question of Genocide – The Nigeria-Biafra War 1967–1970* (New York: Routledge, 2018), 329–59.
Ciba, Michèle, 'Conspiracy, Persecution and Terror: Harry Potter in a Post-9/11 World', in Marion Gymnich et al., eds, '*Harry – Yer a Wizard*': *Exploring J.K. Rowling's Harry Potter Universe* (Baden-Baden: Tectum, 2017), 121–32.
Cinquegrani, Mattia, 'The Rebirth of Death: Representation of Loss in Television Series', in Nate Hinerman and Mary Ruth Sanders, eds, *Care, Loss and the End of Life* (Oxford: Inter-Disciplinary Press, 2016), 37–47.
Clements, Jonathan, and Helen McCarthy, 'Sailor Moon', in *The Anime Encyclopedia: A Century of Japanese Animation* (New York: Stone Bridge Press, 2015), 711–12.
Cline, Ernest, *Ready Player One* (New York: Ballantine Books-Penguin Random House, 2011).
Cline, Ernest, *Ready Player Two* (New York: Ballantine Books-Penguin Random House, 2020).
*Coco*, dir. Lee Unkrich (Los Angeles, Disney, 2017).
Coleridge, Samuel Taylor, 'The Rime of the Ancyent Marinere', in R. L. Brett and A. R. Jones, eds, *Lyrical Ballads* (London: Routledge, 1991), 9–35.
Collective for Radical Death Studies, 'About', The Collective for Radical Death Studies, 2023. <https://www.radicaldeathstudies.com/our-mission>. Accessed 28 October 2023.

Compagnone, Vanessa, and Marcel Danesi, 'Mythic and Occulist Naming Strategies in Harry Potter', *NAMES*, 60/3 (2012), 127–34.

Conrich, Ian, 'Puzzles, Contraptions, and the Highly Elaborate Moment: The Inevitability of Death in the Grand Slasher Narratives of the *Final Destination* and *Saw* Series of Films', in Wickham Clayton, ed., *Style and Form in the Hollywood Slasher Film* (New York: Palgrave Macmillan, 2015), 106–17.

Conway, Deanne, *Mother, Maiden, Crone* (St Paul: Llewellyn Books, 1994).

Cooper, Ayanni C. H., '"There Is More to Me Than Just Hunger": Female Monsters and Liminal Spaces in *Monstress* and *Pretty Deadly*', in Samantha Langsdale and Elizabeth Rae Coody, eds, *Monstrous Women in Comics* (Jackson: University of Mississippi Press, 2020), 51–66.

Corbin, Caroline Mala, 'Terrorists Are Always Muslim but Never White: At the Intersection of Critical Race Theory and Propaganda', *Fordham Law Review*, 86/2 (2017), n.p.

*Corpse of Anna Fritz, The* [El cadáver de Anna Fritz], dir. Hèctor Hernández Vicens (Paris: Splendor Films, 2015).

Corrigan, Maureen, '"Jane Eyre" Meets "Dracula" in This Sharp, Inventive "Mexican Gothic" Tale', *National Public Radio* (text-only version), 9 July 2020. <https://text.npr.org/889365673>. Accessed 15 September 2022.

*Cove, The*, dir. Louie Psihoyos (Beverley Hills: Participant Media, 2009).

'Covid-19 India Timeline', *The Wire*, n.d. <https://thewire.in/covid-19-india-timeline>. Accessed 17 June 2023.

Creed, Barbara, 'Dark Desires: Male Masochism in the Horror Film', in Steven Cohan and Ina Rae Hark, eds, *Screening the Male: Exploring Masculinities in Hollywood Cinema* (New York: Routledge, 1993), 118–33.

Crettaz, Bernard, *Cafe's mortels* [Death Cafés] (Genève: Labor et Fides, 2010).

*Cthulhu*, dir. Grant Cogswell (Washington: Arkham Northwest Productions, 2007).

D'Souza, Dinesh, *Life after Death: The Evidence* (Washington: Regnery Publishing, 2009).

*Dagon*, dir. Stuart Gordon (Barcelona: Castelao Pictures, 2001).

Dalrymple, Theodore, 'In the Asylum', *City Journal*, Summer 2005. <https://www.city-journal.org/article/in-the-asylum>. Accessed 13 April 2022.

Daly, Jennifer, *Deconstructing Zombies of Capitalism: The Walking Dead and New Views of American Zombies* (New York: Montclair State University, 2016).

Das, Purnaprajna, ed., *Sri Kalki Purana*, trans. Bhumipati Das (Mathura: Jai Nitai Press, 2006).

DaShareZone, 'All Social Media Platforms Openly Support White Supremacy', Facebook, 7 August 2018. <https://www.facebook.com/dasharezone/photos/924600964403120>. Accessed 23 May 2021.

DaShareZone, 'Just Walk Out', Facebook, 12 May 2019. <https://www.facebook.com/dasharezone/photos/1092512044278677/>. Accessed 23 May 2021.

## Bibliography

DaShareZone, 'What the Fuck Is the Human Condition?' Facebook, 11 July 2018. <https://www.facebook.com/dasharezone/photos/897121457151071>. Accessed 23 May 2021.

Davies, Cath, 'Technological Taxidermy: Recognising Faces in Celebrity Death', *Mortality*, 15/2 (2010), 138–53.

Davis, Therese, *The Face on the Screen: Death, Recognition and Spectatorship* (Bristol: Intellect, 2004).

Davison, Carol Margaret, 'Introduction to the Corpse in the Closet: The Gothic, Death, and Modernity', in Carol Margaret Davison, ed., *The Gothic and Death* (Manchester: Manchester University Press, 2017), 1–18.

*Dawn of the Dead*, dir. George Romero (Los Angeles: United Film Distribution Company, 1978).

*Day After Tomorrow, The*, dir. Roland Emmerich (Los Angeles: Twentieth Century Fox, 2004).

De Quincy, Thomas, *Suspiria de Profundis* (1845; New York: Dover Publications, 2019).

*Deadgirl*, dir. Marcel Sarmiento and Gadi Harel (Orland Park: Dark Sky Pictures, 2008).

Deardorff, Daniel, *The Other Within: The Genius of Deformity in Myth, Culture and Psyche* (Ashland: White Cloud Press, 2004).

Death Café, n.d. <https://deathcafe.com/>. Accessed 31 May 2023.

*Death Stranding*, dir. Hideo Kojima (Tokyo: Sony Interactive Entertainment, 2019).

*Death Takes a Holiday*, dir. Mitchell Leisen (Los Angeles: Paramount Pictures, 1934).

DeConnick, Kelly Sue, Emma Ríos, Jordie Bellaire and Clayton Cowles, *Pretty Deadly: The Bear* (Portland: Image Comics, 2016).

DeConnick, Kelly Sue, and Emma Ríos, Jordie Bellaire and Clayton Cowles, *Pretty Deadly: The Rat* (Portland: Image Comics, 2020).

DeConnick, Kelly Sue, Emma Ríos, Jordie Bellaire and Clayton Cowles, *Pretty Deadly: The Shrike* (Portland Image Comics, 2014).

*Deepwater Horizon*, dir. Peter Berg (Santa Monica: Summit Entertainment, 2016).

Delchamps, Vivian, '"A Slight Hysterical Tendency" Performing Diagnosis in Perkins Gilman's "The Yellow Wallpaper"', in Johanna Braun, ed., *Performing Hysteria: Images and Imaginations of Hysteria* (Leuven: Leuven University Press, 2020), 105–24. doi:<https://doi.org/10.2307/j.ctv18dvt2c.9>.

DeLillo, Don, *White Noise* (New York: Penguin, 1984).

Derrida, Jacques, *Aporias* (Stanford: Stanford University Press, 1993).

Devine, Kristin, 'Is Supernatural Sexist?', Ordinary Times, 14 November 2019. <https://ordinary-times.com/2019/11/14/is-supernatural-sexist/>. Accessed 10 August 2023.

Dickerson, Kelly, 'Stephen Hawking Says, "God Particle" Could Wipe Out the Universe', *Live Science*, 8 September 2014. <https://www.livescience.com/47737-stephen-hawking-higgs-boson-universe-doomsday.html>. Accessed 3 September 2022.

Doka, Kenneth J., 'Disenfranchised Grief', *Bereavement Care*, 18/3 (1999), 37–9.

Doka, Kenneth, *Disenfranchised Grief: Recognizing Hidden Sorrow* (Maryland: Lexington Books, 1989).
Douglas, Mary, *Natural Symbols: Explorations in Cosmology* (London: Barrie & Rockliff, 1970).
Douglas, Mary, *Purity and Danger: An Analysis of Concept of Pollution and Taboo* (1966; London: Routledge, 2002).
Douglas, Mary, *Risk and Blame: Essays in Cultural Theory* (1992; London: Routledge, 1996).
Douglas, Mary, and Aaron Wildavsky, *Risk and Culture: An Essay on the Selection of Technological and Environmental Dangers* (Berkeley: University of California Press, 1983).
*Dracula*, dir. Tod Browning (Los Angeles: Universal Studios, 1931).
Drzazga, Grazyna, and Magda Stroinska, 'The Grammatical Gender of Death: A Textual and Discourse Approach', *Tekst i Dyskurs*, 5 (2012), 205–21.
Duru, Austine, 'Shades of Gray: Nigeria-Biafra War, U.S. Diplomatic Stance, and the Conscience of the American Nation', in Chima Korieh, ed., *New Perspectives on the Nigeria-Biafra War: No Victor, No Vanquished* (London: Lexington Books, 2021), 91–108.
Edmundson, Melissa, 'Introduction', in Melissa Edmundson, ed., *The Gothic Tradition of Supernatural: Essays on the Television Series* (Jefferson: McFarland, 2016), 1–15.
Elliott, Edward Bishop, *Horae Apocalypticae*, Vol. I, 5th ed. (London: Seely, Jackson and Halliday, 1862).
Emily, Exorcising, 'Supernatural: A History of Violence Against Women', The Geekiary, 16 May 2015. <https://thegeekiary.com/supernatural-a-history-of-violence-against-women-2/24763#:~:text=Alaina%20Huffman%20discussed%20how%20Supernatural,and%20Felicia%20Day%20said%20she/>. Accessed 7 August 2023.
Emmons, Alex, "White Knights", in The Intercept, October 12, 2017. <https://theintercept.com/2017/10/12/before-charlottesville-was-in-the-spotlight-police-arrested-their-most-prominent-critic-in-the-middle-of-the-night/>. Accessed 28 October 2023.
Erik-Soussi, Magda, 'The Western *Sailor Moon* Generation: North American Women and Feminine-Friendly Global Manga', in Casey Brienza, ed., *Global Manga: 'Japanese' Comics without Japan?* (Farnham: Ashgate, 2015), 23–44.
Estok, Simon C., 'Theorising the EcoGothic', *Gothic Nature*, 1 (2019), 34–53.
Estok, Simon C., 'Theorizing in a Space of Ambivalent Openness: Ecocriticism and Ecophobia', *ISLE: Interdisciplinary Studies in Literature and Environment*, 16 (2009), 203–25.
Evans, Jabari Miles, Alexis R. Lauricella, Drew P. Cingel, Davide Cino and Ann Wartella, 'Behind the Reasons: The Relationship between Adolescent and Young Adult Mental Health Risk Factors and Exposure to Season One of Netflix's *13 Reasons Why*', *Frontiers in Human Dynamics*, 9 June 2021. <https://www.frontiersin.org/articles/10.3389/fhumd.2021.600146/full>. Accessed 6 June 2023.

Ezeigbo, Akachi, 'Biafran War Literature and Africa's Search for Social Justice', in Ifi Armadiume and Abdullahi An-Na'im, eds, *The Politics of Memory: Truth, Healing and Social Justice* (London: Zed Books, 2002), 56–67.

Ezedike, Edward Uzoma, 'The Concept of Human Person in African Ontology: A Critical Reflection on the Igbo Notion of Man', *African Research Review*, 13 (2019), 131–7.

Fabian, Ann, *The Skull Collectors: Race, Science, and America's Unburied Dead* (Chicago: University of Chicago Press, 2010).

Fahey, Tracy, 2013. <https://gothicise.weebly.com/>. Accessed 7 June 2023.

'Fate, n.', Def. 3.a. *OED Online*. Oxford University Press. December 2023. <https://doi.org/10.1093/OED/9738000072>. Accessed 22 April 2024.

'Fate, n.', Def. 3.b. *OED Online*. Oxford University Press. December 2023. <https://doi.org/10.1093/OED/9738000072>. Accessed 22 April 2024.

Fangasm, 'Lisa Berry on Supernatural, Playing Death and Getting Excited about Wayward Sisters', Fangasm, 14 December 2017. <https://fangasmthebook.com/2017/12/14/lisa-berry-on-supernatural-playing-death-and-getting-excited-for-wayward-sisters/>. Accessed 14 August 2023.

Fehrle, Johannes, 'Zombies Don't Recognize Borders: Capitalism, Ecology, and Mobility in the Zombie Outbreak Narrative', *American Studies*, 61 (2016), 527–44.

Ferguson, Christopher J., '13 Reasons Why Not: A Methodological and Meta-Analytic Review of Evidence regarding Suicide Contagion by Fictional Media', *Suicide and Life Threatening Behavior*, 49 (2019), 1178–86.

Fernandez, Ingrid, 'Necro-Transcendence/Necro-Naturalism: Philosophy of Life in the Works of Ralph Waldo Emerson', in Adriana Teodorescu, ed., *Death Representations in Literature: Forms and Theories* (Newcastle upon Tyne: Cambridge Scholars Publishing, 2015), 117–37.

*Final Destination*, dir. James Wong (Burbank: New Line Cinema, 2000).

*Final Destination, The*, dir. David R. Ellis (Burbank: New Line Cinema, 2009).

*Final Destination 2*, dir. David R. Ellis (Burbank: New Line Cinema, 2003).

*Final Destination 3*, dir. James Wong (Burbank: New Line Cinema, 2006).

*Final Destination 5*, dir. Steven Quale (Burbank: New Line Cinema, 2011).

*Fire at Sea*, dir. Gianfranco Rosi (Rome: Stemal Entertainment, 2016).

*First Purge, The*, dir. Gerard McMurray (Los Angeles: Blumhouse Productions, 2018).

*Forever Purge, The*, dir. Everardo Valerio Gout (Los Angeles: Blumhouse Productions, 2021).

Foucault, Michel, 'Die Heterotopien', in Michael Bischoff, ed., *Die Heterotopien. Der utopische Körper. Zwei Radiovorträge* (Berlin: Suhrkamp, 2013), 7–36.

Foucault, Michel, *The History of Sexuality*. Vol. I: *An Introduction*, trans. Robert Hurley (trans. 1976; New York: Vintage Books, 1990).

Foucault, Michel, *Society Must Be Defended: Lectures at the Collège de France, 1975–76* (London: Penguin, 2004).

Free-Thinker, 'If Race Is Real, Then How Many Races Are There?' Stormfront.org, 27 December 2019. <https://www.stormfront.org/forum/t1296959-6/>. Accessed 15 November 2020.

Freud, Sigmund, 'Creative Writers and Day-Dreaming', in James Strachey, ed., *The Standard Edition of the Complete Psychological Works of Sigmund Freud: Jensen's "Gradiva" and Other Works*, Vol. 9 [1906–8] (London: Random House, 2001), 141–54.

Freud, Sigmund, 'The Uncanny [1919]', in David Mcliontock, ed., *The Uncanny* (London: Penguin Classics, 2003), 121–62.

Frohlich, Dennis Owen, 'Evil Must Be Punished: Apocalyptic Religion in the Television Series *Death Note*', *Journal of Media and Religion*, 11/3 (2012), 141–55.

Froula, Anna, 'Prolepsis and the War on Terror: Zombie Pathology and the Culture of Fear in *28 Days Later* …', in Jeff Birkenstein, Anna Froula and Karen Randel, ed., *Reframing 9/11: Film Popular Culture and the War on Terror* (New York: Continuum, 2010).

Ganguli, Kisari Mohan, *The Mahabharata of Vyasa*, mahabharataonline.com, n.d. <https://www.mahabharataonline.com/translation/>. Accessed 21 August 2023.

Gautier d'Agoty, Jacques Fabien, *Anatomie générale des viscères en situation, de grandeur et couleur naturelle, avec l'angeologie, et la neurologie de chaque partie du corps humain* (Paris: Le sieur Gautier, 1752).

*Geostorm*, dir. Dean Devlin (Los Angeles: Warner Bros, 2017).

Ghosh, Amitav, *Uncanny and Improbable Events* (London: Penguin, 2016).

Ghosh, Ritu et al., 'Understanding Social Problems during Lockdown and Its Relationship to Perceived Stress – An Online Survey Among Adult Residents of India', *Journal of Family Medicine and Primary Care*, 10/10 (2021). doi: 10.4103/jfmpc.jfmpc_2519_20.

Ghosh, Sankhayan, 'Anurag Basu on Ludo: "Chaos Is My Thing"', *Film Companion*, 21 November 2020. <https://www.filmcompanion.in/interviews/ludo-movie-netflix-anurag-basu-on-ludo-chaos-is-my-thing-abhishek-bachchan-pankaj-tripathi-aditya-roy-kapur>. Accessed 4 June 2023.

*Ghosts*, dir. Nick Broomfield (London: Film4, 2006).

*Ghost Whisperer, The*, dir. John Gray (Los Angeles: ABC Studios/CBS Television Studios, 2005–10).

Giannini, Erin, 'Toxic Masculinity', in Simon Bacon, ed., *Toxic Cultures: A Companion* (Oxford: Peter Lang, 2022), 91–8.

Gibson, Margaret, 'Death and Grief in the Landscape. Private Memorials in Public Space', *Cultural Studies Review*, 17/1 (2011), 146–61.

Gilbert, Sophie, 'What Went Wrong with 13 Reasons Why?', *The Atlantic*, 4 May 2017. <https://www.theatlantic.com/entertainment/archive/2017/05/13-reasons-why-controversy/525237/>. Accessed 4 August 2022.

Gilroy, Paul, *The Black Atlantic: Modernity and Double Consciousness* (Cambridge: Harvard University Press, 1993).
Girl, Interrupted, directed by James Mangold, Columbia Pictures: 1999.
Godden, Salena, 'Interview', The Death Studies Podcast, hosted by B. Michael-Fox and R. Visser, December 2022. <www.thedeathstudiespodcast.com>. Accessed 6 June 2023.
Godden, Salena, *Mrs Death Misses Death* (Edinburgh: Canon Gate, 2021).
Godden, Salena, *Springfield Road* (London: Unbound, 2014).
Goh, Katie, *The End: Surviving the World through Imagined Disasters* (Edinburgh: 404 Ink, 2021).
Goodwin, Sarah Webster and Elizabeth Bronfen, eds, *Death and Representation* (Baltimore: John Hopkins University Press, 1993).
Gould, Madelyn, Patrick Jamieson and Daniel Romer, 'Media Contagion and Suicide among the Young', *American Behavioral Scientist*, 46/9 (2003), 1269–84.
Graetz, J. M., 'The Origin of Spacewar!', in Van Burnham, ed., *Supercade: A Visual History of the Videogame Age: 1971–1984* (Cambridge: MIT Press, 2003), 42–9.
Green, Amy, *Longing, Ruin, and Connection in Hideo Kojima's Death Stranding* (Abingdon: Routledge, 2022).
Greene, Heather, *Lights, Camera, Witchcraft: A Critical History of Witches in American Film and Television* (Woodbury: Llewellyn Publications, 2021).
Greene, Richard, and K. Silem Mohammad, 'A New Lease of Life for the Undead', in Richard Greene and K. Silem Mohammad, eds, *Zombies, Vampires and Philosophy* (Chicago: Open Court, 2010).
Guthke, Karl S., *The Gender of Death: A Cultural History in Art and Literature* (Cambridge: Cambridge University Press, 1999).
Haddad, Vanessa L., 'Zombie Video Games, Eros, and Thanatos: Expressing and Exploring the Life and Death Drives through Video Gameplay', in Stephen J. Webley and Peter Zackariasson, eds, *The Playful Undead and Video Games: Critical Analyses of Zombies and Gameplay* (Abingdon: Routledge, 2020), 99–111.
Haig, Matt, *The Midnight Library* (Edinburgh: Canongate, 2020).
Hallam, Elizabeth, and Jenny Hockey, *Death, Memory and Material Culture* (Oxford: Berg, 2001).
Hallam, Elizabeth, Jenny Hockey and Glennys Howarth, *Beyond the Body: Death and Social Identity* (London: Routledge, 1999).
Handa, Devendra, 'Two Interesting Yama Images from Osian', *East and West*, 33/1/4 (1983), 53–6.
Hartman, Saidiya, 'Venus in Two Acts', *Small Axe*, 12 (2008), 1–14.
Hay, Mark, 'Is the Capitol Rioters' Skull-Mask Fetish Fashion or Fascist?' *Daily Beast*, 23 January 2021. <https://www.thedailybeast.com/is-the-capitol-rioters-skull-mask-fetish-fashion-or-fascist>. Accessed 14 August 2022.

Hegyi, Pál, *Lovecraft Laughing: Uncanny Memes in the Weird* (Szeded: Americana eBooks, 2019).
Heller-Nicholas, Alexandra, *Masks in Horror Cinema: Eyes without Faces* (Cardiff: University of Wales Press, 2019).
Hendriksen, William, *More Than Conquerors: An Interpretation of the Book of Revelation* (Grand Rapids: Baker's Book House, 1939).
*His House*, dir. Remi Weekes (London: BBC Filvfms, 2020).
Hittner, James B. 'How Robust Is the Werther Effect? A Re-examination of the Suggestion-Imitation Model of Suicide', *Mortality*, 10/3 (2005), 193–200.
Hohman, Zachary P., and Michael A. Hogg, 'Fear and Uncertainty in the Face of Death: The Role of Life after Death Group Identification', *European Journal of Social Psychology*, 41 (2011), 751–60.
Holbein, Hans, *Dance of Death* (Lyons: Treschsel Brothers, 1538).
*House of Dracula*, dir. Erle C. Kenton (Universal City: Universal Pictures, 1945).
Howarth, Glennys, *Death and Dying: A Sociological Introduction* (Cambridge: Polity Press, 2007).
Howson, Alexandra, *The Body in Society: An Introduction* (Cambridge: Polity Press, 2004).
Hubner, Laura, Marcus Leaning and Paul Manning, 'Introduction', in Laura Hubner, Marcus Leaning and Paul Manning, eds, *The Zombie Renaissance in Popular Culture* (London: Palgrave Macmillan, 2015).
*Impossible, The*, dir. J. A. Bayona (Madrid: Telecinco Cinema, 2012).
Ingber, Sasha, 'Neo-Nazi James Fields Gets 2nd Life Sentence for Charlottesville Attack', NPR.org, 8 January 2019. <https://www.npr.org/2019/07/15/741756615/virginia-court-sentences-neo-nazi-james-fields-jr-to-life-in-prison>. Accessed 9 January 2021.
Irele, Abiola, 'Narrative History and the African Imagination', *Narrative*, 1(1993),156–72.
Jackson, Maurice, 'The Black Experience with Death', in Richard Kalish, ed., *Death and Dying: Views from Many Cultures* (New York: Baywood Publishing Company, 1977).
Jacobsen, Michael Hvidd, 'Thoughts for the Times on the Death Taboo: Trivialization, Tivolization, and Re-domestication in the Age of Spectacular Death', in Adriana Teodorescu and Michael Hviid Jacobsen, eds, *Death in Contemporary Popular Culture* (Oxon: Routledge, 2020), 15–37.
Jacobson, Sansea L., 'Thirteen Reasons to Be Concerned about *13 Reasons Why*', *Pitzburg Post-Gazette*, 14 May 2017. <https://onlinelibrary.wiley.com/doi/abs/10.1002/cbl.30220>. Accessed 4 August 2022.
*Jaws*, dir. Steven Spielberg (Universal City: Universal Pictures, 1975).

Juul, Jesper, 'Fear of Failing? The Many Meanings of Difficulty in Video Games', in Bernard Perron and Mark J. P. Wolf, eds, *The Video Game Theory Reader 2* (Abingdon: Routledge, 2009), 237–52.

Kaldahl, Jeffrey, 'On Life after Death: A Chaplain's View on the Process of Dying', *Journal of Pastoral Care & Counseling*, 73/1 (2019), 49–51.

Kamin, Leon, 'Behind the Curve', *Scientific American*, 272/2 (1995), 99–103.

Karel, John (@jjjjjohn), 'Nobody's Free Until Everybody's Free', Instagram, 4 July 2019. <https://www.instagram.com/p/BzghCznHrYW/>. Accessed 23 May 2021.

Karpinski, Kelsi, 'Women in Refrigerators: "Supernatural" and the Trauma of Female Characters', Study Breaks, 2 August 2021. <https://studybreaks.com/tvfilm/women-in-refrigerators-supernatural-female-characters/>. Accessed 5 August 2023.

Keen, Ernest, 'Paranoia and Cataclysmic Narratives', in Theodore R. Sarbin, ed., *Narrative Psychology: The Storied Nature of Human Conduct* (New York: Praeger, 1986), 174–90.

Kehl, Karen A., 'Moving toward Peace: An Analysis of the Concept of a Good Death', *American Journal of Hospice & Palliative Medicine*, 23/4 (2006), 277–86.

Kelly, Caitlin, 'Supernatural Star Misha Collins Calls Show "Gratuitously Misogynistic"', Hypable, 14 May 2013. <https://www.hypable.com/supernatural-misha-collins-misogyny/>. Accessed 6 August 2023.

Kerrigan, Michael, *The History of Death* (New York: Sterling Publishing, 2017).

Klein, Naomi, *The Shock Doctrine* (London: Penguin, 2008).

Kochhar, Anuraj Singh et al., 'Lockdown of 1.3 Billion People in India during Covid-19 Pandemic: A Survey of Its Impact on Mental Health', *Asian Journal of Psychiatry* (December 2020). doi: 10.1016/j.ajp.2020.102213.

Kojima, Hideo, *The Creative Gene: How Books, Movies, and Music Inspired the Creator of Death Stranding and Metal Gear Solid* (San Francisco: VIZ Media LLC, 2021).

Kojima, Hideo, 'A Message from Studio Founder, Hideo Kojima', Kojima Productions, 13 May 2022. <https://www.kojimaproductions.jp/en/company>. Accessed 3 September 2022.

Kojima Productions, *The Art of Death Stranding* (London: Titan Books, 2020).

Kolbert, Elizabeth, 'Civilization and Extinction', in Greta Thunberg, ed., *The Climate Book* (London: Penguin, 2022), 11–15.

Komatsu, Kazuhiko, *Introduction to Yōkai Culture: Monsters, Ghosts and Outsiders in Japanese History*, trans. Hiroko Yoda and Matt Alt (Tokyo: Japan Publishing Industry Foundation for Culture, 2017).

Kosmina, Brydie, *Feminist Afterlives of the Witch, Popular Culture, Memory, Activism* (Cham: Palgrave, 2023).

Kosonen, Heidi, 'The Death of the Others and the Taboo: Suicide Represented', *Thanatos*, 1 (2015), 25–56.

Kosonen, Heidi, 'Gendered and Contagious Suicide: Taboo and Biopower in Contemporary Anglophone Cinematic Representations of Self-Willed Death',

Jyväskylä dissertations, Jyväskylä, 2020a. <http://urn.fi/URN:ISBN:978-951-39-8313-0>. Accessed 4 August 2023.

Kosonen, Heidi, 'Suicide, Social Bodies and Danger: Taboo, Biopower and Parental Worry in Films *Bridgend* (2015) and *Bird Box* (2018)', *Journal of Somaesthetics*, 6/2 (2020b), 48–63.

Koudounaris, Paul, *Memento Mori: The Dead Among Us* (London: Thames & Hudson, 2022).

Kundu, Devaleena, 'The Aesthetics of Corpses in Popular Culture', in Adriana Teodorescu and Michael Hviid Jacobsen, eds, *Death in Contemporary Popular Culture* (Oxon: Routledge, 2019), 103–15.

Kurth-Voigt, Lieselotte E., 'Existence after Death in Eighteenth-Century Literature: Prolegomena to a Study of Poetic Visions of the Beyond and Imaginative Speculations about Continued Life in a Future State', *South Atlantic Review*, 52/2 (1987), 3–14.

Lacan, Jacques, *Das Seminar, Buch X: Die Angst* (Wien: Turia+Kant, 2010).

Lacassagne, Aurélie, 'War and Peace in the *Harry Potter* Series', *European Journal of Cultural Studies*, 19/4 (2016), 318–34.

Lady Geek Girl and Friends, 'Is Supernatural: Sexist?', 23 November 2012. <https://ladygeekgirl.wordpress.com/2012/11/23/is-supernatural-sexist/>. Accessed 12 August 2023.

Laksmanan, Karthik, 'Game Theory: Why Ludo King Has Become Such a Rage during the Coronavirus Lockdown', News 18, 24 April 2020. <https://www.news18.com/news/india/game-theory-why-ludo-king-has-become-such-a-rage-during-the-coronavirus-lockdown-2591531.html>. Accessed 4 June 2023.

*Land of the Lustrous*, dir. Takahiko Kyōgoku (Tokyo: Orange Co., 2017).

Langley, M. C. et al., 'Bows and Arrows and Symbolic Displays 48,000 Years Ago in South Asian Tropics', *Science Advances*, 6 (July 2020), 24.

Laranjeira, Carlos, Maria Anjos Dixe, Ana Querido and Jennifer Moran Stritch, 'Death Cafes as a Strategy to Foster Compassionate Communities: Contributions for Death and Grief Literacy', *Frontiers in Psychology*, 13 (2022), 1–5.

Lee, Jason, *Nazism and Neo-Nazism in Film and Media* (Amsterdam: Amsterdam University Press, 2018).

Lester, G. A., 'The Literary Activity of the Medieval English Heralds,' *English Studies*, 71, 3 (1990), 222–29.

Levin, Judith, *Japanese Mythology* (New York: Rosen Central, 2008).

Levy, Steven, *Hackers: Heroes of the Computer Revolution, [1984]* (London: Penguin, 2001).

*Life of Pi*, dir. Ang Lee (Los Angeles: Fox 2000 Pictures, 2012).

Limpár, Ildikó, *The Truths of Monsters: Coming of Age with Fantastic Media* (Jefferson: McFarland, 2021).

Loadenthal, Michael, Samantha Hausserman and Matthew Thierry, 'Accelerating Hate: Atomwaffen Division, Contemporary Digital Fascism, and Insurrectionary Accelerationism', in James Bacigalupo, Kevin Borgeson and Robin Maria Valeri, eds, *Cyberhate: The Far Right in the Digital Age* (Maryland: Lexington Books, 2022).

Loidl, Sonja, 'Constructions of Death in Young Adult Fantastic Literature', *International Research in Children's Literature*, 3/2 (2010), 176–89.

Longerich, Peter, *Heinrich Himmler: Biographie* (Munich: Pantheon Verlag, 2010).

Luckhurst, Roger, *Zombies: A Cultural History* (London: Reaktion Books, 2015).

*Ludo*, dir. Anurag Basu (New Delhi: T-Series Films, 2020).

Lukáč, Tomáš, 'Deadpool – Anti-Hero, Trickster? Both, Neither?', MA dissertation, Masaryk University, Faculty of Arts, 2019. <https://theses.cz/id/w1juol/>. Accessed 9 March 2023.

Lutz, Deborah, 'The Dead Still Among Us: Victorian Secular Relics, Hair Jewelry, and Death Culture', *Victorian Literature and Culture*, 39/1 (2011), 127–42.

MacDonald, Keza, and Jason Killingsworth, *You Died: The Dark Souls Companion* (Cardross: BackPage Press, 2016).

Manning, Shaun, 'Pepe the Frog Is Dead: Creator Kills the White Supremacist-Hijacked Icon', CBR.com, 6 May 2017. <https://www.cbr.com/pepe-frog-creator-kills-white-supremacist-icon/>. Accessed 15 November 2020.

Marin, Louis, 'Montaignes Tomb, or Autobiographical Discourse', *Oxford Literary Review*, 4/3 (1981), 43–58.

Marsh, Ian, *Suicide: Foucault, History and Truth* (Cambridge: Cambridge University Press, 2010).

Marshall, Elizabeth, 'Borderline Girlhoods: Mental Illness, Adolescence, and Femininity in *Girl, Interrupted*', *Lion and the Unicorn*, 30/1 (2006), 117–33.

Maslin, Mark, *Climate Change: A Very Short Introduction* (London: Oxford University Press, 2021).

Mbembe, Achille, 'Necropolitics', trans. Libby Meintjes, *Public Culture*, 15/1 (2003), 34. doi: 10.1215/08992363-15-1-11.

Mbiti, John, African Religions and Philosophy [1969], 2nd ed. (London: Heinemann, 1989)

McKee, Patricia, 'Racialization, Capitalism, and Aesthetics in Stoker's *Dracula*', in *NOVEL: A Forum on Fiction*, 36/1 (Autumn 2002), 42–60.

Mckenna, Mark, 'What Film Is Your Film Like? Negotiating Authenticity in the Distributive Seriality of the Zombi', in Mark Mckenna and William Proctor, eds, *Horror Franchise Cinema* (New York: Routledge, 2022).

McLeod, Ken, 'Visual Kei: Hybridity and Gender in Japanese Popular Culture', *Young*, 21/4 (2013), 309–25.

McNelly, David, *Monsters of the Market: Zombies, Vampires, and Global Capitalism* (Boston: Brill, 2011).

*Mediterranea*, dir. Jonas Carpignano (Culver City: Audax Films, 2015).

*Meet Joe Black*, dir. Martin Brest (Los Angeles: Universal Pictures, 1998).

*Meg, The*, dir. Jon Turteltaub (Burbank: Warner Bros. Pictures, 2018).

Memmott, Carol, '"Mexican Gothic" Is a Creepy, Intoxicating Mystery That's Almost Impossible to Put Down', *Washington Post*, 30 June 2020. <https://www.washingtonpost.com/entertainment/books/mexican-gothic-is-a-creepy-intoxicating-mystery-thats-almost-impossible-to-put-down/2020/06/30/e6f974f2-ba02-11ea-8cf5-9c1b8d7f84c6_story.html>. Accessed 15 September 2022.

Menzies, Robert, *The Circle of Human Life* (Edinburgh: Myles Macphail, 1847).

Meyer, Matthew, 'Shinigami', Yokai.com, 2023. <https://yokai.com/shinigami/>. Accessed 6 June 2023.

Meyer, Morgan, and Kate Woodthorpe, 'The Material Presence of Absence: A Dialogue between Museums and Cemeteries', *Sociological Research Online*, 13/5 (2008), n.p.

Miles, Lizzy, and Charles Corr, 'Death Cafe: What Is It and What We Can Learn from It', *OMEGA*, 75 (2015), 151–65.

Miller, Cassie, '"There Is No Political Solution": Accelerationism in the White Power Movement', *Southern Poverty Law Center*, 23 June 2020. <https://www.splcenter.org/hatewatch/2020/06/23/there-no-political-solution-accelerationism-white-power-movement>. Accessed 5 September 2022.

Miller, Cassie, and Carroll Rivas, Rachel, 'The Year in Hate and Extremism 2021' Southern Poverty Law Center, 9 March 2022. <https://www.splcenter.org/20220309/year-hate-extremism-report-2021>. Accessed 1 August 2022.

Minois, Georges, *History of Suicide: Voluntary Death in Western Culture* (Baltimore: John Hopkins University Press, 1999).

Mithen, Steven, 'The Hunter-Gatherer Pre-History of Human and Animal Relations', Anthropozoos 12:4 (1995), 194–204.

Mohammad, K. Silem, 'Zombies, Rest, and Motion: Spinoza and the Speed of the Undeath', in Richard Greene and K. Silem Mohammad, eds, *Zombies, Vampires and Philosophy* (Chicago: Open Court, 2010).

Montesano, Marina, 'Adam's Skull', in Barbara Baert, Anita Traninger and Catrien Santing, eds, *Disembodied Heads in Medieval and Early Modern Culture* (Leiden: Brill, 2013), 15–30.

Mukherjee, Souvik, *Video Games and Storytelling: Reading Games and Playing Books* (Basingstoke: Palgrave Macmillan, 2015).

Mulvey, Laura, *Death 24x a Second Stillness and the Moving Image* (London: Reaktion, 2006).

Mulvey, Laura, *Visual and Other Pleasures* (Basingstoke: Macmillan, 1989).

Murphy, Carole, 'Rivers of Blood, Sea of Bodies: An Analysis of the Media Coverage of Migration and Trafficking on the High Seas', in Jon Hackett and Sean Harrington, eds, *Beasts of the Deep: Sea Beasts and Popular Culture* (East Barnet: John Libbey Publishing, 2018), 154–70.

Murrow, Edward R., This I Believe: The Personal Philosophies of One Hundred Thoughtful Men and Women, New York: Simon & Schuster, 1952.
Nabofa, Michael Y., 'Blood Symbolism in African Religion', *Religious Studies*, 21 (1985), 389–405.
Napier, Susan, '*Death Note:* The Killer in Me Is the Killer in You', *Mechademia*, 5 (2010), 356–60.
Nash, David, *The Prussian Army, 1808–1815* (London: Almark Publishing, 1972).
Neill, Sarah Elaine, 'A Familiar Soundscape: Existentialism, Winchester Exceptionalism and the Evolution of Death in Supernatural', in Amanda Taylor and Susan Nylander, eds, *Death in Supernatural: Critical Essays* (Jefferson: McFarland, 2019), 52–60.
Neumann, Iver B., 'Naturalizing Geography: Harry Potter and the Realms of Muggles, Magic Folks, and Giants', in Daniel H. Nexon and Iver B. Neumann, eds, *Harry Potter and International Relations* (Lanham: Rowman & Littlefield, 2006), 157–75.
Newitz, Annalee, *Pretend We're Dead: Capitalist Monsters in American Pop Culture* (London: Duke University Press, 2006).
*Night of the Living Dead*, dir. George Romero (Los Angeles: Continental Distributing, 1968).
Nitchi, Magdalena, 'Something's Rotten in High Place: *Mexican Gothic*', *ImaginAtlas*, 31 October 2021. <https://imaginatlas.ca/mexican-gothic-silvia-moreno-garcia/>. Accessed 15 September 2022.
*Noah*, dir. Darren Aronofsky (West Hollywood: Regency Enterprises, 2014).
Northwestern, 'Exploring How Teens, Young Adults and Parents Responded to 13 Reasons Why', Report by Northwestern: Center on Media and Human Development, March 2018. <https://13reasonsresearch.soc.northwestern.edu/netflix_global-report_-final-print.pdf>. Accessed 4 August 2023.
*Nosferatu*, dir. F. W. Murnau (Berlin: Prana-Film, 1922).
Novak, Peter, 'Division of the Self: Life after Death and the Binary Soul Doctrine', *Journal of Near-Death Studies* 20/3 (2002), 143–89.
Noyes, Deborah, *Encyclopedia of the End: Mysterious Death in Fact, Fancy, Folklore, and More* (Boston: Houghton Mifflin, 2008).
Nünning, Vera, and Ansgar Nünning, 'Produktive Grenzüberschreitungen: Transgenerische, intermediale und interdisziplinäre Ansätze in der Erzähltheorie', in Vera Nünning and Ansgar Nünning, eds, *Erzähltheorie transgenerisch, intermedial, interdisziplinär* (Trier: WVT Wissenschaftsverlag Trier, 2002), 1–22.
Nwoye, Chine, 'Igbo Cultural and World View: An Insider's Perspective', *International Journal of Sociology and Anthropology*, 3 (2011), 304–17.
Nyamundi, George D., 'Corporeality as Ideological Trope in African Drama', *Revue LISA/LISA e-journal* [Online], Writers' Corner, 2 March 2015. <http://journals.openedition.org/lisa/7179>. Accessed 6 June 2023.

O'Connor, Alice, 'Soma Launches Safe Mode with Friendlier Monsters', *Rock Paper Shotgun*, 1 December 2017. <https://www.rockpapershotgun.com/soma-safe-mode-update-released>. Accessed 3 September 2022.

O'Suilleabhain, Sean, *Irish Wake Amusements* (Dublin: Mercier Press, 1967).

Obata, Takeshi, 'How to Draw', in Tsugumi Ohba and Takeshi Obata, eds, *Death Note 13: How to Read* (San Francisco: VIZ Media LLC, 2005).

*Office of Film & Literature Classification*, '*13 Reasons Why*: Our Reasons for the RP18 Classification', 27 April 2017. <https://www.classificationoffice.govt.nz/blog/13-reasons-why/>. Accessed 19 September 2023.

Ohba, Tsugumi, and Takeshi Obata, 'Death Note', *Manga Plus Shueisha*, 2019. <https://mangaplus.shueisha.co.jp/titles/100008>. Accessed 6 June 2023.

Omilion-Hodges, Leah M. et al., '"Context Matters": An Exploration of Young Adult Social Constructions of Meaning about Death and Dying', *Health Communication*, 34/2 (2019), 139–48.

Ondračka, Lubomir, 'Yama', in J. D. Long et al., eds, *Encyclopedia of Indian Religions* (New York: Springer, 2022), 1799–1803.

Onoh, Nuzo, *The Sleepless* (Coventry: Canaan Star Publishing, 2016).

*Open Water*, dir. Chris Kentis (Santa Monica: Lionsgate Films, 2003).

Open Water, directed by Andy Collier and Tor Mian, Lions Gate Films: 2003.

'Ouroboros', *Britannica*, n.d. <https://www.britannica.com/topic/Ouroboros>. Accessed 15 September 2022.

Papineau, David, 'There Is No Trace of Any Soul Linked to the Body', in Michael Martin and Keith Augustine, eds, *The Myth of an Afterlife: The Case against Life after Death* (Lanham: Rowman & Littlefield, 2015), 349–68.

Pandey, Gyanendra, 'Unarchived Histories: The Mad and the Trifling', in Gyanendra Pandey, ed., *Unarchived Histories: The Mad and the Trifling in the Colonial and Postcolonial World* (London: Routledge, 2014), 3–20.

Papp, Zilia, *Anime and Its Root in Early Japanese Monster Art* (Folkestone: Global Oriental, 2010).

Patrick, Bethanne, 'The Twisted Evil of Eugenics Made Real in the Novel "Mexican Gothic"'. *Los Angeles Times*, 26 June 2020. <https://www.latimes.com/entertainment-arts/books/story/2020-06-26/mexican-gothic-sylvia-moreno-garcia-review>. Accessed 15 September 2022.

Penfold-Mounce, Ruth, 'Celebrity Deaths and the Thanatological Imagination', in Adriana Teodorescu and Michael Hviid Jacobsen, eds, *Death in Contemporary Popular Culture* (Oxon: Routledge, 2020), 51–64.

Penfold-Mounce, Ruth, *Death, the Dead and Popular Culture* (Bingley: Emerald Publishing, 2018).

Pengelly, Martin, 'Combative Vivek Ramaswamy Emerges as Surprise Focal Point of GOP Debate', *The Guardian*, 24 August 2023. <https://www.theguardian.com/us-news/2023/aug/23/vivek-ramaswamy-focus-republican-debate>. Accessed 25 August 2023.

Perron, Bernard, *The World of Scary Video Games: A Study in Videoludic Horror* (New York: Bloomsbury Academic, 2018).

Petit, Carolyn, 'Getting Killed by Superman in Fortnite Feels Wrong', Kotaku Au. 13 August 2021. <https://www.kotaku.com.au/2021/08/getting-killed-by-superman-in-fortnite-feels-wrong/>. Accessed 3 September 2022.

Phillips, David P., 'The Influence of Suggestion on Suicide: Substantive and Theoretical Implications of the Werther Effect', *American Sociological Review*, 39/3 (1974), 340–54.

Pickover, Clifford, *Death and the Afterlife: A Chronological Journey from Cremation to Quantum Resurrection* (New York: Sterling Publishing, 2015).

*Pirates of the Caribbean* films, dir. Gore Verbinski, Rob Marshall, Joachim Rønning and Espen Sandberg (Hollywood: Walt Disney Pictures, 2003–17).

Plutarch, Plutarch: Lives of the Noble Grecians and Romans [1996], edited by A. H. Clough, Project Gutenberg, N.D. <https://www.gutenberg.org/cache/epub/674/pg674-images.html>. Accessed 28 October 2023.

Pochapska, Victoria, 'Deadpool and Philosophy: Nihilism, Postmodernism, and the Prison of Irony', Movieweb, 20 June 2022. <https://movieweb.com/deadpool-philosophy-nihilism-postmodernism-irony/>. Accessed 8 March 2023.

*Ponyo*, dir. Hayao Miyazaki (Tokyo: Studio Ghibli, 2008).

Porter, Martin, *Windows of the Soul: Physiognomy in European Culture 1470–1780* (Oxford: Oxford Historical Monographs, 2005).

Porter, Rick, '"Supernatural" by the Numbers: A 15-Year Ratings History', *Hollywood Reporter*, 19 November 2020. <https://www.hollywoodreporter.com/tv/tv-news/supernatural-by-the-numbers-a-15-year-ratings-history-4095007/>. Accessed December 2022.

Prasad, Ajnesh, *Auotethnography and Organization Research: Reflections form Fieldwork in Palestine* (Cham: Palgrave Macmillan, 2019).

*Proof*, dir. Rob Bragin (Atlanta: TNT Original Productions, 2015).

*Purge, The*, dir. James DeMonaco (Los Angeles: Blumhouse Productions, 2013).

*Purge: Anarchy, The*, dir. James DeMonaco (Los Angeles: Blumhouse Productions, 2014).

*Purge: Election Year, The*, dir. James DeMonaco (Los Angeles: Blumhouse Productions, 2016).

Quigley, Claire, 'A Celebration of Fungoid Fiction', Book Riot, 26 August 2016. <https://bookriot.com/a-celebration-of-fungoid-fiction/>. Accessed 15 September 2022.

Quinn, Anthony, 'Ghosts [review]', *The Independent*, 12 January 2007. <http://www.independent.co.uk/arts-entertainment/films/reviews/ghosts-15--none-onestar-twostar-threestar-fourstar-fivestar-431703.htl>. Accessed 20 September 2021.

Quintana, Dolores, 'Decolonizing A Proto-Genre: Author Silvia Moreno-Garcia On *Mexican Gothic*', *Fangoria*, 15 June 2021. <https://www.fangoria.com/original/silvia-moreno-garcia-on-mexican-gothic/>. Accessed 15 September 2022.

Quint Entertainment, 'Anurag Basu's Film with Abhishek, Rajkummar Finally Has a Title', *The Quint*, 27 December 2019. <https://www.thequint.com/entertainment/bollywood/anurag-basu-announces-abhishek-bachchan-rajkummar-rao-ludo-film-release-date#read-more>. Accessed 4 June 2023.

Rabin, Nathan, 'The Bataan Death March of Whimsy Case File #1: Elizabethtown', AV Club, 25 January 2007. <https://www.avclub.com/the-bataan-death-march-of-whimsy-case-file-1-elizabet-1798210595>. Accessed 11 May 2023.

Radcliffe-Brown, Alfred R., 'Taboo', in William A. Lessa and Evon Z. Vogt, eds, *Reader in Comparative Religion: An Anthropological Approach*, 46–56 (1939; New York: Harper & Row, 1979).

Randall, Jason, Nathan Nickel and Ian Colman, 'Contagion from Peer Suicidal Behavior in a Representative Sample of American Adolescents', *Journal of Affective Disorders*, 186 (2015), 219–25.

Rich, Paul B., 'Hollywood and Cinematic Representations of Far-Right Domestic Terrorism in the U.S.', *Studies in Conflict & Terrorism*, 43/2 (2020), 161–82.

Robert, Martin, and Laura Tradii, 'Do We Deny Death? I. A Genealogy of Death Denial', *Mortality* (2019), 247–60. doi: 10.1080/13576275.2017.1415318.

Robertson, Adi, 'Hillary Clinton Exposing Pepe the Frog Is the Death of Explainers', *The Verge*, 15 September 2016. <https://www.theverge.com/2016/9/15/12926976/hillary-clinton-trump-pepe-the-frog-alt-right-explainer>. Accessed 15 November 2020.

Romer, Daniel, 'Reanalysis of the Bridge et al. Study of Suicide Following Release of *13 Reasons Why*', *PLoS one*, 15 (2020). <https://journals.plos.org/plosone/article?id=10.1371/journal.pone.0227545>. Accessed 4 August 2023.

Rosado, Tréza, 'The Generation(s) of Harry Potter: The Boy Wizard and His Young Readers', in Cecilia Konchar Farr, ed., *A Wizard of Their Age: Critical Essays from the Harry Potter Generation* (Albany: State University of New York Press, 2015), 73–81.

Rosenbaum, Thane, *Payback: The Case for Revenge* (Chicago: University of Chicago Press, 2013).

Rowlandson, Thomas, and William Combe, *The English Dance of Death* (London: Rudolph Ackermann, 1815).

Rowling, J. K., 'J.K. Rowling and the Live Chat', Bloomsbury.com, 30 July 2007. >. Accessed 5 January 2023.

Rowling, J. K., *Harry Potter and the Deathly Hallows* (London: Bloomsbury, 2007).

Rowling, J. K., *Harry Potter and the Goblet of Fire* (New York: Scholastic, 2000).

Rowling, J. K., *Harry Potter and the Half-Blood Prince* (New York: Scholastic, 2005).

Rowling, J. K., *Harry Potter and the Order of the Phoenix* (London: Bloomsbury, 2003).

Rowling, J. K., *Harry Potter and the Philosopher's Stone* (London: Bloomsbury, 2000).

Rowling, J. K., *Harry Potter and the Sorcerer's Stone* (London: Scholastic, 1997).
Ryan, Marie-Laure, *Possible Worlds, Artificial Intelligence, and Narrative Theory* (Bloomington: Indiana University Press, 1991).
*Sacrifice*, dir. Andy Collier and Tor Mian (London: Hydra Films, 2020).
Saddington, John, *The Representation of Suicide in the Cinema*. Dissertation submitted for the degree of PhD, University of York, 2010. <http://etheses.whiterose.ac.uk/14223/1/550372.pdf.>. Accessed 4 August 2023.
*Sailor Moon*, Season 1, dir. Jun'ichi Satô (Japan: DIC Entertainment and Optimum Productions, 1995).
Saiya, Nilay, 'Confronting Apocalyptic Terrorism: Lessons from France and Japan', *Studies in Conflict & Terrorism*, 43/9 (2020), 775–95.
Sappol, Michael, 'Art, Science and the Changing Conventions of Anatomical Representation', in Joanna Ebenstein, ed., *Death: A Graveside Companion* (London: Thames & Hudson, 2017), 50–2.
Sarbin, Theodore R., 'The Narrative as a Root Metaphor for Psychology', in Theodore R. Sarbin, ed., *Narrative Psychology: The Storied Nature of Human Conduct* (New York: Praeger, 1986), 3–21.
*Saving Hope*, dir. Malcolm MacRury and Morwyn Brebner (Toronto: Entertainment One/Bell Media, 2012–17).
Sawday, Jonathan, *The Body Emblazoned: Dissection and the Human Body in Renaissance Culture* (London: Routledge, 1995).
Sayles, Justin, 'We're Watching More True Crime Than Ever. Is That a Problem?' The Ringer, 9 July 2021. <https://www.theringer.com/tv/2021/7/9/22567381/true-crime-documentaries-boom-bubble-netflix-hbo>. Accessed 18 January 2022.
Schell, Jennifer, 'The Annihilation of Self and Species: The Ecogothic Sensibilities of Mary Shelley and Nathaniel Hawthorne', in Carol Margaret Davison, ed., *The Gothic and Death* (Manchester: Manchester University Press, 2017), 103–15.
*Seaspiracy*, dir, Ali Tabrizi (London: A.U.M. Films, 2021).
Sedgwick, Mark, 'Introduction', in Mark Sedgwick, ed., *Key Thinkers of the Radical Right: Behind the New Threat to Liberal Democracy* (New York: Oxford Academic, 2019).
'Shachath', American Horror Story Fandom, n.d. <https://americanhorrorstory.fandom.com/wiki/Shachath>. Accessed 6 June 2023.
Pinker, Steven, *The Better Angels of our Nature* (London: Penguin, 2012).
*Shallows, The*, dir. Jaume Collet-Serra (Culver City: Columbia Pictures, 2016).
Sharf, Zack, 'Michael Moore Says "Fear" Is to Blame for American Gun Violence', *Indiewire*, 22 December 2015. <https://www.indiewire.com/2015/12/michael-moore-says-fear-is-to-blame-for-american-gun-violence-43009/>. Accessed 12 January 2022.

Shepherd, Rowena, and Rupert Shepherd, *1000 Symbols* (New York: Thames & Hudson, 2002).
Sheppard, W. Anthony, *Revealing Masks: Exotic Influences and Ritualized Performance in Modernist Music Theater* (Berkeley: University of California Press, 2001).
Shilling, Chris, *The Body and Social Theory* (London: Sage, 1993).
*Sinking of Japan, The*, dir. Shinji Higuchi (Tokyo: Dentsu, 2006).
Skeem, Jennifer et al., 'Psychopathic Personality and Racial/Ethnic Differences Reconsidered: A Reply to Lynn (2002)', *Personality and Individual Differences*, 35/6 (2003), 1439–62.
Skehan, Jaelea, 'Six Reasons Why I'm Concerned about a TV Series', Everymind.org, 19 April 2017. <https://everymind.org.au/news/six-reasons-why-im-concerned-about-a-tv-series.>. Accessed 4 August 2022.
Socrates, Ebo, 'Death in Igbo African Ontology', *SKHID*, 3 (2019), 22–8.
*Spacewar!*, dir. Steve Russell (Cambridge: Tech Model Railroad Club, 1962).
Spengler, Oswald, *The Decline of the West*, Vol. 1 & 2, Arthur Helps and Helmut Werner, eds, trans. Charles F. Atkinson (1918–22; New York: Oxford University Press, 1991).
Stack, Steven, and Barbara Bowman, 'Suicide Motives in 61 Works of Popular World Literature and in Comparison, to Film', in Steven Stack and David Lester, eds, *Suicide and the Creative Arts* (New York: Nova Science Publishers, 2009), 113–24.
Stack, Steven, and Barbara Bowman, *Suicide Movies: Social Patterns 1900–2009* (Toronto: Hogrefe, 2012).
Stack, Tim, 'American Horror Story: Ryan Murphy Talks "Dark Cousin"', *Entertainment Weekly*, 29 November 2012. <https://ew.com/article/2012/11/29/american-horror-story-ryan-murphy-dark-cousin-exclusive/>. Accessed 15 December 2022.
Stack, Tim, 'American Horror Story: Ryan Murphy Teases Season 3', *Entertainment Weekly*, 3 January 2013. <https://ew.com/article/2013/01/03/american-horror-story-ryan-murphy-the-name-game-exclusive/>. Accessed 20 December 2022.
Stapley, Garth, '"This Is a Huge Victory". Oakdale White Supremacist Revels after Deadly Virginia Clash', Modesto Bee, 14 August 2017. <https://www.modbee.com/news/article167213427.html>. Accessed 13 March 2021.
Steiner, Franz Baerman, 'Taboo', in Jeremy Adler and Richard Fardon, eds, *Franz Baerman Steiner Selected Writings*, Vol. I: *Taboo, Truth and Religion* (1956; New York and Oxford: Berghahn Books, 1999).
Steizinger, Johannes, 'Why the Ideology of the "New Right" Is So Dangerous', The Conversation, 2 November 2022. <https://theconversation.com/why-the-ideology-of-the-new-right-is-so-dangerous-192833>. Accessed 12 August 2023.
Stobbart, Dawn, *Videogames and Horror: From Amnesia to Zombies, Run!* (Cardiff: University of Wales Press, 2019).
Stojilkov, Andrea, 'Life(and)Death in Harry Potter: The Immortality of Love and Soul', *Mosaic: A Journal for the Interdisciplinary Study of Literature*, 48/2 (2015), 133–48.

Stoker, Bram, *Dracula* (1897; Oxford: University of Oxford Press, 1996).
*Supernatural*, Season 5, Episode 21, 'Two Minutes to Midnight', dir. Phillip Sgriccia (Burbank: Warner Bros. Television, 2010).
*Supernatural*, Season 6, Episode 11, 'Appointment in Samarra', dir. Mike Rohl (Burbank: Warner Bros. Television, 2010).
*Supernatural*, Season 7, Episode 1, 'Meet the New Boss', dir. Phillip Sgriccia (Burbank: Warner Bros. Television, 2011).
*Supernatural*, Season 9, Episode 1, 'I Think I'm Gonna Like It Here', dir. John F. Showalter (Burbank: Warner Bros. Television, 2013).
*Supernatural*, Season 10, Episode 23, 'Brother's Keeper', dir. Phillip Sgriccia (Burbank: Warner Bros. Television, 2015).
*Supernatural*, Season 11, Episode 2, 'Form and Void', dir. Phillip Sgriccia (Burbank: Warner Bros. Television, 2015).
*Supernatural*, Season 12, Episode 9, 'First Blood', dir. Robert Singer (Burbank: Warner Bros. Television, 2017).
*Supernatural*, Season 13, Episode 5, 'Advanced Thanatology', dir. John F Showalter (Burbank: Warner Bros. Television, 2017).
*Supernatural*, Season 13, Episode 19, 'Funeralia', dir. Nina Lopez-Corrado (Burbank: Warner Bros. Television, 2018).
*Supernatural*, Season 14, Episode 10, 'Nihilism', dir. Amanda Tapping (Burbank: Warner Bros. Television, 2019).
*Supernatural*, Season 15, Episode 18, 'Despair', dir. Richard Speight Jr (Burbank: Warner Bros. Television, 2020).
*Supernatural*, Season 15, Episode 19, 'Inherit the Earth', dir. John F. Showalter (Burbank: Warner Bros. Television, 2020).
Svoboda, Michael, 'Cli-fi on the Screen(s): Patterns in the Representations of Climate Change in Fictional Films', *WIRES Clim Change*, 7 (2016). 43–64.
Takeuchi, Naoko, *Pretty Guardian Sailor Moon: Eternal Edition*, Vol. 1 & 2 (New York: Kodansha Comics-Kodansha USA Publishing, 2018).
*Taqdeerwala*, dir. K. Murali Mohana Rao (Hyderabad: Suresh Productions, 1995).
Tatz, Simon, '13 Reasons Why – Suicide the Last Taboo', *Australian Medicine*, 29/10 (2017), 11.
*The Collective for Radical Death Studies*, 2020–present. <https://radicaldeathstudies.com/>. Accessed 1 October 2022.
*Thing, The*, dir. John Carpenter (Universal City: Universal Pictures, 1882).
*Thing, The*, dir. Matthijs van Heijningen Jr (Universal City: Universal Pictures: 2011).
Thomas, Simon, 'Ars moriendi – The Art of Dying', 2013. <http://bav.bodleian.ox.ac.uk/news/ars-moriendi-the-art-of-dying>. Accessed 8 June 2023.

Thorson, James A., and F. C. Powell, 'Life, Death, and Life after Death: Meaning of the Relationship between Death Anxiety and Religion', *Journal of Religious Gerontology*, 8/1 (2008), 41–56.
*Tidal Wave*, dir. J. K. Youn (Seoul: C.J. Entertainment, 2009).
*Titanic*, dir. James Cameron (Century City: 20th Century Fox, 1997).
Toolis, Kevin, *My Father's Wake: How the Irish Teach Us to Live, Love and Die* (London: Weidenfeld & Nicholson, 2017).
Tradii, Laura, and Martin Robert, 'Do We Deny Death? II. Critiques of the Death-Denial Thesis', *Mortality*, 24/4 (2019), 201–17. doi: 10.1080/13576275.2017.1415319.
Tripathi, Khyati, 'Interview', The Death Studies Podcast, hosted by B. Michael-Fox and R. Visser, 21 October 2021. <www.thedeathstudiespodcast.com>. Accessed 6 June 2023. doi: https://doi.org/10.6084/m9.figshare.16843690>.
Troyer, John, Technologies of the Human Corpse, Cambridge: MIT, 2020.
*True North*, dir. Steve Hudson (London: Ariel Films, 2006).
Twindle, Hedley, 'As Others Feel Pain in Their Lungs: Albert Camus' *The Plague*', *English Studies in Africa*, 64 (2021), 24–40.
*Twister*, dir. Jan de Bont (Los Angeles: Warner Bros, 1996).
Ue, Tom, and James Munday, *The Worlds of Ernest Cline's Ready Player One* (New York: Routledge, forthcoming).
University College Dublin (UCD), 'Language Use & Design: Conflicts & Their Significance: Prof. Naom Chomsky, YouTube, April 4, 2013. <https://www.youtube.com/watch?v=iR_NmkkMmO8>. Accessed 28 October 2023.
Upchurch, H. E., 'The Iron March Forum and the Evolution of the "Skull Mask" Neo-Fascist Network', *Combating Terrorism Center at Westpoint*, December 2021. <https://ctc.westpoint.edu/the-iron-march-forum-and-the-evolution-of-the-skull-mask-neo-fascist-network/>. Accessed 1 September 2022.
*Vaah! Life Ho Toh Aisi!*, dir. Mahesh Manjrekar (Mumbai: Aavishkaar Films, 2005).
Varghese, Roy Abraham, *There Is Life after Death: Compelling Reports from Those Who Have Glimpsed the Afterlife* (Franklin Lakes: New Page Books, 2010).
Vaught, Louis Allen, *The Practical Character Reader* (Chicago: Vaught, 1902).
Visser, Renske, 'Mrs Death Misses Death', Dead Good Reading, 17 May 2021. https://www.deadgoodreading.com/blog/mrs-death-misses-death. Accessed 1 October 2022.
Voas, David, and Mark Chaves, 'Religion Is in decline in the West, and America Is No Exception', United States Politics and Policy, 5 September 2016. <https://blogs.lse.ac.uk/usappblog/2016/09/05/religion-is-in-decline-in-the-west-and-america-is-no-exception/>. Accessed 28 January 2022.
Wagner, Anna, and Christian Schwarzenegger, 'A Populism of Lulz: The Proliferation of Humor, Satire, and Memes as Populist Communication in Digital Culture', in Christina Holtz-Bacha and Benjamin Krämer, eds, *Perspectives on Populism and*

*the Media: Avenues for Research* (Baden-Baden: Nomos Verlagsgesellschaft, 2020), 313–32.
Walcott, Derek, 'The Sea Is History', poets.org, 2007. <https://poets.org/poem/sea-history>. Accessed 20 September 2021.
Wald, Priscilla, *Contagious: Cultures, Carriers, and the Outbreak Narrative* (Durham: Duke University Press, 2008).
Walter, Tony, Jane Littlewood and Michael Pickering, 'Death in the News: The Public Invigilation of Private Emotion', *Sociology*, 29/4 (1995), 579–96.
Walvin, James, 'Dust to Dust: Celebrations of Death in Victorian England', *Historical Reflections/Réflexions Historiques*, 9/3 (1982), 353–71.
Warren, Craig A., 'Patriotism as Institutional Racism: The Purge and the Fugitive Slave Act', *Film & History*, 50/1 (2020), 29–40.
*Waterworld*, dir. Kevin Reynolds (Universal City: Universal Pictures, 1995).
*Wave, The*, dir. Roar Uthaug (Oslo Fantefilms, 2015).
Webb, Jen, and Byrnand, Samuel, 'Some Kind of Virus: The Zombie as Body and as Trope', in Sarah Juliet Lauro, ed., *Zombie Theory: A Reader* (London: University of Minnesota Press, 2017).
Waller, Gregory A., *The Living Undead: Slaying Vampires and Exterminating Zombies* (Chicago: University of Illinois Press, 2010).
West, Alexandra. *The 1990s Teen Horror Cycle: Final Girls and a New Hollywood Formula* (Jefferson: McFarland, 2018).
Wetmore Jr, Kevin J., Post-9/11 Horror in American Cinema, New York: Continuum, 2012.
*When the Levee Breaks: A Requiem in Four Acts*, dir. Spike Lee (New York: HBO, 2006).
Wickham, Glynne, The Medieval Theatre, Cambridge: Cambridge University Press, 1987.
Wilson-Tagoe, Nana, 'Reading towards a Theorization of African Women's Writing: African Women Writers within Feminist Gynocriticism', in Stephanie Newell, ed., *Writing African Women: Gender, Popular Culture and Literature in West Africa* (London: Zed Books, 2017), 11–28.
Wittkower, Rudolf, and Margot Wittkower, *Born under Saturn: The Character and Conducts of Artists: A Documented History from Antiquity to the French Revolution* (New York: W.W. Norton, 1969).
Wolterbeek, Marc, 'Grim Reapers and Shinigami: Personifications of Death in Comics and Manga', *International Journal of Comic Art*, 18/1 (2016), 297–330.
Woodthorpe, Kate, 'Private Grief in Public Space: Interpreting Memorialisation in the Contemporary Cemetery', in Jenny Hockey, Carol Komaromy and Kate Woodthorpe, eds, *The Matter of Death – Space, Place and Materiality* (Basingstoke: Palgrave Macmillan, 2010), 117–32.
World Health Organization, 'Dementia', 20 September 2022. <https://www.who.int/news-room/fact-sheets/detail/dementia>. Accessed 21 August 2023.

Wright, Handel Kashope, *A Prescience of African Cultural Studies: The Future of Literature in Africa Is Not What It Was* (New York: Peter Lang, 2004).

Wu, Mingren, 'Shinigami: The Grim Reaper and God of Death in Japanese Folklore', Ancient Origins, 2019. <https://www.ancient-origins.net/myths-legends/shinigami-grim-reaper-japanese-folklore-006072>. Accessed 6 June 2023.

Zimerman, Aline Zimerman, Arthur Caye, André Zimerman, Giovanni A. Salum, Ives C. Passos and Christian Kieling, 'Revisiting the Werther Effect in the 21st Century: Bullying and Suicidality among Adolescents Who Watched *13 Reasons Why*', *Journal of the American Academy of Child & Adolescent fPsychiatry*, 57/8 (2018), 610–3.

Žižek, Slavoj, *Mehr-Genießen: Lacan in der Populärkultur* (Wien: Turia+Kant, 1992).

# Notes on Contributors

KATARZYNA ANCUTA is a lecturer at the Faculty of Arts, Chulalongkorn University, Thailand. Her research interests oscillate around the interdisciplinary contexts of contemporary Gothic/horror, currently with a strong Asian focus. Her recent publications include contributions to *The Edinburgh Companion to Globalgothic* (2023), *Folk Horror: New Global Pathways* (2023), *The Transmedia Vampire* (2021), *The New Urban Gothic* (2020) and *B-Movie Gothic* (2018). Katarzyna has also co-edited two collections: *Thai Cinema: The Complete Guide* (2016) and *South Asian Gothic: Haunted Cultures, Histories and Media* (2022).

SIMON BACON is a writer and film critic based in Poznań, Poland. He has written and edited over thirty books on various subjects including *Gothic: A Reader* (2018), *Horror: A Companion* (2019), *Eco-Vampires* (2020), *The Anthropocene and the Undead* (2022), *Nosferatu in the 21st Century* (2023), *1000 Vampires on Screen Vols 1 & 2* (2023) and *The Palgrave Handbook of the Vampire* (2024). Simon is also the series editor of *Vampire Studies: New Perspectives on the Undead* and can be contacted at: baconetti@gmail.com.

REBECCA BOOTH holds an MA in Film Studies from the University of Southampton, United Kingdom. In addition to contributing essays to collections such as *Toxic Cultures: A Companion* (2022), *Tonight, on a Very Special Episode: When TV Sitcoms Sometimes Get Serious: Volume 2: 1986–1998* (2020) and *Lost Girls: The Phantasmagorical Cinema of Jean Rollin* (2017), she is the co-editor of *Scared Sacred: Idolatry, Religion and Worship in the Horror Film* (2020) and *Filtered Reality: The Progenitors and Evolution of Found Footage Horror* (2023).

KATARZYNA BRONK-BACON is an assistant professor in the Faculty of English at the Adam Mickiewicz University, Poznan, Poland, where she teaches the history of English literature. Katarzyna is the editor of *'Autumnal Faces': Old Age in*

*British and Irish Dramatic Narratives* (2017) and *'Experienc'd Age Knows What for Youth Is Fit'? Generational and Familial Conflict in British and Irish Drama and Theatre* (2019). She is also the author of *'And Yet I Remember': Ageing and Old(er) Age in English Drama between 1660 and the 1750s*, which is the result of a research grant project titled 'Embodied Sites of Memory? Investigations into the Definitions and Representations of Old Age and Ageing in English Drama between 1660 and 1750' (Polish National Science Centre).

OCTAVIA CADE is a speculative fiction writer from New Zealand. Her academic work has appeared in a number of venues, including *Horror Studies*, *Interdisciplinary Literary Studies*, *Supernatural Studies* and anthologies from Routledge and McFarland, amongst others. She's had close to seventy short stories published in markets including *Clarkesworld*, *Asimov's* and *Fantasy & Science Fiction*. She was the 2023 writer in residence at Canterbury University, and her latest book, the 2023 collection *You Are My Sunshine and Other Stories*, is available from Stelliform Press.

CATH DAVIES is a senior lecturer at the Cardiff School of Art and Design, Cardiff Metropolitan University, United Kingdom. She contributes to an interdisciplinary module of Contextual/Critical Studies that nurtures undergraduate and postgraduate students' enthusiasm for materiality, somatic unruliness and grotesque embodiment. The aesthetics of dissolution permeate her research interests, including studies on posthumous stardom, fabric, bodily framing and corporeal disintegration. Cath's PhD thesis titled 'Discourses of Dissolution: Designing the Deceased in Visual and Material Culture' has also been published in the year 2021.

TRACY FAHEY, PhD, is a writer and academic at LSAD, TUS. Recent books are the British Fantasy Award nominated collection *I Spit Myself Out* (2021) and the novella *They Shut Me Up* (2023). She has been awarded writing residencies in Ireland, Greece and Finland, and, in 2023, a Saari Fellowship by the Kone Foundation.

GEMMA FILES is a Canadian horror writer, journalist and film critic. Her short story titled 'The Emperor's Old Bones' won the International Horror

Notes on Contributors

Guild Award for Best Short Story of 1999. Five of her short stories were adapted for the television series *The Hunger*.

PHIL FITZSIMMONS is currently an independent researcher and consultant in education and organisational learning. Prior to this, he was the head of education (Alphacrucis University College Sydney, Australia), assistant dean-research (Faculty of Education, Business and Science, Avondale University, Australia), director of research (San Roque Research Institute, California) and senior lecturer (University of Wollongong, Australia). Phil's current research interests include Australian Gothic literature, popular culture and adolescent spirituality.

MARK FRYERS is a lecturer in Film and Media at the Open University. His thesis, 'British National Identity and Maritime Film and Television, 1960–2012', examined the intersection of the maritime sphere, identity formation and visual culture. Mark has contributed numerous peer-reviewed articles to the *Journal of Popular Television*, *Gothic Nature* and *Revenant* in addition to essays in numerous edited collections on topics ranging from environmentalism, gender and the costume drama to global animation and folklore.

MARIA GIAKANIKI is an independent scholar and co-owner/editor-in-chief of Ars Nocturna, a small publishing house in Athens, Greece. She has co-edited the short story anthology *Bending to Earth: Strange Stories by Irish Women* (2019), and contributed a chapter to *The Streaming of Hill House: Essays on the Haunting Netflix Adaption* (2020). She has also published chapters in *The Palgrave Handbook of Steam Age Gothic* (2021) and *The Palgrave Handbook of Gothic Origins* (2021).

RACHEL GRANT holds a BA in Open Arts & an MFA in Creative Writing. She lives in the United Kingdom and has just finished a novel about childhood trauma and the supernatural. Her short story, 'The Birthday Party', was published by *Popshot Quarterly* in 2022. Rachel resides in the southwest of England, and her academic interests include the uncanny, the macabre, fairy tales and folklore.

RAE HARGRAVE received their master's degree in literature from Virginia Tech in May 2021 where they studied Celtic mythology in pop culture and queerness in anime. They are now an independent researcher, continuing their study of anime through various pop culture lenses. Rae works as a copywriter for a marketing agency and lives with their partner and two cats in Southwest Virginia.

DAVE JEFFERY is the author of eighteen novels and novellas, two collections and numerous short stories. His *Necropolis Rising* series and yeti adventure *Frostbite* have both featured on the Amazon #1 bestseller list. His YA work features the Beatrice Beecham supernatural adventures. Dave is also the creator of the *A Quiet Apocalypse* series which has received worldwide critical acclaim. Actively involved in the Horror Writers Association (HWA), Jeffery is a mentor on the HWA Mentorship Scheme for which he was awarded Mentor of the Year in 2023, and he is also co-chair of the HWA Wellness Committee.

HEIDI KOSONEN is a postdoctoral researcher at University of Jyväskylä, Finland. Heidi defended her doctoral dissertation, which focused on suicide cinema from the perspectives of taboo and biopower, in fall 2020, and she has since been working on several projects at the University of Jyväskylä, and University of Winnipeg, Canada. Heidi has published bilingually on suicide cinema and television (including case studies on productions such as *13 Reasons Why*, *Bird Box*, *Bridgend*, *Midsommar*, *The Moth Diaries*, *The Fall*, *Vanilla Sky* and *Unfriended*), taboo, biopower, death and mourning as well as other affective phenomena in contemporary culture, including disgust and hate speech.

LAURA R. KREMMEL is Assistant Professor of English at Niagara University, New York, United States. Her published work focuses on Gothic studies, the medical humanities, history of medicine and British Romanticism. She is the author of *Romantic Medicine and the Gothic Imagination: Morbid Anatomies* (2022) and is coeditor of *The Palgrave Handbook to Horror Literature* (2018).

ŁUCJA LANGE holds a PhD in Sociology, specialising in thanatology and contributes to the topic of therapy through photography and drama as an activist and researcher. Her scientific interests focus on diversity issues, gender studies, animal studies and death studies. Łucja also researches subjects such as human-animal relations, one health and degrowth and is also part of the Polish collective called the Institute of the Good Death.

ILDIKÓ LIMPÁR is a senior lecturer at Pázmány Péter Catholic University, Budapest, Hungary. She teaches and researches contemporary literature with a special focus on fantasy and monster narratives. Ildikó's academic book *The Truths of Monsters: Coming of Age with Fantastic Media* (2021) discusses the use of monsters as literary tools addressing life challenges in coming-of-age fantasy and science fiction. She is also the editor of *Displacing the Anxieties of Our World: Spaces of the Imagination* (2017) and a Hungarian anthology of essays titled *Monster Studies* (2021).

ANNA LÜSCHER is a doctoral researcher at the University of Konstanz, Germany, supervised by Professor Silvia Mergenthal. Her dissertation investigates genre via liminality, using E. T. A. Hoffmann, Conan Doyle and J. K. Rowling's works as examples. She co-initiated a collaborative writing project for doctoral students and is a doctoral caucus member. She holds MAs in English and German literature from the University of Newcastle, Newcastle-upon-Tyne, and the University of Konstanz, respectively. Her research interests are spatial theory, narratology, Romanticism and speculative fiction.

ROBERT MCLAUGHLIN is the Digital Centre Manager at South Staffordshire College, specialising in media and film theory with an emphasis on industry contextualisation, business and marketing. His academic areas of research are in media theory where he has written academic papers on VHS Culture, hauntlogy and children's horror. He has published a monograph though Auteur / Liverpool University Press focusing on Stephen Spielberg and Tobe Hoopers 1982 classic Poltergeist and has written extensively about films animation, horror and cult television having work cited in The Guardian, Daily Express and Forbes on areas focusing on the weird and unusual side of film and television.

JACK MCCORMACK-CLARK is a New Zealand academic currently completing his PhD at AUT, New Zealand. He specialises in nineteenth-century literature and history which is where his interest in the Gothic originated. Jack has always been passionate about popular culture, fantasy and science fiction, as he feels stories are unique to humanity and express greater truths of our experience, histories and cultures. Through his passion and his interest in storytelling, Jack continues to avidly research to further understand how stories shape our existence.

JAMES T. MCCREA is an early career researcher with broad thematic interests in iconologies of death and dying as well as materialities of the corpse. Working from a background in visual culture and funerary archaeology, James is currently working on a doctorate thesis encompassing a history of the animated skeleton in British culture. His independent research projects range from examining depictions of graveyards, catacombs and other burial grounds in video games to semiotic explorations of goth and no-wave subcultures of the 1980s.

BETHAN MICHAEL-FOX, FRSA, SFHEA, teaches at the Open University, where she is an honorary associate in the School of English and Creative Writing. Her research focuses on the representation of death in popular culture. Before going part-time to raise a family, Beth was a senior lecturer in the School of Education and English at the University of Bedfordshire, United Kingdom. Beth is managing editor for the academic journal *Mortality*, social media manager for the Open Access journal *Revenant: Critical and Creative Studies of the Supernatural* and co-host of *The Death Studies Podcast*.

JENNIFER MORAN STRITCH is a lecturer at TUS in Limerick, Ireland, where she is also the principal investigator of the Loss and Grief Research Group, part of Social Sciences ConneXions Research Institute at TUS. A certified thanatologist, Jennifer co-hosted the first Death Café event in the Limerick area in 2015 and continues to host virtual and in-person Death Café events today.

LISA MORTON is a screenwriter, author of non-fiction books and prose writer whose work was described by the American Library Association's *Readers'*

*Advisory Guide to Horror* as 'consistently dark, unsettling, and frightening'. She is a six-time winner of the Bram Stoker Award®, the author of four novels and over 150 short stories, and a world-class Halloween and paranormal expert. Lisa lives in Los Angeles.

DEBADITYA MUKHOPADHYAY is Assistant Professor of English at Manikchak College, affiliated with the University of Gourbanga, India. Popular literature and films, myths, adaptations and theatre are his areas of interest. Debaditya's research articles have been published in the peer-reviewed journals such as *Muse India*, and *DUJES*. He has recently contributed chapters to the collections *Parenting Through Pop Culture* (2020), *Excavating Indiana Jones* (2020), *Critical Insights: Life of Pi* (2020) and *Children and Childhood in the Works of Stephen King* (2020).

W. SCOTT POOLE is Professor of History at the College of Charleston, South Carolina, United States. He is the author of the 2022 *Dark Carnivals: Modern Horror and the Origins of America Empire* as well as award-winning nonfiction works such as the Stoker-nominated Lovecraft biography titled *In the Mountains of Madness* and *Monsters in America*.

CATHERINE PUGH completed her PhD at the University of Essex, United Kingdom, and is now a writer and independent scholar. Primarily writing about horror and science fiction across cinema, television and theatre, she is particularly fascinated by ideas of monstrosity and mental illness versus literary madness. Catherine's research interests concern disability, mental illness/'madness', metamorphic monsters and horror landscapes. She has contributed to various collections including *At Home in the Whedonverse: Essays on Domestic Space, Place and Life*; *Politics of Race, Gender, and Sexuality in The Walking Dead: Essays on the Television Series and Comics*; *Vying for the Iron Throne: Essays on Power, Gender, Death and Performance in HBO's Game of Thrones* as well as to online journals including *Studies in Gothic* Fiction and *Aeternum: The Journal of Contemporary Gothic Studies*.

KRISTY STRANGE is a PhD student at the University of Westminster. She holds an MLitt in The Gothic Imagination from the University of Stirling as well as a BA in both English Literature and Applied Psychology from Bishop's University. Her research examines ecofeminist and ecogothic presentations of the Anthropocene in contemporary Climate Fiction by women. She also has a keen interest in the nautical Gothic.

TOM UE is Assistant Professor in English of the Long Nineteenth Century at Cape Breton University, Editor of the *Journal of Popular Film and Television*, and Advisory Editor of *The Complete Letters of Henry James* (University of Nebraska Press). He is the author of *Gissing, Shakespeare, and the Life of Writing* (Edinburgh University Press, forthcoming) and *George Gissing* (Liverpool University Press, forthcoming); and the editor of *George Gissing, The Private Papers of Henry Ryecroft* (Edinburgh University Press, forthcoming). Tom is an Honorary Research Associate at University College London and a Fellow of the Royal Historical Society.

RENSKE VISSER is a postdoctoral researcher at the University of Oulu, Finland. Her research interests include ageing and dying and how place shapes end-of-life experiences. Renske holds a PhD in social and policy sciences from the Centre for Death and Society at the University of Bath. She has conducted research on parental bereavement in young adulthood, homemaking in later life, ageing in secure psychiatric hospitals and cancer care in prison. Renske has a blog entitled 'Dead Good Reading' where she reviews books on all things death. She also is co-host of *The Death Studies Podcast*.

STEPHANIE WEBER obtained her doctoral degree in comparative literature from the University of Vienna, Austria, in 2019. Her dissertation deals with the uncanny quality of freak characters and uncanny narrative strategies in postmodern literature. She is currently an independent scholar whose research interests focus on tattoos, body studies, psychoanalysis and narratology.

KEVIN J. WETMORE, JR, is the author of over a dozen books, including *Post-9/11 Horror in American Cinema (2012)*, *Eaters of the Dead: Myths and Realities of Cannibal Monsters (2021)*, and *The Theology of Battlestar Galactica (2012)*, as well as over a 100 book chapters, journal articles and essays, on topics from ghosts on the Japanese stage to African Adaptation of Greek tragedy to Shakespeare in graphic novels. He is also a twice-Bram Stoker Award-nominated editor of books such as *Uncovering Stranger Things (2019)* and *The Streaming of Hill House (2020)*. He is an actor, director and fight choreographer who lives and works in Los Angeles.

CARL WILSON is co-editor of the forthcoming *Routledge Companion to Superhero Studies*. He is also a contributing guest writer for the Eisner-nominated comic book publishers Fanbase Press. He has chapters recently published or forthcoming in the area of transmedia convergence, including the many iterations of Nosferatu in video games, the representation of women in Batman games, the comic book contexts of Catwoman and the digital legacy of various Supermen.

NICOLA YOUNG is an independent scholar whose key research interests are the intersections between philosophy, religion and film. Her published work includes contributions to *Breaking Down Joker: Violence, Loneliness, Tragedy* (2022) and *The Undead in the 21st Century: A Companion* (2022). She has also published in *Transnational Cinemas, Fantasy/Animation* and the *Journal of Popular Television*.

# Index

absurd 168, 171, 194, 196, 249–50
acceptance xviii, 24, 54, 59, 65, 71, 84, 187, 251, 282–4
ageing 4, 27
afterlife 2–4, 10, 20, 64, 79–80, 84–6, 89, 95–6, 106, 108, 113, 126, 130, 187, 194, 210, 212, 226–31, 275, 277
alien 6, 21, 98, 151, 183, 233, 235–40
alienation 96
Alzheimer's 17, 22, 267
angel 46, 50, 76, 109
    Angel of Death 2, 20, 181–3
Anthropocene 12, 143, 145, 147, 149–50
apocalypse xx, 2, 13, 15, 20, 22, 30, 32, 33, 101, 102, 135, 141, 143, 151, 171–3, 175–6, 178, 191
autopsy xiv, 71–5, 77, 231
avoidance xvii, 59

battle xvi, xvii, 14, 22, 45, 105, 106, 118, 140, 172, 178, 188, 196, 203, 206, 264
belief 33, 38, 57, 61–2, 64–6, 72, 75, 79, 81, 84, 96, 101, 131, 196–7, 263
*Bible, The* 55, 67, 75, 141, 165
bullet 250
bully xiii, 100
burial xiii, 133, 155, 165

cadaver 19, 46, 71, 75, 225, 227–9, 231
cannibal xiii, 31, 34, 36
capitalism 21, 24, 31, 66, 135, 139–40, 147–8, 218
    disaster capitalism 143, 147–8
chaos 10, 22, 48, 62, 178, 191, 249–50

Church 33, 198
climate change xiv, 4, 5, 10–12, 20–1, 141, 143–7, 149–50, 220, 288, 294
collective xiv, xviii, 12, 24, 72, 108, 129, 143, 148–50, 155, 205, 215, 260
communicate 80, 91, 129, 152, 155, 166–9, 202
community xiii, 1, 5, 8, 45, 54, 62, 64, 73, 91, 126–7, 129, 132, 139, 144, 164–5, 210, 234, 272, 276
computer 4, 8–9, 11, 24, 132, 135, 149, 236, 238
    computer game 99, 105
contagion xiv, xvi, 3, 7, 8, 14–17, 22–3, 167, 233, 237, 239–42, 254–6, 260–1
coronavirus 11, 14, 17, 22–3, 233, 240–2
costume 97, 138, 173–4
crucifixion 164–5
cult 7, 10, 101–2, 194, 200, 203–5

dance 186, 200–1, 246, 276
Dance of Death 3, 166–7, 192
Day of the Dead 24, 128, 130, 226–8, 281–4
dead xv, xvii–xx, 3, 23, 33, 36, 42, 54, 56, 62, 64, 72–7, 84, 88–90, 195–7, 106–8, 125, 127, 142, 152–3, 157, 166–7, 173, 204, 212–3, 221, 225–31, 241, 244, 246, 248, 256–7, 284
Deadpool 194–6
Death
    assisted death 17
    Death Café 21, 125–33
    death mask 110
    premature death 155

sudden death xiii, xvii, 7, 89
deathly 66
deceased 55, 83, 108, 110, 117, 127, 210, 225–31
deity 65, 66, 243, 249
dementia 17, 22–3, 263, 265–7
desire xiii, xx, 34, 36, 45, 51, 67, 73, 77, 88–92, 101, 113, 146–7, 149, 178, 185, 295–6, 210–1, 256, 258, 266, 271–2, 277
despair 102, 173, 210, 256
destiny 65, 172
devil 7, 76, 135, 139, 142, 185–7
disability 63–4
disaster 5, 21, 39, 141, 143–50, 283–4
discrimination 10, 46, 50–1, 218
disease 1, 3, 11, 14–17, 23, 33, 71, 73, 205, 233–42, 260, 263, 265, 267, 283
disguise 174–5, 200, 204
double 10, 66, 96, 135, 139, 179

ecology 11, 20–1, 151, 159, 226, 291
economics xi, 10, 17, 63, 144, 147, 149, 156–7, 163, 226, 264
empower 111, 128, 204, 207, 211–12, 227, 268
end of life 13, 20, 37–8, 67, 89, 90, 134, 136–8, 140
environment 1, 7, 9–10, 18–19, 21–2, 56, 62, 81, 116, 249, 283
environmental 8, 11, 14, 20, 148, 151–3, 155, 158–60, 163, 248
erotic xix, 3, 205, 256, 278
ethnicity 17, 138, 172–4
evil 6, 16, 19, 33, 45–6, 66, 96, 118, 154, 182, 184, 199, 203–4, 206
existence 13, 15, 29, 39, 48, 50, 55, 71, 72, 80–2, 90, 103–4, 110, 142, 144, 152–3, 156, 166, 192, 200, 202, 206, 227, 234, 241, 275

existential 49, 231
exploitation 12, 50, 138, 141, 144, 147–9, 154, 200, 204, 214
extremism 1, 4–8, 11, 12–14, 17, 21–2, 29, 31–6, 169, 171–4, 176, 178–9

faith 2, 16, 47, 65, 132, 184–7, 189
famine xviii, 2
fantastic xiv, 39, 64, 80, 91, 141, 151, 153, 172, 189, 203, 205
fantasm 88, 90, 92–3
fantasy xix, 35, 45, 91, 101, 135, 183, 199
feminine 2, 7, 65–7, 72–7, 115, 199, 204–6
Four Horsemen 2
funeral 40, 64, 110, 127–8, 130–1, 181, 195, 270–1, 275, 282

gender 17, 46, 49, 51, 73, 97, 152, 199, 204, 217–8, 221, 256, 261
ghost xx, 30, 53–5, 80, 84, 88, 109, 137–42, 152
God 38, 45–6, 50, 84, 95–6, 104, 109, 152–3, 157, 172, 183–4, 186–7, 189, 191, 193, 244, 245
'GOD' 175–6
Goddess 62, 65, 67, 96, 99, 101, 191, 199–200
Gothic 29, 63, 125, 129, 136, 138, 153, 156–7, 199–200
grave xv, xviii–xix, 38, 41, 153, 155, 199, 210
graveyard 3, 31, 228, 282
grief 45, 83, 126–9, 132, 216, 221, 257, 276, 278
grim reaper 2, 7, 10, 16, 20, 37, 41, 46–51, 95–7, 101, 104, 109–10, 111, 209–14, 218

haunt xv, xix, 74, 102, 138–9, 144, 149, 152, 186, 202, 204, 267
Heaven 4, 45, 79–80, 111, 172, 194, 249

*Index*

Hell 45, 80, 108, 172, 173, 184, 186–7, 211
hero 57–9, 137, 191–3, 246, 249, 256, 266
heroine 200, 204
horror xviii, 5, 29, 31, 37, 40, 43, 95, 98–9, 111–2, 125, 136, 140, 142, 151, 153, 155–6, 171, 173, 175, 183, 189, 199, 203, 206, 233, 237, 247, 270, 274, 283

identity 10, 14, 17, 21–3, 62, 64, 66, 81, 112, 139–40, 147, 162–3, 173, 186, 204, 221, 225–8, 231, 263, 265–7, 283
ideology 7, 9, 12, 14, 31, 33, 62, 64, 148, 161, 165, 170, 172, 174, 176, 178, 217–18, 284
imagination xiv, xvi–xvii, xx, 1, 5, 7, 16, 35, 63, 80, 83, 97, 99, 114, 144–5, 177, 209, 211, 220, 225–6, 231, 233, 243, 251–2, 255, 257, 260–1, 269–71, 275
immortality 20, 46, 58, 72–3, 113, 145, 183–4, 195, 244
incarnation 46, 48, 49–50, 66, 115, 120, 228
internet 5, 8–11, 161, 164, 167

judgement 2, 22, 101, 172, 184, 187, 210, 244, 248–9
justice xix, 99, 104, 169, 209–10, 212, 214, 220, 227

Karma 248–9
kill xv, xvi, 13, 34–5, 39–50, 55, 58, 63–4, 66–7, 77, 80, 96, 99, 102–3, 111, 115, 138, 144, 161–2, 171–2, 176, 183–4, 191–2, 200, 204–6, 213, 241, 250–1, 264, 273
killer 30, 37, 39, 101, 140, 162, 199

life xv, xviii, 2–3, 10, 12–13, 17–21, 23–4, 33, 35, 37–9, 41–2, 47–8, 55–62, 64–5, 67, 72, 74, 80–2, 84, 87–93, 95, 101, 103–4, 107, 109, 112, 127–9, 127–8, 132, 138, 142, 150, 152–7, 165, 172, 181–7, 192–3, 195–6, 199, 202, 204, 207, 211, 213, 218, 219, 227, 230, 239–40, 242–9, 251, 260, 271, 274–6, 280
 cycle 144, 153
 expectancy xvii
 forms 144, 157, 233, 263
 giving 199, 218–9
 saving xvi
 span xv, 99, 103
 story 93, 97, 99–102
 style 149
 time xiv
 writing 87, 89, 91–3
loss 10, 17, 23, 55, 64, 82, 112, 128–9, 132, 138, 178, 186, 196, 220–1, 226, 230–1, 263–7, 271, 276, 278, 283
love 1, 34, 45–6, 49, 55, 57, 77, 84, 96, 113, 115–7, 119, 131, 193–7, 210–1, 213, 226–7, 229, 241, 244, 250, 253, 256–8, 265, 267, 271, 281

magic 56, 59, 80, 85, 118, 209
martyr 57, 256
masculinity 20, 72, 73, 77, 217–9, 256
mask xix, 13, 15, 22, 97, 109–10, 132, 173–5, 177–9, 241
maternal 205, 221
matriarch 183, 199–200, 204, 206
medical xvii, 1, 20, 43, 73, 79–82, 84–5, 129, 167, 233–4, 261, 284
medicalise 16, 19, 72, 235, 253, 255, 258–60, 262
memento mori 2, 10, 125–6, 128–31, 133, 161, 192, 269, 271–2, 275–6, 280
memorial xviii, xx, 226–30

memory xviii, xix, 23, 63, 67, 82–3, 88–9, 114–5, 131–2, 139, 154, 206, 236–41, 263–7, 279, 283
mental health 9, 17, 22–3, 153, 199, 254, 259–62
merciless 37
mercy 77, 141, 203
*Mexican Gothic* (2020) xiv, 21, 151–7
misogyny 50–1, 155
monster xiii, xviii, 3, 5–7, 10–12, 18, 29–31, 33, 36, 98–9, 109, 140, 186
  Frankenstein's xiii–xiv, xviii, 31, 36, 99, 109
monstrosity 151, 200
monstrous 4–5, 22, 31, 65, 182, 237
morality xx, 38, 49, 100, 139–40, 160–1, 183–4, 186–7, 199, 203, 210, 212, 214
  amoral 46, 52, 20
  immoral 59
mortal xvii, 144, 184, 226, 229, 244–6, 248, 264
mortality xiii, 21, 46, 48, 71, 77, 115, 126, 128, 130, 132–3, 14t, 161, 183, 212, 225, 229, 242, 256, 275, 278
mummy 31, 36, 270
murder xiv, xvii, 37, 47, 57, 66, 76, 88, 97, 176–7, 248, 266
myth 2, 39, 41–2, 56, 67, 86, 129, 154, 156, 171, 189, 199, 243–5, 248–9, 256, 274, 278

natural xviii, 9, 14, 37–8, 41, 47–8, 61–2, 111, 143–4, 148–9, 155, 214, 241, 265
nature xiv, 2, 5–6, 8–9, 11–12, 15, 22–3, 30–1, 48, 51–2, 56, 62, 80–1, 85, 99, 112, 142–7, 149, 167, 170, 204–6, 221, 234, 237, 248–9, 253–4, 26t, 267, 269, 273, 283
necromancy 256–8, 261–2

normal 16, 59, 65, 83, 89, 93, 117, 149, 164, 205, 215, 221, 252, 278
  new xi, 1, 16, 23, 243–52
nightmare xiii, xiv, xx, 202
nostalgia 1, 257

ordinary 99, 184, 278
origin 6, 9, 15–16, 19, 21, 39, 90, 95, 108, 128, 170, 206, 235, 239, 241, 244, 248, 264, 267, 269, 283
originality 46, 107, 165, 169, 266

pain 17, 41, 43, 55, 67, 107, 119, 132, 210, 270, 276, 277, 283
pandemic xi, xvii, 1, 3–5, 8, 13–18, 22–3, 36, 84, 188, 221, 233, 236, 237, 239, 241–3, 251–2, 269, 275, 283
parasite 31, 98, 139, 149, 202, 204–6
patriarchy 62, 152–6, 203, 217–8
personification 2, 37–8, 41, 71–2, 96, 140, 171, 174, 185, 191–3, 199, 209, 215, 217, 219–21, 243
phantom 135, 235
philosophy 41, 45, 47–8, 71, 106, 112, 167, 248, 260, 276
plague xviii, 33, 132, 202, 234, 241
politics xiv, xv, xviii–xx, 1, 4, 8, 12–15, 19, 21–2, 31–2, 64, 135, 140–1, 148–9, 153, 161–2, 164–6, 168, 170–6, 178–9, 188, 200, 206, 215, 217, 221
  bio 164
  necro xix, 215
populist 4, 5, 8, 12–14, 21, 168
posthuman 152
posthumous 89, 225, 227–8, 230–1, 253, 270
power xviii–xix, 12–14, 19–20, 22, 49–50, 61, 66, 73, 76–7, 82, 95–6, 99, 103, 116, 118, 131, 146–7, 147–56, 164, 172–3, 178–9, 185, 193, 195–6, 200, 203–6, 211, 218–9, 246

Index 327

bio 258, 260
less 168
powerful 3, 41, 113–5, 118, 127–8, 178, 187, 199, 201, 203–5, 215, 219, 221
precarity 73, 142, 206, 229
predetermination 41, 49, 107
prediction 173, 282
privilege 3, 12, 140, 153, 156
prophecy 36, 39, 178, 246, 256
purgatory 80, 108, 185

queer 215

rebirth 21, 70, 151–7, 204, 206
reborn 115–6, 153
religion xiii, xv, xviii, 3–5, 14, 32–3, 62, 71, 79–81, 101, 127, 171, 181, 185–7, 204–5
remembrance xx, 2, 225–8, 282
resurrect 20, 48, 62, 64, 105, 113, 119, 166, 273, 277
revenge 11, 22, 76, 156, 199, 212
  eco- 21
ritual 24, 63–4, 75–7, 104, 128, 202, 204, 209, 227–9, 270, 272, 283
romanticising 23, 192, 253, 255–8, 261–2
roulette 19

sacrifice 46–7, 57–8, 64–5, 77, 103, 140, 155, 204–5
sadistic 41, 43
Satan 184, 186–7
science 4, 11–12, 15, 19–20, 32, 72, 80–5, 112, 148, 152, 162, 164, 184, 235–7, 259, 241
scythe 2, 38, 47–8, 96–7, 101, 192, 215
skeleton xiv, xv, 2–3, 9, 38, 46, 72, 76, 96–8, 108–10, 128, 161–4, 166–72, 175, 191–2, 211, 215, 226, 228–9, 231, 283

skull xviii, 3, 21, 97, 99, 125, 128, 130–1, 161–6, 169, 173, 178, 195, 272, 281–3
social media 8, 20, 48, 162, 168–9, 260–70, 276, 279–80
society xviii, 1, 3, 5, 12, 14, 19, 21, 23, 62, 73, 132, 143–4, 148, 164, 179–80, 200, 207, 210, 2280, 251–2
soul 2, 31, 64, 80–2, 84, 96–7, 106–8, 113, 117–8, 146, 175, 186, 195, 204, 219, 229, 244, 246, 263, 281
spectre 12, 38, 81, 145, 170–1, 183–4, 187, 189, 257, 284
spirit 10, 62–4, 66–7, 75, 96–7, 130, 152, 204, 218, 226, 282, 284
spiritual 62, 64, 71, 80–1, 84, 127
suffer xv–xvi, xviii, 17, 37, 43, 50, 65–6, 77, 108, 112, 116, 138, 154, 156, 203, 206, 212, 221, 229, 249, 256
suicide xiv, 7, 12–13, 74, 96–7, 110, 183, 211, 221, 253–62
supernatural 13, 67, 76, 81–2, 101, 155, 183, 187, 199–200, 203–4, 207, 214, 235
superstition 91
symbiosis 153, 155
symbolic 5, 31, 35, 49, 64–5, 72, 93, 140, 145, 154, 172–4, 179, 255
symbolism xviii, 20–1, 32–5, 45, 56–7, 71, 75, 88, 103, 109, 127, 137, 187, 193, 199, 206, 236, 238, 241–2, 247, 275, 283

technology xv–xvi, 1, 3–5, 8–11, 16, 19–20, 36, 69, 71, 111, 141, 147, 181, 188, 226, 236–7, 283
terror xiv, 4–8, 10, 16, 18–19, 27, 29, 34–6, 41, 57, 59, 109, 172–3, 188, 215
transcend 77, 81, 83, 112, 153, 196
transgender 73

trauma  xviii, 1, 5–6, 19, 29, 61–3, 74, 86–7, 204–5, 212, 226, 270, 286

undead  7, 31, 34–5, 66, 107, 109, 111, 154, 270, 280
underworld  64, 96, 199, 244
unnatural  36, 58, 97, 145, 152, 155

vampire  13, 15, 30, 36, 80, 154, 232–6, 238
vengeance  34–6, 144–5, 155, 209, 211–2, 214
violence  xviii, 7, 13, 19–20, 22, 37–43, 97, 101, 110, 140, 145, 148, 162, 170, 172, 174–5, 194–5, 196, 200, 203, 249–51, 263, 266

war  xv–xix, 2, 7, 19, 57, 59, 61–4, 105, 112, 140, 165, 203, 209–10, 239, 273
 culture  12, 14, 21
 on terror  4, 16, 18, 27, 36
warfare  xv–xvi, 3, 5–7, 210, 236
weapon  xiv–xviii, 47, 99, 109, 114–5, 147, 195
weaponise  101, 143, 147, 164
werewolf  30, 235
witch  75, 83–5, 199–200, 202–6
 doctor  64, 66
 trials  72, 75–6

zombie  3–4, 7, 13–15, 18, 29–36, 80, 97, 153

## Genre Fiction and Film Companions

Series Editor: Simon Bacon

The *Genre Fiction and Film Companions* provide accessible introductions to key texts within the most popular genres of our time. Written by leading scholars in the field, brief essays on individual texts offer innovative ways of understanding, interpreting and reading the topics in question. Invaluable for students, teachers and fans alike, these surveys offer new insights into the most important literary works, films, music, events and more within genre fiction and film.

We welcome proposals for edited collections on new genres and topics. Please contact baconetti@googlemail.com or oxford@peterlang.com.

### Published Volumes

The Gothic
Edited by Simon Bacon

Cli-Fi
Edited by Axel Goodbody and Adeline Johns-Putra

Horror
Edited by Simon Bacon

Sci-Fi
Edited by Jack Fennell

Monsters
Edited by Simon Bacon

Transmedia Cultures
Edited by Simon Bacon

Shirley Jackson
Edited by Kristopher Woofter

Toxic Cultures
Edited by Simon Bacon

*Magic*
Edited by Katharina Rein

The Undead in the 21st Century
Edited by Simon Bacon

The Deep
Edited by Marko Teodorski and Simon Bacon

Death in the 21st Century
Edited by Katarzyna Bronk-Bacon and Simon Bacon

www.ingramcontent.com/pod-product-compliance
Ingram Content Group UK Ltd.
Pitfield, Milton Keynes, MK11 3LW, UK
UKHW021253180426
11947UKWH00010B/763